Internal Medicine
Handbook for Clinicians
Resident Survival Guide

Elbert S. Huang, M.D.
Fellow, General Internal Medicine
Massachusetts General Hospital

W. H. Wilson Tang, M.D.
Fellow, Cardiology
Cleveland Clinic Foundation

David S. Lee, M.D.
Fellow, Cardiology
Cleveland Clinic Foundation

Carey Conley Thomson, M.D.
Fellow, Pulmonary/Critical Care Medicine
Massachusetts General Hospital

Melissa A. Fischer, M.D.
Fellow, Ambulatory Care Medicine
VA Palo Alto Healthcare System
Stanford University

Scrub Hill Press, Inc.
46 S. Glebe Road #301
Arlington, VA 22204
www.scrubhillpress.com

The opinions expressed in this book represent a broad range of opinions of the authors. These opinions are not meant to represent a "standard of care" or a "protocol" but rather a guide to common clinical conditions. Use of these guidelines are obviously influenced by local factors, varying clinical circumstances, and honest differences of opinion.

The indications and dosages or all drugs in this book have been recommended in the medical literature and conform to all the practices of the general medical community. The medications described do not necessarily have specific approval by the Food and Drug Administration for use in the diseases and dosages for which they are recommended. The package insert for each drug should be consulted for use and dosage as approved by the FDA. Because standards for usage change, it is advisable to keep abreast of revised recommendations, particularly those concerning new drugs.

Publisher: Scrub Hill Press, Inc.
Editorial Production: Silverchair Science + Communications
Cover design: Christopher Carbone

Editorial offices:
Scrub Hill Press, Inc.
46 S. Glebe Road #301
Arlington, VA 22204
e-mail: johndavidgordon@erols.com
www.scrubhillpress.com
Member of the American Medical Publishers Association

*To the past, current, and future medicine house staff at Stanford,
and to those who have taught us the art of healing*

The authors thank the following publishers for permission to reproduce material in this book:

New England Journal of Medicine
American Heart Association
Lippincott Williams & Wilkins
American Medical Association
Stanford Coagulation Laboratory
McGraw-Hill
American College of Physicians
W. B. Saunders
Elsevier Science
Abbott Laboratories
American Family Physician
Stanford Transfusion Service
Chapman & Hall
Hippokrates Verlag
Stanford Health Services Department of Nephrology
University of Chicago Press
Stanford Clinical Microbiology/Virology Laboratory
Plymouth Press
Stanford Hospital and Clinics
Arthritis Foundation
Palo Alto Medical Foundation
Hospital Medicine
American College of Cardiology
Stanford Health Services Department of Pathology
British Journal of Hospital Medicine
American Academy of Pediatrics

Contents

Foreword   *xi*
    Kelley Skeff, M.D., Ph.D.
Preface   *xii*

1. CARDIOLOGY   1

Valvular Heart Disease   1
Other Valvular Heart Disease   4
Congenital Heart Diseases: Adult Diagnosis   5
Dynamic Auscultation Maneuvers   6
Prosthetic Valves   7
Electrocardiogram (ECG)   8
ECG Presentation of Clinical Syndromes   10
Wolff-Parkinson-White Syndrome   11
Wide Complex Tachycardia   12
Narrow Complex Rhythm   14
Atrial Fibrillation   15
Syncope   18
Pacemakers   20
Coronary Imaging   21
American Society of Echocardiography 16-Segment Model of Left Ventricle   22
Coronary Artery Diseases   23
Classification of Myocardial Infarction   24
ECG Changes in Myocardial Infarction   25
Acute Coronary Syndrome: Unstable Angina   26
Thrombolytic Therapy   30
Adjunctive Medical Therapy in Myocardial Infarction   31
Nonmedical Therapeutic Interventions in Myocardial Infarction   32
Complications of Myocardial Infarction   33
Cardiogenic Shock: Pharmacologic Interventions   34
Revascularization   35
Coronary Artery Bypass Grafting (CABG)   37
Stress Testing   38
Heart Failure   39
Management of Systolic Heart Failure   40
Pulmonary Hypertension   42
Hypertensive Crisis (Emergency)   43
Pharmacologic Management of Hypertensive Crisis   44
Aortic Dissection   45
Hemodynamic Monitoring: Pulmonary Artery Catheter   46
Pulmonary Artery Pressures in Various Forms of Shock   47
Coronary Care Unit Formulas   48
Pressors   49

2. PULMONARY

2. PULMONARY   50

Respiratory Distress   50
Respiratory Support: Oxygen   51
Bilevel Intermittent Positive Pressure (BIPAP) and
    Noninvasive Positive Pressure Ventilation (NIPPV)   52
Mechanical Ventilation   53
Asthma/COPD Exacerbation   56
NAEPP Classification of Asthma Severity   57
Inhaled Steroids   58
Pulmonary Embolism (PE)   59
Heparin Sliding Scale   60
Hemoptysis   61
Pleural Effusion   62
Pulmonary Function Testing   64

3. RENAL   65

Urinalysis   65
Proteinuria   66
Nephrotic Syndrome   66
Hematuria   66
Special Urine Tests   67
Urine Electrolytes and Functional Tests and When to Use Them   68
Functional Tests and When to Use Them   69
Renal Imaging Techniques and When to Use Them   70
Hypernatremia   71
Hyponatremia   72
Syndrome of Inappropriate Antidiuresis (SIAD)   74
Hyperkalemia   75
Hypokalemia   77
Hypercalcemia   78
Hypocalcemia   80
Hyperphosphatemia   81
Hypophosphatemia   81
Hypermagnesemia   82
Hypomagnesemia   82
Acid-Base Primer   83
Evaluation of Metabolic Acidosis   84
Renal Tubular Acidosis   85
Evaluation of Metabolic Alkalosis   86
Acute Renal Failure   87
Drugs Associated with Renal Failure   88
Hepatorenal Syndrome   89
Rhabdomyolysis and Pigment Nephropathy   89
Chronic Renal Failure   90
Nephrolithiasis   91

4. GASTROENTEROLOGY   **92**

Bedside Diagnosis: Abdominal Pain
Gastrointestinal Endoscopy
Gastrointestinal Functional Tests
Gastrointestinal Bleeding: Acute Management
Nausea and Vomiting   98
Acute Diarrhea   99
Clostridium Difficile Colitis   99
Constipation   101
Pancreatitis   102
Cirrhosis and Chronic Hepatitis   103
Acute Hepatitis   106
Fulminant Hepatic Failure   109

5. HEMATOLOGY   **110**

Peripheral Blood Smear   110
Red Blood Cell Indices   111
Hematology Coagulation Tests   112
Coagulation Cascade   113
Heparin Sliding Scale   114
Low-Molecular-Weight Heparin (LMWH)   114
Warfarin   116
Hypercoagulable States   118
Evaluation of a Bleeding Patient   119
Anemias   120
Etiologies of Thrombocytopenia   121
Pancytopenia   121
Transfusions   122
Transfusion Reactions   123
Thrombocytopenic

6. ONCOLOGY   **126**

Evaluation of the Cancer Patient   126
Tumor Markers   127
Recommended Antiemetics   129
Side Effects of Chemotherapy   128
Oncologic Emergencies   129
Cancer Statistics   130
Non–Small Cell Lung Cancer: TNM Classification   132
Breast Cancer: TNM Classification   133
Colorectal Cancer: TNM Classification   134
Prostate Cancer: TNM Classification   136

7. INFECTIOUS DISEASE   **138**

Stanford Adult Parenteral Antimicrobial Dosing Guidelines   138
Vancomycin and Aminoglycoside Monitoring   141

CONTENTS

Single Daily Aminoglycoside Dosing | 142
Fever and Rash Differential Diagnosis | 143
Fever of Unknown Origin | 144
Severe Soft-Tissue Infections | 148
Endocarditis | 149
Meningitis | 151
Community-Acquired Pneumonia | 153
Urinary Tract Infections | 155
Treatment Regimens for Urinary Tract Infections | 156
Vaginitis | 157
Pelvic Inflammatory Disease | 158
Transplant Infections | 161
Human Immunodeficiency Virus and Acquired Immunodeficiency Syndrome | 162
Tuberculosis Treatment | 165
Antibiotic Sensitivities | 167

8. NEUROLOGY — 172

Dermatomes | 172
Peripheral Nerves | 174
Glasgow Coma Scale | 175
Increased Intracranial Pressure | 176
Coma: Correlating Examination Findings with Level of Brain Dysfunction | 177
Transient Insomnia ("Sleeper") | 178
Altered Mental Status (Δ-MS) | 178
Alcohol Withdrawal | 180
Dementia | 182
Folstein Mini-Mental Status Examination | 182
Weakness: Differential Diagnosis of Acute or Subacute Onset | 183
Guillain-Barré Syndrome | 184
Emergency Headache Evaluation | 185
Migraine Headache | 186
Stroke and Thrombolytics | 188
Quick Guide to Aphasia | 190
Seizures | 191
Status Epilepticus | 192
Acute Pain | 193

9. ENDOCRINOLOGY — 195

Common Screening Tests in Endocrine Disorders | 195
Thyroid Disease | 197
Thyroid Nodule Evaluation | 197
Thyrotoxicosis | 198
Myxedema Coma | 198
Adrenal Crisis | 199
Diabetic Ketoacidosis | 201
Hyperosmolar Nonketotic Coma | 202
Insulin Therapy | 203

CONTENTS

10. RHEUMATOLOGY — 205

Joint Examination — 205
Common Patterns of Joint Involvement in Various Arthritides — 208
Arthrocentesis and Steroid Injection for Idiots — 209
Joint Fluid Analysis — 210
Synovial Fluid Analysis — 215
Immunologic Tests — 217
Systemic Lupus Erythematosus — 218
Rheumatoid Arthritis — 218
Gout — 219
Vasculitis — 220

11. NUTRITION — 221

Nutritional Requirements — 221
Total Parenteral Nutrition (TPN) — 222
Enteral Nutrition — 223
Nutritional Feeding Formulation Chart — 224

12. OUTPATIENT — 226

Health Care Maintenance — 226
Hypertension — 227
Hypercholesterolemia — 229
Outpatient Diabetes Mellitus Guidelines — 230
Travel Medicine — 231
Smoking Cessation — 232
Oral Contraception — 233
Menopause and Hormone Replacement Therapy (HRT) — 234

13. CONSULTATIVE MEDICINE — 235

Ten Commandments for Effective Medical Consultation — 235
Preoperative Evaluation: Cardiovascular — 236
Stepwise Approach to Preoperative Cardiac Assessment — 237
Preoperative Evaluation: Pulmonary — 240
Perioperative Management: Anticoagulation — 242
Perioperative Management: Antimicrobial Prophylaxis — 244
Endocarditis Prophylaxis — 245

14. TOXICOLOGY — 246

Benzodiazepine Overdose — 246
Benzodiazepine Withdrawal — 246
Opioid Overdose — 247
Opioid Withdrawal — 247
Acetaminophen Overdose — 248
Acetaminophen Nomogram — 249
Aspirin Overdose — 250
Tricyclic Antidepressant Overdose — 251
Anaphylaxis — 252

ix

CONTENTS

15. CLINICAL PHARMACOLOGY 253
Composition of Commonly Used Intravenous Solutions 253
Monitoring Guidelines for Drugs Commonly Used in the Intensive Care Unit 254
Drugs and Liver Disease Patients 256
Considerations for Drug Dosage Adjustments in Liver Disease 256
Nonantibiotic Drug Dosage Adjustments in Renal Failure 257
Drug Interactions with Digoxin 259
Drug Interactions with Theophylline 259
Drug Interactions with Cyclosporine 260
Drug Interactions with Coumadin 260
Selected Clinical Manifestations of Adverse Drug Reactions 261

16. EVIDENCE-BASED MEDICINE 266
How to Use an Article About Therapy or Prevention 266
How to Use Articles About Diagnostic Tests 267
Fagan's Nomogram 269

17. RADIOLOGY 270
Chest Radiology: Chest X-Ray 270
Gastrointestinal Radiology: Specialized Imaging Protocols 271
Specialized Radiologic Procedures Preparation (Stanford Protocol) 272

18. PROCEDURES 273
Procedure: Central Venous Line 273
Procedure: Lumbar Puncture 275
Procedure: Thoracentesis 276
Procedure: Paracentesis 277

19. ADVANCED CARDIOPULMONARY LIFE SUPPORT 278
Selected ACLS Drugs 278
Ventricular Fibrillation/Pulseless Ventricular Tachycardia 279
Pulseless Electrical Activity Algorithm 280
Asystole Algorithm 281
Bradycardia Algorithm 282
Tachycardia Algorithm 283

20. RESOURCES 284
Normal Laboratory Values 284
Local Resources 293
Personal Local Resources 294
Personal Resources: Subspecialty Consultants 295
Personal Resources 296
Internet Resources 297

SUBJECT INDEX 299

DRUG INDEX 311

Foreword

The role of a house officer is complex. Residents and interns have responsibilities that represent the essence of academic medicine: care of patients, teaching of colleagues and self, and a dedication to continued acquisition and discovery of new knowledge. These tasks require that these physicians not only are committed and knowledgeable but also have effective resources.

The authors of the *Internal Medicine Survival Guide* have addressed the need for effective resources. They have collected a broad spectrum of information to assist house staff, students, and faculty in their professional roles as physicians and teachers. The information in this text is designed to fill the needs of busy physicians. It is literature based, easily retrievable, and distilled to represent core knowledge that can facilitate comprehensive patient care and education. By expanding the available resources, this text makes an important contribution that will assist house officers, students, faculty, and ultimately the patients they serve.

Kelley M. Skeff, M.D., Ph.D.
Professor of Medicine and Residency Program Director
Stanford University Medical Center

Preface

The relevant information physicians need to practice medicine comes from disparate sources: handbooks, textbooks, articles, Web sites, patients, and words of wisdom from more experienced physicians. As interns at Stanford University Medical Center, we began to consolidate the core of this data in one place so we could travel lightly and practice efficiently. We wanted useful information that was easy to read with bleary eyes. And most important, we wanted up-to-date references to understand the evidence behind the practice.

Although this handbook was created from the perspective of the house officer, we feel that even seasoned clinicians will find it a useful aide in the practice of medicine. All of us continue to refer to this manual to review the standards of care for common medical problems. This book is not designed to replace traditional textbooks or the latest research, and we happily admit that we stand on the shoulders of many physicians before us.

We owe our greatest debt to current and past Stanford house staff who helped to shape the original handbook and have put it to real use. Drs. Paul Eckburg, Gail Pyle, Sandy Ramirez, Lisa Shieh, and Heather Wakelee contributed several of the original sections. Many others have played an important role in the creation of this handbook.

George Waltuch, M.D., and the Stanford Community of Internists were instrumental in providing the initial financial support for this project. Our thanks also go to Dr. Kelley Skeff, our program director, mentor, and teacher, and all the staff in the Department of Medicine at Stanford.

A sincere thanks to all the reviewers for the various versions of the handbook: Drs. Paul Ford, Mark Genovese, Scott Hall, Ed Klofas, Rick Kraemer, Felix Lee, Jaime Lopez, Jeff Loutit, Laura Nicholson, Peter Rudd, Steve Ruoss, Alan Yuen, Eddie Atwood, Stefan Chin, Rajinder Chitkara, John Day, Richard Lafayette, Scott Lee, Jason Marx, Peter Pompei, George Triadafilopoulos, Byron Wilson, and others who offered their help anonymously.

Special thanks to Elizabeth Willingham and Lisa Cunningham at Silverchair for their endless patience. Bill Gillespie of Scrub Hill Press provided computer graphics support. Finally, we must recognize Dr. John Gordon of Scrub Hill Press, who made the publication of this work a reality.

Elbert S. Huang, M.D.
W. H. Wilson Tang, M.D.
David S. Lee, M.D.
Carey Conley Thomson, M.D.
Melissa A. Fischer, M.D.

1. Cardiology

VALVULAR HEART DISEASE (N Engl J Med 337:32, 1997; ACC/AHA Guidelines—Circulation 98:149, 1998)

Aortic Stenosis (Cardiol Clin 16:353, 1998; Am Heart J 132:408, 1996; Chest 113:1109, 1998)

Symptoms	Average untreated 50% survival	(Circulation 38(Suppl 5):V-61, 1968)
Angina	5 years	
Syncope	3 years	
Heart failure	2 years	

Physical Examination
- **Murmur:** Early harsh ejection (crescendo-decrescendo) murmur at right upper sternal border to carotid (peaks later if severe); ↑with legs up, squat; ↓with Valsalva, hand grip, standing; unchanged with respiration; faint diastolic murmur at upper left sternal border (*Gallavardin's phenomenon*: murmur disappears over sternum, reappears in apex)
- **Heart sounds:** Soft S_1, soft A_2, paradoxical split S_2 (softer S_2 if severe), apical S_4
- **Exam:** Narrow pulse pressure, a waves, *pulsus parvus et tardus* (poor and delayed carotid upstroke), prominent point of maximal impulse

Grading (American Heart Association 1998)

	Valve area	Gradient	Echo follow-up (AHA recommended)
Mild	>1.5 cm^2		Every 5 years
Moderate	1.0–1.5 cm^2		Every 2 years
Severe/critical	Area ≤1.0 cm^2	>50 mm Hg*	Every 6–12 months, cath†

*Lower gradient may also represent severe aortic stenosis in lower cardiac output; some references noted area <0.7–0.8 cm^2 as critical aortic stenosis.

†Indications for cath: (1) coronary angiography before aortic valve repair in patients with coronary risks, (2) assessment of severity of stenosis in symptomatic patients planning for surgery, or with inconclusive noninvasive test results, or (3) discrepancy between clinical findings regarding severity of stenosis or need for surgery.

Management
- **Observe** if asymptomatic; refer when symptomatic or with gradient >30 mm Hg.
- **Medical:** Careful diuretics and nitrates (preload/afterload dependent), endocarditis prophylaxis; use of ACE inhibitors and stress testing is controversial.
- **Surgical replacement:** Symptomatic, bypass/valvular/aortic surgery (≥ moderate aortic stenosis), systolic dysfunction, ventricular tachycardia, valve area <0.6 cm^2, hypotension in exercise test. Balloon aortic valvotomy if surgical replacement contraindicated.

continued

CARDIOLOGY

Chronic Mitral Regurgitation (*Cardiol Clin* 16:421, 1998; *Am Heart J* 135:925, 1998; *Mayo Clin Proc* 72:1034, 1997; *Curr Probl Cardiol* 23:202, 1998)

Symptoms
- Dyspnea
- Heart failure
- Palpitations

Physical Examination
- **Murmur:** Loud, harsh, holosystolic blowing; high-pitched murmur at apex to axilla; ↑with squat, hand grip; ↓with amyl nitrite
- **Heart sounds:** ↓S_1, wide split S_2 ($P_2 >A_2$), left S_3 (S_4 if acute)
- **Exam:** Displaced hyperdynamic PMI, apical systolic thrill, parasternal heave

Management
- **Observe** if none-to-mild symptoms and ejection fraction >60%; yearly exam and echocardiogram
- **Medical:** Digoxin, ACE inhibitor (acute: nitroprusside ± inotropic agents, balloon pump)
- **Surgical replacement:** Symptomatic, LVEF <60% (RV <30%) end-systolic minor-axis diameter >45 mm, end-systolic volume index >50 ml/m^2 (emergent surgery in heart failure, flail leaflet), ?atrial fibrillation
- **Acute mitral regurgitation** (*Am J Med* 78:293, 1985): usually has ↑atrial V-wave with normal left atrial compliance and smaller chamber sizes than chronic; prompt surgical repair warranted.

Mitral Stenosis (*Cardiol Clin* 16:375, 1998; *Curr Probl Cardiol* 23:130, 1998)

Symptoms
- Dyspnea
- Hoarseness (Ortner's syndrome)
- Heart failure
- Mitral face
- Hemoptysis
- Palpitations (atrial arrhythmias)

Physical Examination
- **Murmur:** Low mid-diastolic rumble, best at left sternal border (LSB)/apex especially at left lateral decubitus, ↑in expiration, left lateral, exercise; ↓in inspiration (A_2-P_2 snap), presystolic crescendo
- **Heart sounds:** ↑S_1, narrow/↑S_2 widens with standing, opening snap (↓A_2 snap interval if severe)

Management
- **Observe** yearly if asymptomatic with valve area ≥1 cm^2 (stress test if area <1 cm^2); refer if atrial fibrillation, pulmonary hypertension, symptomatic (valve area <1.5 cm^2)
- **Medical:** Diuretics, rate control, and anticoagulation in atrial fibrillation
- **Surgical management:** Pulmonary hypertension (pulmonary artery systolic pressure ≥60 mm Hg), heart failure, atrial fibrillation, valve area <1.5 mm^2 (gradient ≥6 mm Hg)

Chronic Aortic Regurgitation   (*Cardiol Clin* 16:463, 1998; *JAMA* 281:2231, 1999)

Symptoms
- Heart failure
- Syncope
- Angina

Physical Examination
- **Murmur:** High-pitched, diastolic, blowing, decrescendo murmur at LSB; ↑with forward lean, squat, hand grip, Austin Flint murmur (low-pitched diastolic rumble)
- **Heart sounds:** Soft S_1, left S_3
- **Exam:** Left displaced PMI, bisferiens, and bounding pulse

Physical Signs
- Quincke's (capillary pulsations)
- Palmar click (abrupt flushing in systole)
- Landolfi's (pupillary pulses)
- Corrigan's (supraclavicular/carotid artery pulses)
- Traube's (double pistol shot sound over femoral artery)
- Duroziez's (to-and-fro diastolic bruit over femoral artery)
- Water-hammer (abruptly collapsing high-pitched pulse)
- Bisferiens pulse (double systolic arterial pulses)
- Hill's (popliteal artery pressure ≥1–40 mm Hg higher than brachial artery pressure)
- Müller's (uvula pulses)
- de Musset (head-bob, "yes-yes" sign)
- Rosenbach's (liver pulses)

Management
- **Medical management and follow** yearly if end-systolic left ventricle <55 mm Hg (2-year follow-up if <40 mm Hg) and ejection fraction >55%; refer if symptomatic or worsening systolic dysfunction (follow every 6 months)
- **Medical:** Vasodilators for afterload reduction (nifedipine, ACE inhibitor)
- **Surgical replacement:** Symptomatic, LVEF <55%, end-systolic LV >55 mm Hg, end-diastolic LV >65 mm Hg

Rheumatic Fever   (*JAMA* 268:2069, 1992; *Lancet* 349:935, 1997)

Diagnosis *(Jones' Criteria, Revised 1992)*
- One major and three minor, or two major
- Supporting evidence of antecedent group A streptococcal infection:
  Throat culture
  Rapid strep antigen test
  ↑ASO titer >1:600

Major criteria		Minor criteria	
Carditis	Erythema marginatum	Arthralgia	↑ESR
Polyarthritis	Subcutaneous nodules	Fever	↑C-reactive protein
Chorea		↑Acute phase reactants	↑PR interval

Management
- Supportive
- Endocarditis prophylaxis

3

CARDIOLOGY

OTHER VALVULAR HEART DISEASE

Hypertrophic Obstructive Cardiomyopathy (HOCM) [or Idiopathic Hypertrophic Subaortic Stenosis (IHSS)]
(*Am J Coll Cardiol* 33:1071, 1999)

- **Murmur:** Systolic ejection murmur at right upper sternal border to carotids; ↑with standing and Valsalva; ↓with squat, hand grip, leg up
- **Heart sounds:** Left S_4 (triple ripple PMI)
- **Exam:** Bisferiens pulse (double pulse, two palpable systolic peaks)

Pulmonary Stenosis
- **Murmur:** Systolic ejection murmur best heard at left upper sternal border, radiates to back and neck, ↑after Valsalva release, ↓with inspiration
- **Heart sounds:** ↓A_2, wide split S_2, ↓P_2, right-sided S_4, pulmonic click
- **Exam:** ↑a wave, right parasternal lift

Tricuspid Regurgitation
- **Murmur:** Pansystolic, blowing murmur (localized to LSB; ↑with inspiration, leg up
- **Heart sounds:** Paradoxical ↑S_2, right S_3
- **Exam:** ↑v wave, ↑y descent, ↑jugular venous pulsations ("no-no" sign), weak apex, (RV hypertrophy)

Mitral Valve Prolapse
- Midsystolic click at apex, ↑S_1, ↑with stand and Valsalva, ↓with squat
- Endocarditis prophylaxis if valvular regurgitation and/or thickened leaflets present

Pulmonary Regurgitation
- **Murmur:** High-pitched (low in congenital) diastolic rumble at left upper sternal border (Graham-Steel murmur); ↑with inspiration, ↓with squat, hand grip, leg up
- **Heart sounds:** Decrescendo after loud P_2
- **Exam:** RV hypertrophy

Tricuspid Stenosis
- **Murmur:** High-pitched mid-diastolic murmur at left lower sternal border; ↑with inspiration, leg up
- **Exam:** ↑a wave

CONGENITAL HEART DISEASES: ADULT DIAGNOSIS
(ACC/AHA Guidelines—Circulation 90:2180, 1994)

Atrial Septal Defect (ASD)
- **Types:** ostium secundum (most common), ostium primum (may involve mitral/tricuspid rings), sinus venosus defects (superior or inferior).
- **Exam:** Ejection murmur across pulmonic valve, diastolic flow "rumble" murmur across tricuspid valve area, widely split and split S_2, parasternal impulse.
- **Tests:** Increased pulmonary marking in X-ray, rSr' in V_1 with left axis in ECG.
- **Sequelae:** pulmonary hypertension, right-to-left shunt, heart failure, atrial arrhythmias, emboli
- **Management:** surgical repair when pulmonary-to-systemic blood flow ratio ≥1.8:1 or right ventricular dilation.

Ventricular Septal Defect (VSD)
- **Murmur:** Harsh, pansystolic murmur at fourth left intercostal space with thrill, ↓ with valsalva, handgrip.
- **Heart sounds:** Delayed S_2, diastolic flow murmur with S_3 occasionally, P_2 coincident with A_2 if large VSD, ↑a and v waves, hyperkinetic apex, laterally displaced apical pulse and prominent parasternal impulse, cardiomegaly with biventricular hypertrophy in x-ray/ECG.
- **Sequelae:** left-to-right shunt, endocarditis, progressive aortic regurgitation (supracristal VSD), heart failure, pulmonary hypertension and reversal shunt (Eisenmenger's).
- **Management:** endocarditis prophylaxis, surgical repair when pulmonary-to-systemic blood flow ratio ≥1.5:1 and more favorable outcome when pulmonary vascular resistance <7.5 Woods unit, S_AO_2 ≥90%.

Patent Ductus Arteriosus (PDA)
- **Murmur:** Continuous "machinery" murmur enveloping S_2, especially beneath left clavicle in second intercostal space, widened arterial pulse pressure, hyperdynamic apical impulse.
- **Tests:** Left ventricular hypertrophy in ECG, prominent pulmonary artery and left atria, occasionally calcified ductus.
- **Sequelae:** pulmonary hypertension, endoarteritis.
- **Management:** endoarteritis prophylaxis, surgical ligation if progressive pulmonary hypertension or endoarteritis.

Other Congenital Cardiac Diseases
- **Congenital valvular diseases:** bicuspid aortic stenosis/regurgitation, pulmonary stenosis
- **Coarctation of aorta:** secondary hypertension.
- **Ebstein's anomaly:** tricuspid regurgitation, paroxysmal atrial tachycardia.
- **Tetralogy of Fallot** (right ventricular outflow tract obstruction + VSD + RV hypertrophy + overriding aortic root): cyanosis.
- **Right ventricular dysplasia:** arrhythmias.

CARDIOLOGY

DYNAMIC AUSCULTATION MANEUVERS (N Engl J Med 318:1572, 1998; Curr Probl Cardiol 13:675, 1988)

Maneuver	Physiology	Murmurs affected
Left lateral decubitus	↑Exercise, ↑flow	↑MS, ↑left murmur
Standing (squat vice versa)	↓VR, ↓CO, ↑LVEF	↑IHSS/MVP, ↓others
Inspiring (expire vice versa)	↑RV filling, ↑VR	↑Right murmur, ↓innocent, ↓rate, ↓MR
Müller's (suck to closed nares 10s)	↓RV filling, ↓PVR	↓Right murmur, AS, IHSS, VSD
Valsalva (expire to closed glottis 20s)	↓VR/AL/CO, ↑LVEF	Narrow S_2, ↑IHSS/MVP, ↓others
Passive leg raise (40–60 degrees)	↑VR	Widen S_2, ↑S_3, ↓IHSS/MVP, ↓others
Isometric hand grip	↑AL, ↑CO	↑MR, ↑VSD
Bending over	↓Chamber distance	↑AR, ↑pericardial rub
Arterial occlusion (BP cuff)	↑Aortic impedence	↑AR, ↑MR, ↑VSD
Amyl nitrite ("reverse hand grip")	↓AL/LV volume, ↑VR/LVEF	↑AS, MS, PS, IHSS, TS, TR; ↓VSD, MR, AR, not PR

MS = mitral stenosis; VR = venous return; CO = cardiac output; IHSS = idiopathic hypertrophic sub-aortic stenosis; MVP = mitral valve prolapse; PVR = pulmonary vascular resistance; AL = afterload; MR = mitral regurgitation; AR = aortic regurgitation; AS = aortic stenosis; PS = pulmonic stenosis; TS = tricuspid stenosis; TR = tricuspid regurgitation; PR = pulmonic regurgitation.

PROSTHETIC VALVES *(N Engl J Med 335:407, 1996; Cardiol Clin 16:505, 1998; Mayo Clin Proc 73:665, 1998)*

Anticoagulation

INR	Indications*
2.5–3.5	Low-risk patients with bileaflet tilting-disk (e.g., St. Jude Medical), high-risk patients with all bioprosthesis
3.0–3.9	Low-risk patients with single tilting-disk (e.g., Björk-Shiley)
4.0–4.9	Low-risk patients with caged-ball (e.g., Starr-Edwards), ≥1 prostheses, high-risk patients with all mechanical valves

High-risk patient = afibrillation, prior embolus, left atrial thrombus, severe LV dysfunction.
*For low-risk bioprosthetic heterograft, warfarin (3 months, INR 2–3), then optional ASA.

Murmur Characteristics

Type of Valve	Aortic Prosthesis		Mitral Prosthesis	
	Normal Findings	Abnormal Findings	Normal Findings	Abnormal Findings
Caged-Ball (Starr-Edwards)		Aortic diastolic murmur Decreased intensity of opening or closing click		Low-frequency apical diastolic murmur High-frequency holosystolic murmur
Single Tilting-Disk (Björk-Shiley or Medtronic-Hall)		Decreased intensity of closing click		High-frequency holosystolic murmur Decreased intensity of closing click
Bileaflet Tilting-Disk (St. Jude Medical)		Aortic diastolic murmur Decreased intensity of closing click		High-frequency holosystolic murmur Decreased intensity of closing click
Heterograft Bioprosthesis (Hancock or Carpentier-Edwards)		Aortic diastolic murmur		High-frequency holosystolic murmur

Source: Reprinted with permission from *N Engl J Med* 335:410, 1996. Copyright © 1996 Massachusetts Medical Society. All rights reserved.

CARDIOLOGY

ELECTROCARDIOGRAM (ECG) (Adapted from W Hancock. *Synopsis of Criteria for ECG Interpretation.* Stanford University Hospital ECG Laboratory, 1998.)

Standardization

For paper speed 25 mm/second, 1 mm = 0.04 seconds (x-axis) = 1 mV (y-axis)

Rate

- For each large box (5 mm) interval → 300-150-100-75-60-50-43-38-33-30 bpm
- **6-second method:** rate = number of beats in 6 seconds (full 12-lead) × 10

Interval

P-wave <0.1 second (pos I, II; neg R)
- PR interval: 0.12–0.20 second
- QRS interval: 0.05–0.10 second (pos I, II, V_5, V_6; neg R, V_1)
- T wave: positive in I and V_6, negative in R
- QTc interval: 0.34–0.42 second (rate-related, 40% of R-R interval)

Axis

Normal: −30 degrees to +100 degrees or upright I and III
- **Left axis deviation** (−30 degrees to −90 degrees, upright I/downward aVF)
    → in left bundle branch block, left anterior fascicular block, Wolff-Parkinson-White syndrome, hyperkalemia, COPD, RV ectopy, MI, LV hypertrophy
- **Right axis deviation** (+100 degrees to −90 degrees, downward I/downward aVF)
    → in COPD, RV hypertrophy, right bundle branch block, left posterior vascicular block, dextrocardia, LV or RV ectopy, Wolff-Parkinson-White syndrome, lateral infarction, RV strain (pulmonary embolism)

Hypertrophy

- **Left atrial enlargement:** $P(V_1)$ ≥1 mm and ≥0.04 second, P(II) >1.1 second
    Ancillary: left axis of terminal P forces (negative III), P notched but not widened
- **Right atrial enlargement:** P(II, III, F) >2.4 mm and peaked
    Ancillary: initial P(I, II) pos 1.5 mm

LV hypertrophy	RV hypertrophy
$R(V_5, V_6) + S(V_1)$ >35 mm	QRS >75 degrees
R(I) + S(III) >25 mm	$R/S(V_1)$ >1, or $R(V_1)$ or R' (V_1) >6 mm, or $R/S(V_6)$ <1
R(L) >11 mm	
$S(V_3)$ + R(L) >18 mm (women) or >28 mm (men)	

Ancillary: intrinsicoid deflection (V_1) >0.04 second, secondary ST-T changes

Bundle Branch Block

QRS interval ≥0.12 second, incomplete branch block if QRS 0.10–0.12 seconds.
- **Left anterior fascicular block (LAFB):** QRS <45 degrees and <0.12 second, q(I, aVL), rS(II, III, aVF)
- **Left posterior fascicular block (LPFB):** QRS >90 degrees and <0.12 second, qR(II, III, aVF), rS(I, aVL)
- **Left bundle branch block (LBBB):** QRS >0.12 second, monophasic/slurred/notched R(I, V_5, V_6), no Q, ST/T change opposite QRS
- **Right bundle branch block (RBBB):** QRS >0.12 second, R(V_1) peak >0.05 second, wide S(I, V_5, V_6)
- **RBBB + LAFB:** RBBB criteria, first 0.06 second of QRS >–30 degrees, absent Q(II, III, F)
- **RBBB + LPFB:** RBBB criteria, first 0.06 second of QRS >+90 degrees, rS(I), qR(II, III)

Nodal Block

- **Sinus pause:** Abrupt increase/constant P-P interval of 150%
- **SA Mobitz I (Wenckebach):** Abrupt increase P-P interval of <50%, preceded by short P-P
- **SA Mobitz II:** Abrupt increase P-P interval 100%, P-P interval in whole-number ratio
- **First-degree AV block:** P precedes QRS 1:1, PR interval >0.2 second
- **Second-degree AV block:** Regular PP, ≥2 consecutive AV conduction then non-conducted P

    Mobitz I/Wenckebach: PR progressively longer until drop beat
    Mobitz II: PR constant in conducted beats, with nonconducted beats
- **Advanced:** Regular P-P interval, ≥2 consecutive nonconducted P (2:1 = every other beat)
- **Third-degree/complete AV block:** AV independent, A-rate >V-rate, no P conducted when expected

CARDIOLOGY

ECG PRESENTATION OF CLINICAL SYNDROMES

- **Hyperkalemia:** Mild: T wave narrow and peaked; Severe: widened QRS (non-specific)
- **Hypokalemia:** T wave amplitude small or absent, U wave amplitude increased
- **Hypercalcemia:** ↓ST interval, normal T wave duration
- **Hypocalcemia:** ↑ST interval, normal T wave duration
- **Pulmonary embolus:** Sinus tachycardia, $S_1Q_3T_3$, right axis deviation, RV strain
- **Digitalis toxicity:** ST depression ≤2 mm, T wave inversion ≤3 mm, ST concave upscoop, ↓QT interval, AV block
- **Quinidine toxicity:** Widened QRS, ST depression, T wave inversion, ↑QTc (1.5 × normal)
- **Acute pericarditis:** ST elevation (aVR, V_1, III, aVL) ≥1 mm, ST↑ >25% R amplitude, PQ↓
- **Myocardial injury:** ST↑ ≥1 mm, ST↑ straight/convex up
- **COPD:** Low voltage (limb), QRS 60–120 degrees, P >60 degrees, P wave inversion in aVL, S wave in precordial leads, R wave in V_5 >5 mm

DIAGNOSTIC ECG FINDINGS

- **Low voltage** [peak-to-peak QRS <5 mm (limb) or <10 mm (chest)]: in obesity, myxedema, COPD, effusion/tamponade, infiltrative disease (e.g., amyloid, sarcoid, tumor)
- **Long QT:** in congenital heart defects, hypokalemia, hypomagnesemia, hypocalcemia, drugs (e.g., tricyclic antidepressants, class I or III antiarrhythmics, phenothiazines), ischemia, myocarditis, sinus node disease, neurologic diseases, hypothermia
- **Short QT:** in hypercalcemia, digitalis, hyperthyroidism
- **Tall R(V_1):** in congenital heart defects, right ventricular hypertrophy, RBBB, IHSS, Wolff-Parkinson-White (type A), constrictive pericarditis, posterior infarction
- **Q(I, aVL, V_{4-6}):** In anterolateral infarction, pneumothorax, LBBB, right heart pacing, Wolff-Parkinson-White (type C), IHSS, dextrocardia, infiltrative disease
- **Q(II, III, aVF):** In inferior infarction, Wolff-Parkinson-White (type A/B), IHSS, transposition, cor pulmonale, LBBB, right heart pacing, infiltrative disease
- **Q(V_{1-3}):** Pneumothorax, pectus excavatum, LV hypertrophy, IHSS, Wolff-Parkinson-White (type B), infiltrative disease, trauma
- **T wave inversions:** MI, neurologic, metabolic diseases, pericarditis, drugs (e.g., digoxin, quinidine)

WOLFF-PARKINSON-WHITE SYNDROME *(Am Heart J* 138:403, 1999)

Symptoms
- Palpitations
- Watch for ventricular tachycardia if AV node is blocked (accessory pathway conduction)

Diagnosis

Type A
- PR <0.12 second
- Upright QRS >0.1 second with anterior delta wave V_{1-3}
- Inferior-posterior MI/RBBB-like

Type B
- PR <0.12 second
- QRS >0.1 second with posterior delta wave V_{4-6}, I, aVL, with V_{1-3} showing QS or rS complex, tall V_{4-6}
- Inferior MI/anteroseptal MI/LBBB-like

Management
- Electrophysiology study → ablation.
- Never use AV nodal–blocking agents for rate control; procainamide is OK.

CARDIOLOGY

WIDE COMPLEX TACHYCARDIA

Definitions
- **Ventricular tachycardia:** ventricular rate >120 bpm, QRS >0.12 second
  Duration: Salvos (3–6 beats) vs. nonsustained (>6 beats, <10 seconds) vs.
    sustained (>30 seconds)
  Morphology: Monomorphic vs. polymorphic (bidirection, torsades de
    pointes)
- **Accelerated idioventricular rhythm (AIVR):** QRS >0.12 second, ventricular
  rate 60–120 bpm (idioventricular rhythm if rate <60 bpm)
- **Supraventricular tachycardia with aberrant conduction** (differentiated from
  ventricular rhythm by Brugada criteria; see below)

Brugada Criteria for Wide Complex Tachycardia
(Reproduced with permission from P Brugada et al. A new approach to the differential diagnosis of a regular tachycardia with a wide QRS complex. *Circulation* 83:1649, 1991)

				Sensitivity	*Specificity*
1. Is there absence of RS in ALL precordial leads?	Yes (n = 83)	VT (stop)		21%	100%
No ↓ (n = 471)					
2. Is the R to S interval >100 ms in any one precordial lead?	Yes (n = 175)	VT (stop)		66%	98%
No ↓ (n = 296)					
3. Is there AV dissociation? (capture/fusion beats)	Yes (n = 59)	VT (stop)		82%	98%
No ↓ (n = 237)					
4. Are there morphologic criteria* for VT present in both V_{1-2} & V_6	Yes (n = 68)	VT (stop)		99%	97%
No (n = 169)	Diagnosis of SVT with aberration			97%	99%

*See next page.

Brugada ECG Morphologic Criteria for Wide Complex Tachycardia
(Reproduced with permission from P Brugada et al. A new approach to the differential diagnosis of a regular tachycardia with a wide QRS complex. *Circulation* 83:1649, 1991)

ECG Lead V₁ only

ECG Lead V₆

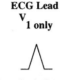

Monophasic R wave

QS or QR

QR or RS

R/S < 1
(seen with LAD)

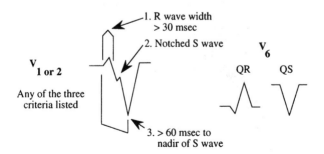

V₁ or 2
Any of the three criteria listed

1. R wave width > 30 msec

2. Notched S wave

3. > 60 msec to nadir of S wave

V₆

QR   QS

CARDIOLOGY

NARROW COMPLEX RHYTHM
- **Sinus rhythm:** P wave precedes QRS configuration 1:1, P wave 0–90 degrees, rate 50–99 bpm
    - **Sinus bradycardia** when rate <50 bpm
    - **Sinus tachycardia** when rate 110–210 bpm
- **Sinus arrhythmia:** Sinus rhythm, vary PP interval >10% (>50% = marked SA)

Narrow Complex Tachycardia
- **Atrial tachycardia with AV block:** Atrial rate 100–260 bpm, ≥2 degrees AV block, changed P morphology, isoelectric interval between P waves
    - *Ancillary: atrial rhythm could be irregular, P wave diminutive*
- **Multifocal atrial tachycardia:** P wave precedes QRS configuration 1:1, >2 P wave morphology, rate >100 bpm
- **Reentrant SVT:** Regular rate 110–240 bpm, QRS configuration same unless aberrancy present, P wave unseen or in ST/T, short PR interval, P wave consistent with retrograde atrial activation
    - Sinoatrial node re-entrant tachycardia
    - Intra-atrial re-entrant tachycardia
    - Atrioventricular node re-entrant tachycardia
- **Junctional rhythm:** Regular basic rhythm, early A-conducted capture/reciprocal beats, retrograde atrial activation or independent rhythm, QRS configuration same unless aberrancy exists; classified as: junctional tachycardia (rate >99 bpm); accelerated junctional rhythm (rate 70–99 bpm); accelerated junctional escape rhythm (rate 60–69 bpm); junctional escape rhythm (rate <60 bpm)
- **Reciprocal beat:** Premature complex occurs in course of a junctional rhythm, retrograde P wave between premature and junctional beat
    - *Ancillary: retrograde V-A conduction usually long in slow junctional rhythm*
- **Capture beat:** Premature complex occurs in course of junctional/idioventricular rhythm, not retrograde P wave between premature and junctional beat
    - *Ancillary: regular atrial rate, AV dissociation except for the captured beats*
- **Atrial flutter:** Atrial rate 200–360 (300s) bpm, no isoelectric interval between waveforms in II, III , F (sawtooth), AV ratio variable, QRS configuration same unless aberrancy exists
    - Type I (typical): atrial rate 250–350 bpm
    - Type II (atypical): atrial rate 350–400 bpm
- **Atrial fibrillation:** atrial rate ill-defined >280 bpm, inconstant rate/morphology, AV ratio varies, irregular ventricular rate, QRS same unless aberrancy present
    - *Ancillary: ventricular rhythm may be regular due to AV block/accelerated junctional/ventricular rhythm*

ATRIAL FIBRILLATION   (*Lancet* 350:94, 1997; *Am J Med* 104:272, 1998; ACC/ AHA Guidelines—*Circulation* 93:1262, 1996)

Fast Facts

- Incidence: 0.5% (ages 50–59 years) to 9% (ages 80–89 years)
- Prevalence: Framingham studies 17.5–21.5/1,000
- Clinical manifestations (*SPAF-III*):

None: 44%	Palpitations: 32%
CHF: 10%	Stroke: 2%
Syncope: 2%	

- Admission indications:

Hypotension	Heart failure
Angina	Structural heart diseases
Comorbidities	Rate uncontrolled with two or more drugs

Common Etiologies of Atrial Fibrillation ("PIRATES")

- **P**ulmonary (COPD/pneumonia, pulmonary embolism, pericardial disease)
- **I**nfarction/infection
- **R**heumatic mitral stenosis (and other valvular diseases: MR, MS, MVP)
- **A**lcohol ("holiday heart syndrome") or **A**trial myxoma
- **T**hyrotoxicosis or **T**heophylline/caffeine
- **E**lectrolyte disturbance (Na$^+$, K$^+$, Ca^{+2})
- **S**ystemic illness (sepsis, malignancy, diabetes mellitus) or **S**tress (postoperative)

Rate Control   (*Ann Intern Med* 125:311, 1996)

Calcium Channel Blockers (in Acute/Chronic Atrial Fibrillation)

- Onset ≥15 minutes
- **Diltiazem:** 0.25 mg/kg (10–20 mg) IVP (2 minutes), repeat 0.35 mg/kg (25 mg) IVP
  Drip: 1–15 mg/hour IV gtt
  Oral (sustained release): 120–240 mg PO qd
- **Verapamil:** 0.15 mg/kg IVP (2 minutes), repeat 0.3 mg/kg IVP (5–10 mg)
  Drip: 5–20 mg/h IV gtt
- Reverse with **calcium gluconate** 10%, 10 mg IV

Beta Blockers (in Acute/Chronic Atrial Fibrillation)

- Especially in hyperadrenergic states, onset ≥10 minutes; do not use in CHF/COPD
- **Metoprolol:** 5 mg IVP (2 minutes) q5min × 3;
  Oral: 25–50 mg PO bid
- **Esmolol:** 500 µg/kg IVP (1 minute), repeat +25–50 µg/kg/minute IV q4min, overall less effective
- **Propranolol** 10–30 mg PO tid–qid, maximum 640 mg/day especially in hyperthyroid AF
- Reverse with **glucagon**

continued

CARDIOLOGY

Digoxin (in Chronic Atrial Fibrillation Rate Control or Before IA Antiarrhythmics)
- Onset ≥5 hours, not effective in acute management, favored in heart failure patients
- **Digoxin:** 0.25–0.50 mg IVP every 6 hours (load 1 g/24 hours)
  Oral: 0.125–0.250 mg PO/IV qd

Anticoagulation for Stroke Prevention
- High risk of atrial thrombus formation secondary to atrial stasis in AF ≥48 hours' duration, requiring anticoagulation before cardioversion
- Stroke risk: 17.5-fold increase with AFib (fourfold increase in lone AFib)
  Incidence of stroke in chronic AF: 5.6–6.9%
  Incidence of stroke in paroxysmal AF: 2.0–6.0%
- Duration
  Postcardioversion requires 3–4 weeks
  Precardioversion (3 weeks) if AFib duration ≥72 hours

Warfarin
For high-risk patients with risk factors for embolic events *(data from SPAF-II)*:
- Age >75
- Cerebrovascular accidents
- Diabetes mellitus
- Heart failure
- Mitral stenosis
- Aneurysm
- Prosthetic valves
- Hypertension
- CAD
- MI
- Intracardiac thrombus
- Hyperthyroidism

Target INR 2–4 *(data from SPAF, SPAF-II, SPINAF, CAFA)*
Ineffective in low dose and with aspirin *(data from SPAF-III)*

Aspirin
- Age <65 without risks *(data from SPAF, SPAF-II)*
- 325 mg PO qd

Cardioversion
Failure Factors
- Age
- Heart failure
- Left atrial enlargement (≥5 cm)
- Hypertension
- Atrial fibrillation duration >1 year
- LV enlargement

Electrical
- Direct current synchronized 100 J → 200 J → 360 J
- Lower stroke risk if no thrombus seen on transesophageal echocardiogram
- Correct electrolytes (potassium, magnesium)

Pharmacological
- Watch for ↑QTc, hypotension, torsades de pointes
- Correct electrolytes before chemical cardioversion (K^+, Mg^{+2})

> Type IA: **Procainamide,** 100 mg IV q10min or 20 mg/minute IV
> Type IC:
>> **Propafenone,** 600 mg PO × 1 (max 1,200 mg, no structural abnormality)
>> **Flecainide,** 100–200 mg PO (max 400 mg/day, no structural abnormality)
> Type III:
>> **Sotalol,** 80 mg PO bid (max 320 mg/day)
>> **Amiodarone,** 600–800 mg/day PO load × 4 weeks, then 200–400 mg/day PO
>> **Ibutilide,** 1 mg (0.01 mg/kg) IVP (10 minutes), may repeat × 1 (max 2 mg)

CARDIOLOGY

SYNCOPE *(Ann Intern Med 126:989, 1997; Ann Intern Med 127:76, 1997)*

Fast Facts
- Incidence:
  - Framingham data: 3.0–3.5%
  - Nursing home residents: 6% annual, 23% lifetime
- Indications for admission:

Structural heart disease	History of arrhythmia
Trauma	Clinical suspicion of acute coronary syndrome
Stroke	

Symptoms or findings	Diagnostic consideration
After sudden pain, unpleasant sight/sound/smell	Vasovagal syncope
During/after micturition, cough, swallow, defecation	Situational syncope
With neuralgia (glossopharyngeal/trigeminal)	Bradycardia/vasodepressor reaction
On standing	Orthostatic hypotension
Prolonged standing	Vasovagal
Well-trained athlete after exertion	Neurally mediated
Changing position (sitting → lying, turning over in bed)	Atrial myxoma/thrombus
Syncope with exertion	Atrial stenosis, pulmonary hypertension, pulmonary embolism, mitral stenosis, IHSS, CAD, neurally mediated
With head rotation, pressure on carotid sinus (collar, shave)	Carotid sinus syncope
With vertigo, dysarthria, diplopia, other neurologic symptoms	TIA, subclavian steal, basilar artery↓
With arm exercise	Subclavian steal
Confusion after episode	Seizure

PACEMAKERS   (*Lancet* 349:41, 1997; *N Engl J Med* 334:89, 1996; *Curr Probl Cardiol* 26:341, 1999)

Natural Pacemakers (bpm)
- SA node: 60–100
- Atrial: 75
- AV node/His-Purkinje: 40–60
- Ventricular: 30–40

Potential Troubleshooting
- Failure to pace

Cause	Solution
Oversensing	Decrease sensitivity
Battery failure	Replace battery

- Failure to sense
- Wire fracture
- Arrhythmia
- Perforation
- Infection

Pacemaker Settings
- Output: Strength of electrical impulse to heart
- Base rate: Frequency of pacing
- Maximal rate: Upper limit for P wave tracking in dual chamber or V pace in single chamber
- Sensitivity: Strength of electrical signal needed from heart for pacemaker to recognize intrinsic activity (usually separate sensitivities for atrium and ventricle)
- A-V interval: Time interval between atrial and ventricular pacing in DDD mode
- Atrial refractory period: Time span after ventricular depolarization that pacemaker will not sense atrial activity (prevents pacemaker mediated tachycardia)

Pacer Modes

Chamber paced	Chamber sensed	Mode of response	Programmable	Antiarrhythmic
V ventricle	V ventricle	T triggered	P programmable	P pacing
A atrium	A atrium	I inhibited	M multi-program	S shock
D dual (V+A)	D dual (V+A)	D/A trigger, V inhibit	C communicate	D dual
S single	O none	O none	R rate modulate	O none
—	S single	R reverse pace (tachy)	O none	—

continued

CARDIOLOGY

Permanent Pacemaker Indications (ACC/AHA Guidelines—*J Am*
Coll Cardiol 31:1175, 1998)

Disorder	American College of Cardiology/American Heart Association indication	Recommended pacing mode
Sinus node dysfunction	I: Sinus node dysfunction with documented symptomatic ↓HR II: Sinus node dysfunction, HR <40 III: No symptoms	AAI if no conduction disease; DDD if AV disease; DDDR if no chronotropic response; DDIR if SVT present
AV block	I: Symptomatic second- and third-degree AV block, asymptomatic third-degree AV block with HR <40, pause >3 seconds II: Asymptomatic Mobitz II second- and third-degree AV block with HR >40 III: First-degree AV block or asymptomatic Mobitz I	DDD if chronotropic competence of sinus node preserved; VVI if no organized atrial activity; DDDR/VVIR if no chronotropic response
Bifascicular/tri-fascicular block	I: With intermittent complete heart block, HR >40, with Mobitz II II: HV intervals >100 ms, pacer-induced infra-HIS or fascicular block with syncope III: Asymptomatic, first-degree AV block	DDD if chronotropic competence of sinus node preserved; VVI if no organized atrial activity; DDDR/VVIR if no chronotropic response
Neurogenic syncope	I: Recurrent carotid sinus syncope, pause >3 seconds II: Syncope with ↓HR by tilt-table III: Syncope with negative tilt-table	DDD or DDI
Cardiomyopathy	II: IHSS refractory to drug therapy III: Dilated cardiomyopathy	DDD if condition refractory to medicines and chronotropic competence of sinus node preserved; DDDR if no chronotropic response

Class I = definite; class II = recommended with some evidence; class III = not recommended with evidence.

CORONARY IMAGING

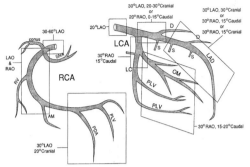

Schematic representation of the right coronary artery (RCA) and left coronary artery (LCA) depicted in the left anterior oblique and right anterior oblique projections, respectively. Approximate frontal and sagittal plane projections and angulations for visualization of various portions of the coronary arteries are indicated. The LCA branches are as noted: SNA = sinus node artery; RV = right ventricular; AM = acute marginal; PDA = posterior descending artery; PLV = posterior left ventricular; LC = left circumflex artery; OM = obtuse marginal; S = septal; D = diagonal; LAD = left anterior descending. Reprinted from CJ Pepine, JA Hill, C Lambert (eds). *Diagnostic and Therapeutic Cardiac Catheterization* (3rd ed). Williams & Wilkins, 1998.)

CARDIOLOGY

AMERICAN SOCIETY OF ECHOCARDIOGRAPHY
16-SEGMENT MODEL OF LEFT VENTRICLE

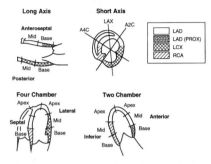

Source: Reproduced with permission from E. Topol (ed). *Comprehensive Cardiovascular Medicine*. Philadelphia: Lippincott–Raven, 1998.

CORONARY ARTERY DISEASES (N Engl J Med 326:242, 1992; Circulation 97:1095, 1998)

Risk Factors and Favorable Factors for Coronary Heart Disease

Definitive risks	Postulated risks	Favorable factors
Age (male >55, female >65)	Intracellular parasites infection (*Chlamydia pneumoniae*, *Mycoplasma*, CMV)	HDL >60
Male gender or estrogen deficiency if female	Immune complex (e.g., lupus)	
Elevated LDL/low HDL cholesterol (<30)	Stress or type A personality	
Smoking (within 3 years)	Low plasma antioxidants	
Hypertension	Physical inactivity	
Family history (first-degree relative, male <55, female <65)	High triglyceridemia/saturated fats; high small, dense LDL	
Diabetes mellitus	Lipoprotein (a)	
Hyperhomocystinemia	High VLDL remnants/IDL	
	Fibrinogen/factor VII	
	Factor V Leiden	

Differential Diagnosis of Chest Pain

Assess *duration* and *reproducibility*.

Cardiac	Gastrointestinal
MI	Gastroesophageal reflux disease
Unstable angina	Esophageal spasm
Pericarditis	Peptic ulcer disease
Aortic dissection	Dyspepsia
CHF	Esophageal rupture

Pulmonary	Miscellaneous
PE	Musculoskeletal
Pneumothorax	Costochondritis
Pneumonia	Rib or sternal fracture
Pulmonary hypertension	Panic attack or anxiety
Pleuritis	Anemia

continued

CARDIOLOGY

Enzymes for Myocardial Ischemia   *(Arch Intern Med 158:1173, 1998)*

Serum marker	Positive	Onset	Peak	Normalize	Sensitivity/ specificity
CK	>170	3–6 hrs	24–36 hrs	3 days	57–88%/93–100%
CK-MB (mass/RI)	>5/5%	4–8 hrs	15–24 hrs	3–4 days	93–100%/94–100%
Myoglobin	>106	2–3 hrs	6–9 hrs	>12 hrs	70%/75–95%
Cardiac troponin I	>0.5*	4–6 hrs	10–24 hrs	7–10 days	100%/>98%
AST	>59	6–8 hrs	24–48 hrs	4–6 days	48–88%/89–97%
LDH-1/ LDH-2	>25/41%	>6 hrs	NA	>3 days	94–99%/61–90%

LDH = lactate dehydrogenase; RI = relative index.
*For diagnosis of myocardial ischemia, cardiac troponin I >2.0 has 100% sensitivity and 98% specificity at Stanford/Palo Alto Veterans Administration Hospital.

CLASSIFICATION OF MYOCARDIAL INFARCTION
Killip and Kimball   *(Am J Cardiol 20:457, 1967)*

Class	Heart failure signs	Mortality
I	No heart failure	3–5%
II	Tachycardia, basilar rales, S_3	12–15%
III	Tachycardia, S_3, rales above scapular tip, pulmonary edema	25–30%
IV	Hypotension, clammy extremities, mental status changes, oliguria	75–85%

Forrester et al.   *(N Engl J Med 295:1356, 1404, 1976)*

Class	Wedge pressure	Cardiac index	Mortality
I	≤18	≥2.2	3%
II	>18	≥2.2	9%
III	≤18	<2.2	23%
IV	>18	<2.2	51%

ECG CHANGES IN MYOCARDIAL INFARCTION

Septal
- QS/qR and ST elevation in V_1, V_2 ≥1 mm
- R in V_3 >V_2 >V_1 ≥1 mm

Lateral
- Q/ST elevation in I, L, V_5, V_6 ≥1 mm

Inferior
- Changed Q/ST elevation in II, III, aVF ≥1 mm
- QRS <0.04 seconds
- Q/R in F >1/3
- Slurred/notched Q in aVF
- T wave inversion in aVF
- Q in II

Anterior
- Q/ST elevation in V_3, V_4 ≥1 mm
- R in V_3 <R in V_2
- Slurred/notched Q in V_3, V_4
- T wave inversion in V_3, V_4

Posterior
- Tall R in V_1 <0.04 second
- R/S in V_1 >1 (no RV hypertrophy/RBBB)
- Upright T in V_1
- ST elevation in V_9 (behind lead)
- ST depression in V_1

Right Ventricular Infarct   (*N Engl J Med* 330:1211, 1994)

- ST ↑ in V_3R, V_4R ≥1 mm + inferior infarction criteria
- Right atrial pressure >10 mm Hg and within 1–5 mm Hg of pulmonary capillary wedge pressure (PCWP) (sensitivity 73%/specificity 100%)

CARDIOLOGY

ACUTE CORONARY SYNDROME: UNSTABLE ANGINA

(*Circulation* 97:1195, 1998; *J Am Coll Cardiol* 33:107, 1999; *Circulation* 90:613, 1994)

Basic Facts

- Clinical syndrome falling between stable angina and myocardial infarction
- ECG changes: 30% ST depression, 20% T-wave inversions/pseudonormalization, 4% ST elevation [~30% without ST elevation have non–Q-wave myocardial infarction (NQWMI)]
- High-risk categories:
  - Recurrent/refractory pain
  - Unexplained LV dysfunction
  - Elevated troponin I level
  - Prior myocardial infarction
  - Silent ischemia on Holter (>60 minutes in 24 hours)

Likelihood of Significant Coronary Artery Disease with Symptoms Suggesting Unstable Angina (*Circulation* 90:613, 1994)

High likelihood (0.85–0.99)	Intermediate likelihood (0.15–0.84)	Low likelihood (0.01–0.14)
Prior MI/sudden death/ CAD	Absence of high-likelihood features	Absence of high- to intermediate-likelihood features
Angina, age male ≥60 or female ≥70	Angina, age male <60, female <70	Chest pain, unlikely angina
Hemodynamic/ECG changes	Probable angina, age male ≥60, female ≥70	0–1 risks other than diabetes
Variant angina (pain with reversible ST↑), recurrent	Chest pain ± angina in diabetics or ≥2–3 risks other than diabetes	T flattening/inversion <1 mm in dominant R waves
Definite ST↑↓ ≥1mm	Extracardiac vascular diseases	Normal ECG
Symmetric T inversions in precordial leads	ST↓ 0.05–1 mm or T inversions ≥1 mm in dominant R waves	

Management ("Rule-Out MI")   (Adapted from ACC/AHA Guidelines—*Circulation* 100:1016, 1999)

- Identification: symptoms, ECG changes (ST depression or T-wave inversion), serum markers
- Telemetry for arrhythmia, IV access (observe without IV access if low likelihood)
- Anti-ischemic therapy: establish antiplatelet and adequate beta blockade
  Chew aspirin tablet
  Sublingual or IV nitrates if persistent/recurrent pain
  Beta blockers (titrate to HR 50–60, MAP ≥60 mm Hg while maintaining neurologic and renal function; avoid if second- or third-degree AV block, bronchospasm, systolic BP <90 mm Hg, or impending cardiogenic shock)
- Antithrombotic therapy:
  Unfractionated heparin IV bolus and drip or low-molecular weight heparin (LMWH) SC if persistent/recurrent pain/high likelihood of ischemia
  Consider glycoprotein IIb/IIIa antagonist in conjunction to angiography/angioplasty for high-risk patients (recurrent ischemia, ↓LV function, widespread ECG changes, prior MI)
- Serial monitoring (>48 hours for high likelihood in unit, 24–48 hours for intermediate likelihood)
  Serial ECG for evolution of ECG changes, always consider posterior infarct ("ECG-silent")
  Serial serum markers (CK with MB-fraction q8h × 3, cardiac troponin I, ?myoglobin).
  Right-sided ECG in inferior ischemia to rule out right ventricular infarct.
  If emergent intervention is considered, hold coumadin, metformin, and food.

CARDIOLOGY

Medical Management for Unstable Angina (Adapted from
Circulation 90:613, 1994; *Circulation* 100:1016, 1999; *J Am Coll Cardiol* 33:107, 1999)

Regimen	Dose	Reference Trial(s)
Anti-thrombotic therapy		
Aspirin	160–325 mg PO qd	Meta-analyses (*JAMA* 260:2259,1988; *BMJ* 308:81,1994)
	ASA-intolerant: ticlopidine 250 mg PO bid *(Circulation* 82:17, 1990) or clopidogrel 75 mg PO bid (CAPRIE, *N Engl J Med* 348:1329, 1996), reviewed in *Circulation* 100:1667, 1999	
Heparin	70 U/kg IVb + 15 U/kg/hr gtt	Meta-analysis (*BMJ* 313:652, 1996)
LMWH (reviewed in *Circulation* 98:1575, 1998)		
Enoxaparin	(30 mg IVb) 1 mg/kg SC q12h	ESSENCE (*N Engl J Med* 337:447, 1997)
	→ 40 mg SC q12h × 1 wk	TIMI-11B (*Circulation* 100:1593, 1999) with IVb
Dalteparin	120 IU/kg q12h SC × 5 d	FRISC (*Lancet* 347:561, 1996)
	→7500 IU q12h × 3 mo	FRISC-II (*Lancet* 354:701, 1999)
GP-IIb/IIIa-inhibitors: bolus and IV gtt × 72 hours, usually with heparin/LMWH; reviewed in *Circulation* 100:437,1999		
Abciximab	0.25 mg/kg IVb → 10 mg/min gtt	CAPTURE (*Lancet* 349:1429, 1997)
Lamifiban	300 µg IVb → 5 µg/min gtt	PARAGON (*Circulation* 97:2386, 1998)
Tirofiban	0.6 µg IVb → 0.15 µg/kg/min gtt	PRISM (*N Engl J Med* 378:1498, 1998)
		PRISM-PLUS (*N Engl J Med* 378:1488, 1998)
Eptifibatide	180 µg/kg IVb → 1.3 µg/kg/min gtt	PURSUIT (*N Engl J Med* 339:436, 1998)

Regimen	Dose	Reference Trial(s)
Anti-ischemic therapy		
Nitroglycerin	5–100 µg/min IV gtt	Gold (*Lancet* 346:1653, 1995)
	0.4 mg SL q5min or nitropaste 1–2 inches to chest wall q6h (keep systolic BP >100 mm Hg)	
Beta blocker	Metoprolol 2–5 mg IVb titrate to HR 50–60 bpm → 50 mg PO bid	Meta-analysis (*JAMA* 260:2259,1988)
Diltiazem	Especially in Prinzmetal's angina, NQWMI, or angina despite beta blockade and nitrates	Gibson (*N Engl J Med* 315:423, 1986; *Am J Cardiol* 60:203, 1987) for diltiazem use

LMWH = low-molecular-weight heparin, SL = sublingual, gtt = IV drip, IVb = IV bolus, SC = subcutaneous, SaO$_2$ = oxygen saturation.

Other Therapy (No Evidence Basis)
- Analgesics: morphine sulfate 2–4 mg IV (especially after nitrate therapy), acetaminophen, antacids ("GI cocktail")
- Oxygen (titrate to SaO$_2$ >92%
- Dioctyl sodium sulfosuccinate (DSS), 250 mg PO bid (prevent straining)

Contraindicated/Controversial Therapies in Unstable Angina
- Thrombolytic therapy (UNASEM, TIMI 3A, TAUSA)
- Routine primary angioplasty/coronary stenting (TIMI 2A, VANQUISH, FRISC-II)
- Anti-inflammatory agents (no evidence)

CARDIOLOGY

THROMBOLYTIC THERAPY (*Circulation* 97:1632, 1998; *ACC/AHA Guidelines—Circulation* 100:1016, 1999; *Circulation* 94:2341, 1996)

Indications
- Chest pain: >30 minutes and <12 hours
- No response to NTG
- ≥1 mm ST↑ in two contiguous limb leads
  or ≥2 mm ST↑ in two contiguous precordial leads
  or new LBBB
  LBBB criteria for patients with acute MI (*N Engl J Med* 334:343, 1996):
      ST elevation ≥1 mm concordant to QRS
      ST depression ≥1 mm in V_1, V_2, or V_3
      ST elevation ≥5 mm discordant to QRS

Contraindications

Absolute	Relative
Active internal bleed	CPR >15 minutes
Cerebrovascular accident within 2 months	Uncontrolled hypertension
Trauma or surgery within 10 days	Bleeding disorders
Brain tumor	GI bleed

Protocols
Accelerated tPA (Alteplase)
- In patients with prior streptokinase use, age <75, anterior MI, chest pain <4 hours
- 15 mg IVP, 50 mg (0.75 mg/kg) IV over 30 minutes, then 35 mg (0.5 mg/kg) over next 60 minutes with heparin [GUSTO-1 (*N Engl J Med* 329: 673, 1993)]

Streptokinase
- In patients with age >75 years, nonanterior MI, chest pain 4–12 hours
- 750,000 units IVP over 20 minutes, then 750,000 units over 40 minutes [GISSI-1 (*Lancet* 1:397, 1996), ISIS-2 (*Lancet* 2:349, 1988)]

Reteplase (rPA)
- 10 units IVP over 2 minutes, repeat in 30 minutes [INJECT (*Lancet* 346:329, 1995), RAPID (*Circulation* 91:2725, 1995), RAPID-II (*Circulation* 94:891, 1996), GUSTO-II (*N Engl J Med* 337:1118, 1997)]

Complications
- Intracranial bleed (~0.4% in SK, ~0.7% in tPA, ~0.9% in rPA, 0.9% in TNK-tPA, 1.1% in nPA)
- Hypotension (10% with streptokinase)
- Reperfusion arrhythmia
- Allergic reaction (1–10% in streptokinase, rare in alteplase/reteplase)

Future Thrombolytic Agents in Clinical Trials (Awaiting FDA Approval)
- Lanoteplase (nPA) 120 KU/kg IV over [InTIME (*Circulation* 98:2117, 1998)]
- Tenecteplase (TNK-tPA) according to body weight: 30 mg (≤60 kg), 35 mg (60–69.9 kg), 40 mg (70–79.9 kg), 45 mg (80–89.9 kg), 50 mg (≥90 kg), single bolus over 5–10 seconds [ASSENT-2 (*Lancet* 354:716, 1999)]

ADJUNCTIVE MEDICAL THERAPY IN MYOCARDIAL INFARCTION
(ACC/AHA Guidelines—*Circulation* 100:1016, 1999; *Circulation* 94:2341,1996)

Regimen	Class I	Class IIa	Class IIb	Class III
Oxygen	Pulmonary edema, SaO$_2$ ≤90%	Uncomplicated MI ≤3 hrs	Routine use in uncomplicated MI	—
Nitroglycerin IV	Large anterior MI, ↑BP, persistent/recurrent heart failure/ischemia	—	Uncomplicated MI ≤48 hrs	SBP <90 or HR <50
Aspirin, 160–325 mg	All MI/ischemia, unless intolerant	See note*	—	—
Atropine, 1 mg IVP	SB + ↓BP, ↑PVCs at MI onset, IMI, second- or third-degree AVB, nausea after morphine	IMI + second- or third-degree AVB + Sx (no ↓BP), arrhythmia	IMI + second or third-degree AVB (no Sx)	SB + Sx, second or third-degree AVB
Heparin/ LMWH†	PTCA/CABG	Using altepase, high risk for emboli, non ST↑ MI	Using thrombolytics other than altepase	—
Beta blocker	Thrombolysed <12 hrs, recurrent ischemia, AFib, tachycardia	—	NQWMI	↓LVEF, severe COPD/ asthma
Calcium channel blocker	—	Ongoing ischemia without beta block, rate control	NQWMI, Prinzmetal's	↓LVEF, nifedipine
Magnesium	—	Torsades de pointes, ↓magnesium	High risk	—
ACE inhibitors	LVEF <40%, ST↑, anterior MI (<24 hrs)	LVEF 40–50%, other MI (<24 hrs)	Post-MI with LV dysfunction	—
GPIIb/IIIa inhibitors	—	High risk non-ST↑ MI, refractory ischemia	—	High bleeding risk

SB = sinus bradycardia; AVB = AV block; NQWMI = non–Q-wave MI; LVEF = left ventricular ejection fraction; IMI = inferior MI; PVC = premature ventricular complexes; AFib = atrial fibrillation; Sx = symptoms.
Class I = definite; class IIa = recommended with evidence; class IIb = recommended with little evidence; class III = not recommended with evidence.
*Aspirin-intolerant or allergic patients, substitute with oral ticlopidine 250 mg bid or clopidogrel 75 mg qd, or dipyridamole 75–100 mg qid.
†Recommended unfractionated heparin (UFH) dose is 60 U/kg IV bolus (max 4000 U) followed by 12 U/kg/h IV gtt (max 1000 U/hr) adjusted to aPTT 1.5–2× control (50–70s) for 48 hrs; SC heparin (UFH 7500 U or enoxaparin 1 mg/kg bid) to reduce thrombotic/embolic risk.
Class I = definite; class IIa = recommended with evidence; class IIb = recommended with little evidence; class III = not recommended with evidence.

CARDIOLOGY

NONMEDICAL THERAPEUTIC INTERVENTIONS
IN MYOCARDIAL INFARCTION (ACC/AHA Guidelines—*Circulation* 100:1016, 1999; *Circulation* 94:2341, 1996)

Temporary Pacemaker: Indications

Prophylactic	Therapeutic
New LBBB	Asystole
RBBB + LAFB/LPFB	Mobitz II and third-degree AV block
Alternating block	Bradycardia with hypotension

Pulmonary Artery Catheter

Indications
Hypotension unresponsive to IV fluid
Unexplained ↑HR, ↑RR, ↓Po$_2$, ↓BP
Refractory acidosis
Refractory pulmonary edema
Suspicion for new VSD or mitral regurgitation

Intra-Aortic Balloon Pump

Indications	Contraindications
Cardiogenic shock	Aortic regurgitation
Mitral regurgitation	Aortic dissection
VSD	Severe aorto-iliac/femoral disease
Refractory ischemia/ventricular tachycardia	
Complicated PTCA	

Intra-Aortic Balloon Pump Placement
- Position balloon tip 1–2 cm from aortic knob
- Heparin if >1:2 augment
- ± Antibiotic coverage (cefazolin)
- Watch for decreased platelets and pulse rates
- Inflation starts at dicrotic notch (aortic valve closure)
- Arterial line: prioritize left arm to better monitor balloon pump proximal positioning

---

Implantable Defibrillators

Indications
Ventricular fibrillation or ventricular tachycardia arrest
Inducible sustained or nonsustained ventricular tachycardia
↓Ejection fraction

COMPLICATIONS OF MYOCARDIAL INFARCTION

Left Ventricular Pseudoaneurysm or Aneurysm
- Up to 3 months
- Contained rupture of myocardium versus wall-contained pericardium or thrombus
- ↑Risk of true rupture
- 90% anterior MI
- Treatment: surgery

Left Ventricular Thrombus
- 20%, usually within <5 days of anterior MI
- ↑Risk with atrial fibrillation, ejection fraction <30%, or emboli within 3 months
- Treatment: heparin/coumadin (INR 2–3) for 3 months

Right Ventricular Infarction
- Involving posterior wall or RV, with hypotension
- Treatment: IV fluid resuscitation, pacemaker

Mitral Regurgitation
- Ruptured papillary muscles
- 1%, especially inferior MI (inferoposterior), within 2–7 days, seen in transesophageal echocardiography (TEE)
- Treatment: intra-aortic balloon pump/vasodilators/inotropic agents→emergent surgical repair

Pericarditis
- Acute ≤10%, within 2–4 days
- Infrequently causes tamponade (absolute contraindication for thrombolysis)
- Treatment: NSAIDs
- Dressler's syndrome: immunologic reaction; occurs 1–12 weeks post-MI in 1% of patients; may lead to constriction

Postinfarct Angina
- Reinfarction in 30% after tPA versus 10% after PTCA
- Treatment: heparin, beta blockers, catheter/PTCA/CABG

Free-Wall Rupture
- 1–3%, several days (day 3) post–anterior MI (lateral)
- Shock/electromechanical dissociation/tamponade

Ventricular Septal Rupture
- 1–2%, mostly 3–5 days (up to 14 days)
- In anterior MI (60%), inferior MI (40%)

Arrhythmia
- Reperfusion (transient, no treatment) versus ventricular tachycardia/fibrillation (3–6 months post-MI, structural)
- Treatment: lidocaine/amiodarone versus defibrillator/catheter ablation

Left Ventricular Dysfunction/Cardiogenic Shock
- 5–8% several days post–anterior MI, especially in diabetes mellitus, ejection fraction <35%, elderly
- Treatment: IV fluids, intra-aortic balloon pump, inotropic agents, emergent PTCA/CABG

CARDIOLOGY

CARDIOGENIC SHOCK: PHARMACOLOGIC INTERVENTIONS

(*Ann Intern Med* 131:47, 1999)

Drug effect	Furo-semide	IV nitrates	Dobutamine	Dopamine	ACE inhibitors
Preload	↓	↓	—	↑	↓
Afterload	—	Minimal ↓	Minimal ↓	↑	↓
Sinus tachy-cardia	No	Yes	Minimal	Yes	Minimal

Parameters	Furo-semide	IV nitrates	Dobuta-mine	Dopa-mine	ACE inhibitors
Moderate heart failure (PCWP 20–24)	Yes	Yes	If systolic BP >70	If systolic BP >70, ↓urine	Oral main-tenance
Severe heart fail-ure (PCWP >24, cardiac index >2.5)	Yes	If systolic BP >95	If systolic BP >70	If systolic BP >70	Yes
Cardiogenic shock (systolic BP <95, PCWP >18, cardiac index <2.5)	CI	CI	Yes	Yes, IABP consid-ered	Relative CI
RV infarction	CI	CI	Titrated	Relative CI	CI

Yes = useful; CI = contraindicated; IABP = intra-aortic balloon pump.

Source: Reprinted with permission from MG Khan. *Heart Disease Diagnosis and Therapy: A Practical Approach*. Baltimore: Williams & Wilkins, 1996.

REVASCULARIZATION   *(N Engl J Med 335:129, 1996; Ann Intern Med 125:539, 1997)*

Percutaneous Transluminal Coronary Angioplasty (PTCA, "Balloon")

Acute Complications
- Death (1%)
- Emergent CABG (1–3%)
- MI (2–5%)

Postcatheterization Care   *(Am Heart J 136:S32, 1998; Ann Intern Med 127:458, 1997)*

Chest Pain
- Acute closure (2–7%; one-third within 24 hours; treatment: PTCA/CABG)
- Spasm (NTG drip)

Thrombosis
- Heparin 18–24 hours postoperative in high-risk patients
- ASA/ticlopidine/abciximab (see the section on Cardiac Stenting for dose information)

↑CK/Troponin I: (10–30%)
- ↑Mortality with fivefold increase
- Monitor q8h until ↓CK

Access Complication
- Hemorrhage (compress)
- Pseudoaneurysm
- AV fistula (check with ultrasound)→sandbag/G-clamp (check distal pulses)

Nephropathy (30%)
- Hydration, mannitol
- Normalize 2–7 days

Restenosis (30–50%, recurrent angina 3–9 months)
- Detected by thallium stress test and ECG

Hemodynamic Instability
- Especially with rotational atherectomy
- Management: balloon pump, pacing, NTG

continued

CARDIOLOGY

Cardiac Stenting (Gianturco-Roubin/Palmaz-Schatz)

(*J Am Coll Cardiol* 32:1471, 1998; *Lancet* 351:1943, 1998)

- Subacute stent thrombosis
     Presents as acute MI in 2–14 days
- Restenosis in 3–6 months
- Antiplatelet: ticlopidine (Ticlid), 250 mg bid, or clopidogrel (Plavix), 75 mg qd × 2 weeks + ASA
- Glycoprotein IIb/IIIa inhibitor (*Circulation* 98:2629, 1998)
     May give with heparin/ASA 30 minutes before PTCA up to 12 hours post-PTCA
     Abciximab (ReoPro), 0.25 µg/kg IVb→0.125 µg/kg/minute (max 10 µg/minute) IV gtt × 12 hours [EPIC (*N Engl J Med* 330:956, 1994), EPILOG (*N Engl J Med* 336:1689, 1997) CAPTURE (*Lancet* 349:1429), EPISTENT (*Lancet* 352:87, 1998)]
     Tirofiban (Aggrastat), 10 µg/kg over 3 minutes→0.15 µg/kg/minute IV gtt × 36 hours [RESTORE (*Circulation* 96:1445, 1997)]
     Eptifibatide (Integrilin), 135 µg/kg IV bolus→0.5 µg/kg/minute IV gtt × 24 hours [IMPACT (*Lancet* 349:1422, 1997)]

CORONARY ARTERY BYPASS GRAFTING (CABG)

Indications   [CASS Registry (*Circulation* 92:1629, 1995); ACC/AHA Guidelines—*Circulation* 100:1464, 1999]

- Left main >50% stenosis or equivalent (≥70% proximal left anterior descending and/or circumflex arteries)
- Three-vessel disease (>50% stenosis) and ↓LVEF (<50%)
- Less severe CAD with severe valvular lesions
- Less severe CAD refractory to PTCA or medical management especially with proximal left anterior descending lesions
- Diabetics: CABG advantageous over PTCA, especially left internal mammary artery graft→left anterior descending [BARI (*N Engl J Med* 335:217, 1996)]

PTCA vs. CABG

- CABG has greater relief of angina
- CABG has fewer repeat procedures (left internal mammary artery graft ~15 years, saphenous vein graft ~8 years)
- CABG has no survival advantages over PTCA
- CABG is better than PTCA for left main disease and three-vessel disease with ↓LVEF

Intervention vs. Medical Therapy

- All patients should be treated medically with aggressive treatment of risk factors
- Intervention (PTCA, CABG) is better for patients with three-vessel disease and normal ejection fractions, for symptom relief, and for exercise tolerance
- Either (PTCA or medical therapy) is acceptable for one- or two-vessel disease without proximal left anterior descending disease in symptomatic patients
- Medical therapy is preferred in one- or two-vessel disease without proximal left anterior disease in asymptomatic patients

CARDIOLOGY

STRESS TESTING (*Circulation* 76:653A, 1986; ACC/AHA Guidelines—*Circulation* 96:345, 1997)

Indications for Exercise Testing

Class 1: Clear Indication (Patients with Suspected or Proven CAD)

- Diagnosis: Patients with exercise-related complaints of palpitations, dizziness, or syncope
- Diagnosis: Men with atypical symptoms
- Prognostic assessment and functional capacity evaluation in patients with chronic stable angina or post-MI
- Symptomatic recurrent exercise-induced arrhythmias
- Evaluation after revascularization procedure

Class 2: Test May Be Indicated

- Diagnosis: Women with typical or atypical angina pectoris
- Functional capacity evaluation to monitor cardiovascular therapy in patients with CAD or heart failure
- Evaluation of patients with variable angina
- Follow-up of patients with known CAD
- Evaluation of asymptomatic men more than 40 years old who are in special occupations, who have two or more atherosclerotic risk factors, or who plan to enter a vigorous exercise program

Class 3: Test Probably Not Indicated

- Evaluation of patients with isolated premature ventricular beats and no evidence of CAD
- Multiple serial testing during the course of cardiac rehabilitation program
- Diagnosis of CAD in patients who have pre-excitation syndrome or complete LBBB or are on digitalis therapy
- Evaluation of young or middle-aged asymptomatic men or women who have no atherosclerotic risk factors or who have noncardiac chest discomfort

Contraindications for Exercise Testing

- Unstable angina with recent chest pain
- Untreated life-threatening cardiac arrhythmias
- Severe hypertrophic obstructive cardiomyopathy
- Uncompensated CHF
- Advanced AV block
- Acute myocarditis or pericarditis
- Critical aortic stenosis
- Uncontrolled hypertension
- Acute systemic illness

Ineligible Patients

- Abnormality of baseline ECG (LBBB, LV hypertrophy, digitalis effect)
- Poor exercise tolerance

HEART FAILURE   (*N Engl J Med* 335:490, 1996; *Lancet* 352[Suppl 1]:1, 1998; Action-HF Guidelines—*Am J Cardiol* 83:2A, 1999)

New York Heart Association (NYHA) Classification for Systolic Heart Failure* (*Circulation* 90:644, 1994)

I   Patients with cardiac disease but without resulting limitation of physical activity. Ordinary physical activity does not cause undue fatigue, palpitation, dyspnea, or angina.

II   Patients with cardiac disease resulting in slight limitation of physical activity. They are comfortable at rest. Ordinary physical activity results in fatigue, palpitation, dyspnea, or angina.

III   Patients with cardiac disease resulting in marked limitation of physical activity. They are comfortable at rest. Less than ordinary physical activity causes fatigue, palpitation, dyspnea, or angina

IV   Patient with cardiac disease resulting in inability to carry on any physical activity without discomfort. Symptoms of cardiac insufficiency or of the anginal syndrome may be present even at rest. If any physical activity is undertaken, discomfort is increased.

*New NYHA Functional Classification includes objective assessments: A = no cardiovascular disease; B = minimal cardiovascular disease; C = moderate cardiovascular disease; D = severe cardiovascular disease.

Reversible Etiologies
- Anemia
- Atrial myxoma
- Valvular/congenital heart disease
- Beri-beri
- Obesity
- Thromboembolic disease (PE)
- Thyroid disease
- AV fistula
- Alcohol
- Arrhythmia (tachycardia)
- Paget's disease

Admission Criteria
- Pulmonary edema
- SaO_2 ≤90%
- Systolic BP ≤75 mm Hg
- ↑Hepatic/renal/pulmonary dysfunction
- Cardiac arrest
- Defibrillator (ICD) firing
- MI
- Respiratory distress while sitting
- HR ≥120
- ↓Mentation
- ↑Anasarca
- Symptomatic arrhythmia
- Syncope
- Decompensating, chronic CHF

CARDIOLOGY

MANAGEMENT OF SYSTOLIC HEART FAILURE (ACTION-HF
Guidelines—*Am J Cardiol* 83:1A, 1999)

- Lifestyle modification: cardiac rehabilitation/exercise training, diet control (salt restriction), daily weights, cardiac risk reduction (smoking/EtOH cessation, BP/glycemic control), immunization (pneumovax/flu vaccine), avoid NSAIDs and nephrotoxins

Medical Management

Regimen	Start → Target dose	Trials/reference	Considerations
Diuretics (furo-semide/thiaz-ides)	—	—	Closely monitor K/Na
ACE-inhibitor/ AII receptor blockers (ARB)			First-line therapy, use if serum Cr ≤3.0 mg/dl, K ≤5.5 mEq/dL
Captopril	6.25 qd → 50–100 mg tid	SAVE (*N Engl J Med* 327:669,1992)	
Enalapril	5 qd → 10–20 mg bid	SOLVD (*N Engl J Med* 325:293,1991)	
Lisinopril	2.5 qd → 10–40 mg qd	ATLAS (*Circulation* 100:1, 1999)	
Ramipril	1.25 qd → 5–10 mg bid	AIRE (*Lancet* 342:821,1993)	
Losartan	50 qd → 50 mg qd–bid	ELITE (*Lancet* 349:747,1997)	For ACE-intoler-ant*
Beta blocker			
Carvedilol	6.25 qd → 25–50 mg bid	U.S. trial (*N Engl J Med* 334:1349,1996)	Slow titration, watch for ↓HR, ↓BP
Metoprolol-XL	12.5 qd → 50–100 mg qd	MERIT-HF (*Lancet* 353:2001,1999)	
Digoxin	→ 0.125 mg qd–qod	DIG (*N Engl J Med* 336:525,1997)	No need to monitor
Spironolactone	25 qod → 25–50 mg qd	RALES (*N Engl J Med* 341:709,1999)	Watch ↑K, NYHA3+
Hydralazine (H)/nitrates (N)	H: 10 qid → 100 mg qid + N: 10 qid → 40 mg qid	VHeFT-II (*N Engl J Med* 325:303,1991)	For ACE-intolerant (isosorbide dinitrate preferred)
Warfarin	Titrate to INR >2	(*J Am Coll Cardiol* 31:749,1998)	For ↑LV volume, ↓EF
Amiodarone	200–300 mg qd	GEISCA (*Lancet* 344:493,1994)	Refractory arrhythmia
Inotropic agents (dobutamine/milrinone)	—		End-stage heart failure

*Not approved by FDA for heart failure indication; currently recommended for use only in ACEI-intolerant patients; preliminary results from ELITE-II showed no statistically significant difference with captopril on mortality reduction; therefore should not substitute ACE inhibitors

Surgical Management
- Coronary revascularization (CABG) for viable myocardium
- Defibrillator (ICD) placement
- Mechanical assistive devices (*N Engl J Med* 339:1522, 1998; *Circulation* 97:2079, 1998)
- Cardiomyoplasty (*Cardiol Clin* 16:727, 1998)
- Orthotopic heart transplantation (*JAMA* 280:1692, 1998)

CARDIOLOGY

PULMONARY HYPERTENSION (N Engl J Med 336:111, 1997; Chest 104:236, 1993)

Symptoms
- Dyspnea (60%)
- Angina (47%)
- Raynaud's
- Syncope (8%)
- Edema/anasarca

Diagnosis
- Exam: high-pitched blowing systolic murmur, narrow split S_2, loud P_2, right ventricular hypertrophy/tricuspid regurgitation
- ECG with right axis deviation/RV hypertrophy
- Chest x-ray with prominent main pulmonary artery
- Echocardiogram with bubble study
- Pulmonary artery catheterization
- $\dot{V}/\dot{Q}$ to rule out pulmonary embolus
- Pulmonary function tests
- ANA

Differential Diagnosis (Secondary Etiology)
- Parenchymal lung disease
- Congenital
- Thromboembolic (e.g., PE)
- Mediastinal fibrosis
- Foreign body
- Tumor
- Schistosomiasis
- Vasculitides
- Rapeseed oil
- Cocaine
- HIV
- Fen-phen
- Portal hypertension
- Congenital heart disease (shunt)

Management
- Oxygen
- Anticoagulation
- Prostacyclin
- Diuretics
- Oral nifedipine
- Lung transplantation

HYPERTENSIVE CRISIS (EMERGENCY) (N Engl J Med 323:1177, 1990)

Definition
Systolic BP >220 / diastolic BP >120 + end-organ damage
- Visual disturbance
- Change in mental status/encephalopathy
- MI
- Hemolytic anemia
- Headache
- CHF
- Renal failure
- Retinopathy grade 3–4

Hypertensive urgency refers to severe elevations of blood pressure in absence of symptoms or evidence of target organ involvement (usually treated with oral regimen)

Common Etiologies
- Uncontrolled/noncompliant hypertension
- Renal disease (renal artery stenosis)
- Eclampsia
- Drugs (cocaine, methamphetamine, LSD, PCP, diet/cold medications, MAOI with tyramine)
- Drug withdrawal (alcohol, ACE inhibitor, clonidine)
- Pheochromocytoma (↑urine catecholamines)
- Hyperaldosteronism (↓K, ↑PTH)
- Vasculitis
- Cushing's syndrome

Management
- Aim for 25–33% reduction in diastolic BP to 90–100 mm Hg
- No therapy for acute cerebrovascular accident

CARDIOLOGY

PHARMACOLOGIC MANAGEMENT OF HYPERTENSIVE CRISIS (*Drug Safety* 2:99, 1998; *N Engl J Med* 323:1177, 1990)

Drug	Dose (IV)	Onset	Duration	Side effects	Remarks
Nitroprusside (Nipride)	0.3–10.0 µg/kg/min IV gtt	Instant	2–3 mins	Vomiting, cyanide toxicity (>48 hrs)	All indications, fast-acting, needs arterial line
NTG	5–100 µg/min IV gtt	1–2 mins	3–5 mins	Headache, vomiting, tachyphylaxis	Especially for MI, post-CABG, avoid in RV infarction
Diazoxide	50–100 mg IVP, 15–30 mg/min IV gtt	1–5 mins	6–12 hrs	↓BP, MI, vomiting, tachycardia	Long half-life limits use
Hydralazine	10–20 mg IVP q10min	5–15 mins	2–6 hrs	↓BP, tachycardia, headache, vomiting	Especially in eclampsia, reflex tachycardia
Labetalol	20–80 mg IVP, 1–2 mg/min IV gtt	5–10 mins	2–6 hrs	↓BP, AV block, vomiting, wheezing	Pregnancy-safe, especially for head and spine trauma
Phentolamine	5–10 mg IVP prn	1–2 mins	15–60 mins	↑↓BP, tachycardia	Pheochromocytoma
Esmolol	500 µg/kg/min IVP; 50–300 µg/kg/min IV gtt	1–3 mins	1–2 mins	AV block, bronchospasm	Especially aortic dissection, avoid in pheochromocytoma
Enalaprilat	0.625–5.0 mg IVP q6h	15 mins	4–6 hrs	↓BP, angioedema	Scleroderma, renal crisis/CHF
Nicardipine	5–15 mg/hr IV gtt	1–5 mins	30 mins	↓BP, AV block	Convert to PO

AORTIC DISSECTION *(N Engl J Med 328:35, 1993)*

Fast Facts: Stanford Classification
- Type A (proximal)→surgical treatment
- Type B (distal)→medical treatment

Physical Examination
- Check bilateral BP/carotid pulse
- Check radial-femoral lag
- Aortic regurgitation murmur

Diagnosis
- Widened mediastinum on chest x-ray

	Sensitivity	Specificity
Aortography	85–90%	94%
Spiral CT	85–95%	87–100%
MRI	98%	98%
TEE	98%	77–97%

Management

Beta Blockers
- Propranolol, 5 mg IVP→1 mg IVP q5min × 2
- Labetalol, 5–10 mg IV q2min to 10–20 mg/hour→40–120 mg/hr gtt
- Metoprolol, 5 mg IVP q2min × 3→50 mg PO q6h
- Esmolol, 30 mg IVP→3–12 mg/minute gtt

Vasodilators
- Nitroprusside, 20 µg/minute→20–800 µg/minute gtt
- Enalaprilat, 0.625–5.0 mg IV q6h

CARDIOLOGY

HEMODYNAMIC MONITORING: PULMONARY ARTERY CATHETER
(ACC/AHA Guidelines: *J Am Coll Cardiol* 32:840, 1998)

Indications for Pulmonary Artery (Swan-Ganz) Catheter

- MI complicated by hypotension unresponsive to:
    Fluid challenge
    Pressors/intra-aortic balloon pump
    Heart failure
    Questionable tamponade, mitral regurgitation, or wall rupture/ventricular
        septal defect
- Unstable angina with NTG drip
- Identify cardiogenic pulmonary edema:
    Determine if patient requires pre-/afterload and inotropic therapy
    Determine if patient requires diuretics/fluid
- Pulmonary hypertension diagnosis and therapy
- Optimizing PEEP/volume therapy in adult respiratory distress syndrome
- Diagnosis of intracardiac shunt and cardiac tamponade

Normal Right-Sided Pressures

- RA: a wave = v wave = 2–10 mm Hg
- RV = 15–30 mm Hg (systolic)/2–8 mm Hg (diastolic)
- PA = 15–30 mm Hg (systolic)/4–12 mm Hg (diastolic)/9–18 mm Hg (mean)

Normal Left-Sided Pressures

- PCWP/LA = 2–10 (mean), a wave = v wave ~3–12
    PCWP should be < pulmonary artery diastolic pressure
    Mean PCWP should be < mean PAP
- LV = 100–140 (systolic BP)/3–12 (diastolic BP)*
- Aorta = 100–140 (systolic BP)/60–90 (diastolic BP)/70–105 (mean)*

---

*Available only in left-sided catheterization.

PULMONARY ARTERY PRESSURES IN VARIOUS FORMS OF SHOCK

Abnor-mality	RAP	RVEDP	PAD	PCWP	CI	SVR	Comment
Normal	2–10	2–8	8–15	2–10	—	—	—
Hypo-volemic	—	—	—	↓	Varies	↑	—
Cardio-genic	—	—	—	↑	↓	↑	—
Sepsis	—	—	—	N	Varies	↓	—
LV failure	N/↑	N/↑	↑	↑	↓	↑	Large anterior MI
RV infarct	↑	↑	N	N	↓	↑	Inferior MI
Ventricular septal defect	↑	↑	N/↑	N/↑	↓	↑	O$_2$ step up
Acute mitral regurgitation	N/↑	N/↑	↑	↑	↓	↑	V waves
Tamponade	↑	↑	↑	↑	N/↓	↑	—
Free-wall rupture	↑	↑	↑	↑	↓	↑	Pulsus paradoxus

RAP = right atrial pressure; RVEDP = right ventricular end diastolic pressure; PAD = pulmonary artery diastolic; PCWP = pulmonary capillary wedge pressure; SVR = systemic vascular resistance; N = normal.

CARDIOLOGY

CORONARY CARE UNIT FORMULAS

Cardiac Output

$$CO\text{-Fick} = SV \times HR = \frac{\overline{V}O_2}{C(a - \bar{v})O_2 \times 10}$$
4.8–7.6 (liters/min)/m²

$$\approx \frac{125 \text{ ml/min/m}^2 \times BSA \text{ (in m}^2)}{10 \times [1.36 \times (Hgb) \times (SaO_2\% - SvO_2\%)]} \text{ or } \frac{3 \text{ ml/kg} \times \text{weight (in kg)}}{10 \times [1.36 \times (Hgb) \times (SaO_2\% - SvO_2\%)]}$$

Systemic Vascular Resistance

$$SVR = \frac{(MAP - CVP) \times 80}{CO}$$
700–1,600 dynes-sec/cm⁵

Pulmonary Vascular Resistance

$$PVR = \frac{(MPAP - PCWP) \times 80}{CO}$$
30–130 dynes-sec/cm⁵

Cardiac Index

$CI = CO / BSA$
2.4–3.8 (liters/min)/m²

Arterial O₂ Content

Arterial
$O_2 \text{ content} = (1.36 \times Hgb) \times SaO_2 + (PaO_2 \times 0.0031)$
16–22 cc O₂/dl blood

Mixed Venous O₂ Content

Mixed venous
$O_2 \text{ content} = (1.36 \times Hgb) \times SvO_2 + (PvO_2 \times 0.0031)$
12–17 cc O₂/dl blood

AV O₂ Content Difference

$AV \, O_2 \text{ content difference} = CaO_2 - CvO_2$
3.5–5.5 cc O₂/dl blood
$\rightarrow$ >5 implies cardiac shock (low output); <5 implies sepsis

Oxygen Delivery

$\text{Oxygen delivery} = CO \times \text{arterial } O_2 \text{ content} \times 10$
700–1,400 cc/min

Body Surface Area

$$BSA \text{ (m}^2) = \sqrt{[\text{height (cm)} \times \text{weight (kg)} \div 3600]}$$

Shunt Ratio

$$\frac{Q_p}{Q_s} = \frac{(SaO_2 - MvO_2)}{(PvO_2 - PaO_2)}$$
Small if ratio <1.5
Large if >2, R→L <1

48

PRESSORS

Drug	Dose (μg/min)	Target receptor	Inotropy	Chronotropy	Vasoconstriction	Cardiac output	Side effects
Dopamine	0–3	D	0	0	Dilatation	↑	Ventricular arrhythmias
	3–10	β1 >β2	++	++	0	↑	
	>10	α1	0	0	++	↓	
Dobutamine	2–20	β1 >β2	++++	++	0/–	↑↑	Ventricular arrhythmia
Epinephrine	0.02–0.40	α1 = β1 = β2	++++	++++	++++	↑	Ischemia vs. arrhythmias
Norepinephrine (Levophed)	0–16	α1 >β1	++	++	++++	±	Reflex bradycardia
Phenylephrine (NeoSynephrine)	0–300	α1	0	0	++++	↓	Reflex bradycardia
Milrinone	0.375–0.750	cAMP	+++	++	Vasodilation	↑	Tachyarrhythmia, ↓BP

cAMP = cyclic adenosine monophosphate.

2. Pulmonary

RESPIRATORY DISTRESS
Differential Diagnosis
- Heart failure (cardiomyopathy, vascular disease, valvular disease, MI)
- Anaphylaxis
- Noncardiogenic pulmonary edema
- Bronchospasm
- Infection
- Pulmonary hypertension
- Pneumothorax, hemothorax
- Pulmonary embolus
- Mucus plugging
- Upper airway obstruction

Diagnosis
- Vital signs + SaO_2
- Physical examination (crackles/rales, dullness/↓breath sounds, stridor, wheezes, jugular venous distention, murmur, deep venous thrombosis signs, no breath sounds)
- Chest x-ray
- ECG
- Arterial blood gases (ABGs)

Treatment
General
- Oxygen
- Consider intubation versus bilevel intermittent positive pressure (BIPAP)
- Suctioning

Pulmonary Edema
- Lasix (↓afterload and preload)
- Morphine (↓preload/pulmonary pressures)
- Nitrates (↓afterload, ↓pulmonary pressures)
- Oxygen
- Position (elevate head to ↓preload)

Bronchospasm
- Nebulizers/steroids

Anaphylaxis: See page 252

Pneumothorax, Hemothorax, and Pleural Effusion (*Clin Chest Med* 13:92, 1992)
- Chest tube
- Consider pleurodesis or surgery if no improvement and the following indications:

Second pneumothorax	Air leak >7–10 days
Unexpanded with continued air leak	History of contralateral pneumothorax
Bilateral pneumothorax	High risk (e.g., diver, pilot)
Large bullae	Tension pneumothorax
	Undrained hemothorax

Pulmonary Embolus (see Pulmonary Embolus section)

RESPIRATORY SUPPORT: OXYGEN (Marino, *The ICU Book* [2nd ed]. 1998, p. 344)

Fast Facts
- Normal $PaO_2 = 103 - 0.4 \times age$
- **Pulse oximetry:** below 87% Hb saturation is nonlinear (ABG needed especially for change in pH)

Equations
Alveolar-arterial oxygen gradient (A-a gradient) $= PAO_2 - PaO_2$
$$= [FIO_2 (P_B - PH_2O) - PaCO_2/RQ] - PaO_2$$
$$\approx [713 \times (FIO_2)] - PaCO_2/0.8] - PaO_2$$
At sea level and room air: A-a gradient $= 150 - 1.25 \times (PaCO_2) - PaO_2$ (normal ≤15–25)
Oxygen content $= (1.34 \text{ ml } O_2/g \text{ Hgb} \times Hgb \times O_2 \text{ Sat.%}/100) + (PaO_2 \times 0.0003)$

Types of Oxygen Support

Oxygen supply	Liters/minute	FIO$_2$	PaO$_2$ at sea level
Room air		0.21	100
Nasal cannula	1–6	0.4 (↑4%/liter)	227
Venturi mask	1–4	0.5 (0.24–0.5)*	300
Face mask	6–15	0.6 (0.4–0.6)	370
Partial rebreather	5–7	0.8 (0.4–0.8)	512
Non-rebreather	≥15	1.0 (0.4–1.0)	655

- *Venturi mask with O_2 concentration at 24%, 28%, 30%, 35%, 40%, and 50%
- High-flow mask uses two wall outlets and provides FIO$_2$ up to 100%
- Down's flow provides PEEP continuously through respiratory cycle and can supply high FIO$_2$.
- BIPAP provides inspiratory positive airway pressure (IPAP) (pressure support) and expiratory positive airway pressure (EPAP) (PEEP) with oxygen bleed-in (can't usually obtain FIO$_2$ >50%).

PULMONARY

BILEVEL INTERMITTENT POSITIVE PRESSURE (BIPAP) AND NONINVASIVE POSITIVE PRESSURE VENTILATION (NIPPV)

(*N Engl J Med* 325:1824, 1991; *N Engl J Med* 333:817, 1995; *Am J Respir Crit Care Med* 151:1799, 1995)

Fast Facts
- IPAP ≈ to pressure support (PS)
- EPAP ≈ to PEEP

Indications
- Bridge to endotracheal intubation for a patient in respiratory distress due to pulmonary edema, COPD, pneumonia, atelectasis
- Patients with hypercarbia alone are better candidates than those with severe hypoxia
- NIPPV results in lower rates of intubation (31%) versus standard therapy (73%)
- Patient able to talk and eat; more comfortable than intubation
- Less expensive
- Less risk of nosocomial pneumonia
- Easy to administer

Contraindications
- Acute facial trauma or facial deformity
- Agitation or inability to cooperate
- Patient heavily sedated or paralyzed
- Airway secretions, obstruction, or injury
- Risk of aspiration
- Unstable ventilatory drive
- Cardiac dysrhythmias

Initial Settings
- IPAP at 9–10 cm H_2O; EPAP at 5 cm H_2O; titrate the O_2 bled in.
- Adjust mask until it fits without leak
- Nasal mask is better tolerated and has less risk of aspiration/emesis than full-face mask
- May increase IPAP/EPAP at 2- to 3-cm H_2O increments based on ABGs, clinical status
- Follow up ABGs

MECHANICAL VENTILATION (*Am J Med* 99:553, 1995; *N Engl J Med*
330:1056, 1994; *Am J Med* 88:268, 1990)

Indications for Intubation

- Uncorrectable hypoxemia: PaO_2 <55 mm Hg on 100% non-rebreathing system (NRBS)
- Hypercapnia ($PaCO_2$ >55 mg Hg) with acidosis
- Fatigue (RR >35 with ↑$PaCO_2$) and use of accessory muscles
- Airway protection (poor mental status, sedatives/narcotics, upper airway obstruction)
- Pulmonary toilet or procedure
- Shock or sepsis (↓work of breathing and ↑oxygenation to assist in management)

Modes of Ventilation

- **Assist control (AC):** Provides minimum number of fixed-volume breaths, but patient can initiate assisted breaths as well (get set volume with each initiation).
- **Intermittent mandatory ventilation (IMV):** Delivers fixed volume at set rate. Patient can breathe on own (assisted with pressure support) between assisted breaths.
- **Synchronized intermittent mandatory ventilation (SIMV):** Like IMV except provides ventilator breaths synchronized with patient's initiated inspiration.
- **Minimum mandatory ventilation (MMV):** Sets minimum tidal volume and frequency per minute. Patient must meet the minimum minute ventilation (by any combination of frequency and spontaneous tidal volume) while being assisted with a set PS. If patient fails to meet minimum, the machine will meet it for the patient. Can also apply PEEP.
- **Pressure control (PCV):** Presets pressure (not volume) (i.e., the lung inflation will terminate when preset pressure is reached). Volume will vary according to mechanical properties of the lung (↑airway resistance and/or ↓compliance reduce volume delivered).
- **Pressure support (PS):** gives preset pressure with each patient breath (backup SIMV for apnea). At least 5 cm of PS is needed to overcome resistance of endotracheal tube.
- **CPAP/PEEP:** ↑PaO_2 by ↑functional residual capacity. CPAP between mandatory ventilator breaths = PEEP. May induce barotrauma (pneumothorax) or ↓preload, ↓mean airway pressure, and ↓CO. Watch for auto-PEEP in asthmatics, COPD patients.

Initial Ventilator Settings

- Mode: SIMV
- Rate: 10–20 breaths/minute
- Tidal volume: 10–12 cc/kg (600–800 cc) (for ARDS: low tidal volumes of 6–8 cc/kg)
  10 breaths × tidal volume = 7–8 liters/minute (normal only 4–5 liters/minute)
- FIO_2: 100% with taper
- PS: 5–20 cm H_2O (especially with poorly compliant lungs, hypercarbia)
- PEEP: 0–15 cm (start lower) (use extreme caution in asthmatics) *continued*

PULMONARY

Ventilator Adjustment Considerations
Agitation
- Rule out drug or substance withdrawal
- Rule out medications
- Rule out hypoxemia
- Rule out mucus plug
- Rule out/treat pain

Increased PaCO$_2$

Rule out:	Therapy
Obstruction	Suction, bronchodilators
Auto-PEEP	Bronchodilators; increase inspiratory flow rate and/or decrease ventilator rate
Pneumothorax	Chest tube
Cuff leak	Change ETT or increase volume in balloon
Right mainstem intubation	Reposition ETT
Hypoventilation	Increase rate of pressure support or tidal volume

Decreased PaCO$_2$

Rule out:	Therapy
Iatrogenic overventilation	Decrease rate or tidal volume
Increased respiratory drive	Evaluate causes and treat (agitation, pain, fever, CNS event, drug, hypoxia, acidosis, withdrawal)
	May need to sedate, or paralyze if unable to ventilate after correcting

Decreased PaO$_2$

Rule out:	Therapy
Pneumonia	Gram stain, culture, treat; increase PEEP, FiO$_2$
Pulmonary edema	Evaluate etiology and treat; increase PEEP, FiO$_2$; diurese if needed
Pulmonary embolus	Anticoagulate ± IVC filter
Atelectasis	Suction, chest therapy, increase PEEP, rotate positions, adequate tidal volume
Pneumothorax/hemothorax	Chest tube
Mucus plug	Suctioning, chest therapy; increase PEEP/tidal volume/pressure support
Pleural effusion	Thoracentesis; may need chest tube
Right mainstem intubation	Reposition endotracheal tube
ARDS	FiO$_2$,PEEP, lung protective strategy (6–8 ml/kg tidal volume), paralyze, prone, nitric oxide

Increased Airway Pressure

Rule out:	Therapy
Mucus plug	Suction
Bronchospasm	Bronchodilators, steroids, check plateau pressure
Auto-PEEP	Decrease ventilator rate, ±PEEP, treat underlying cause
Right mainstem intubation	Reposition ETT
Pneumothorax	Chest tube
Endotracheal tube cuff herniation	Deflate balloon and then change ETT
Poor compliance/ARDS	Lung protective strategy (6–8 ml/kg tidal volume/PCV); may need to paralyze

Hypotension

Rule out:	Therapy
Steroid withdrawal/adrenal insufficiency	Stress dose steroids after cosyntropin stimulation test
Pneumothorax	Emergently, 14- or 16-gauge angiocath in second intercostal space (midclavicular line) to decompress, then chest tube
Tamponade	Emergent ECG, pericardiocentesis
Myocardial infarction	Evaluate cause and treat for MI
Sepsis	Culture, antibiotics
Auto-PEEP	Decrease ventilator rate, volume (allow the lungs to deflate)
Blood loss	Evaluate source, IV access, fluids, transfuse
Decreased preload on positive pressure ventilation	Fluids

Weaning and Extubation   (Marino, *The ICU Book* [2nd ed]. 1998; *N Engl J Med* 324:1444, 1991)

Weaning Parameters ("WEANS NOW")
- Wakefulness
- Electrolytes
- Acid-base status
- Neurologic state
- Secretions
- Nutrition
- Oxygenation: PaO_2 >60 mm Hg on FIO_2 <0.4, PEEP <5 cm H_2O
- Work of breathing

Modes of Weaning
- **IMV wean:** ↓number of IMV breaths (↓by 2 q1–2h and call house officer if RR>30), then ↓PS, ↓PEEP, T-piece trials
- **Pressure support wean:** For patient only on PS, slowly ↓PS until patient only on PEEP, then ↓PEEP
- **T-piece trials:** Put patient on T-piece for 30 minutes, then assess. Slowly increase time on T-piece and off ventilator. Check ABGs 30 minutes after each change, and check for ↑RR, ↓O₂, agitation

Predictors of Weaning Success
- **Rapid shallow breathing index:** RR/tidal volume ratio <100 success (22% fail)
  - >100 = ventilator dependent (5% weanable)
- **VC** >10–15 ml/kg = success (15% fail)
  - <10–15 ml/kg = ventilator dependent (50–63% weanable)
- **MIP** –30 cm or less (more negative) = success (26% fail)
  - –20 cm or greater (less negative) = ventilator dependent (up to 100% weanable)
- **MV** <10 liter/minute = success (11% fail)
  - >10 liter/minute = ventilator dependent (25% weanable)

Variable	Sensitivity	Specificity	Positive predictive value	Negative predictive value
Frequency/tidal volume ratio	0.97	0.64	0.78	0.95
Maximal inspiratory pressure	1.0	0.11	0.59	1.0
Tidal volume	0.97	0.54	0.73	0.94
Frequency	0.92	0.36	0.65	0.77
Minute ventilation	0.78	0.18	0.55	0.38
Dynamic compression	0.72	0.50	0.65	0.58
Static compression	0.75	0.36	0.60	0.53

PULMONARY

ASTHMA/COPD EXACERBATION (*Chest* 113:235S, 1998; *N Engl J Med* 328:1017, 1993; *Am J Respir Crit Care Med* 160:1079, 1999)

Etiology

Asthma		COPD	
Allergen	Drug-induced	Mucus plugging/secretions	PE
Infections		Infections	Effusion
Noncompliance		Pneumothorax	
		α_1-Antitrypsin deficiency	

Diagnosis

- Chest x-ray
- CBC
- Peak flow (PEFR):
  - Sputum Gram's stain and culture
  - Serial ABGs
  - Beside spirometry/PFTs

    normal: 450–650 liters/minute (male), 350–500 liters/minute (female)

    mild: >300   mild/moderate: 200–300

    moderate/severe: <200   severe: <100

Management

- O_2 (check respiratory drive/hypercarbia): Check HCO_3, ABG for CO_2 retention status
- β-adrenergic agonist (albuterol): Nebulizer 0.5 cc/2.5 cc NS continuous/q1–2h and PRN→q4–6h→metered-dose inhaler
- Ipratropium bromide (Atrovent): Metered dose inhaler 1p q6h or nebulizer unit dose q6h for COPD
- Steroids [methylprednisolone (Solu-Medrol) ± 125 mg IV load followed by 40–60 mg IV q6–8h × 72 hours, then taper; *or* prednisone, 1 mg/kg PO qd, then taper over 5 days to several weeks. In asthmatics and responsive COPD patients, add steroid inhaler before tapering off oral steroids.]
- Antibiotics if severe exacerbation or suspicious of infection
- Controversial: theophylline/aminophylline (used in nocturnal asthma/COPD), magnesium, COPD [pneumococcal vaccine polyvalent (Pneumovax), flu shot]
- Status asthmaticus: continuous albuterol nebulizers, steroids; consider epinephrine 0.1–0.5 mg (0.1–0.5 ml of 1:1,000 solution) SQ or IM; may repeat in 10–15 minutes; *or* 0.1 to 0.25 mg (1–2.5 ml of 1:10,000 solution) IV over 5–10 minutes; may repeat in 5–10 minutes.

Indications for Hospitalization

- Severe shortness of breath and cough, dyspnea on exertion >100 ft
- Prior ICU admission or intubation
- Pulsus paradoxus (>12–20 mm Hg)
- Diaphoresis, cyanosis, respiratory alternans, abdominal paradox
- Altered mental status, arrhythmia, syncope, fragmented speech, exhaustion
- Infection
- Pneumothorax
- HR >120, RR >30
- FEV_1 <750 (40% predicted), PEFR <200 (<25% predicted)
- No improvement >10% on nebulizer treatment
- PO_2 <60, SaO_2 <90%, PCO_2 rising, pH <7.35

NAEPP CLASSIFICATION OF ASTHMA SEVERITY

Category	Character	Night-time symptoms	Lung function	Short-acting medication	Long-acting medication
Severe persistent	Continual symptoms; limited activity; frequent exacerbation	Frequent	FEV_1 or PEF ≤60%; PEF variability >30%	$β_2$ agonist; other medication according to severity of exacerbation (IV/PO steroids, antibiotics, intubation)	High-dose steroid MDI and long-acting $β_2$ agonist MDI or tablets, or SR theophylline and PO steroids
Moderate persistent	Daily symptoms; limited physical activity; frequent exacerbations	>Once/wk	FEV_1 or PEF >60%/<80% of predicted PEF; variability >30%	Short-acting $β_2$ agonist MDI PRN; other medication according to exacerbation (use of $β_2$ agonist daily may indicate ↑long-acting medication)	Steroid MDI (medium dose) or steroid MDI (low to medium dose) + a long-acting $β_2$ agonist, SR theophylline, or long-acting PO $β_2$ agonist
Mild persistent	Symptoms >2×/wk; exacerbations <1×/day; may affect activity	>2×/mo	FEV_1 or PEF ≥80%; PEF variability 20–30%	Short-acting $β_2$ agonist PRN. ↑Use daily may indicate ↑long-acting therapy	One daily medication: either steroid or cromolyn MDI or SR theophylline (not preferred)
Mild intermittent	Symptoms ≤2×/wk; asymptomatic and normal PEF between exacerbations; exacerbations brief	≤2×/mo	FEV_1/PEF ≥80%; PEF variability <20%	Short-acting $β_2$ agonist PRN. Use >2×/wk may indicate need for long-term control therapy	No daily medication

Source: NIH Expert Panel 2. NIH Guidelines Publication #97-4051, August 1997.

PULMONARY

INHALED STEROIDS

Drug	Low dose	Medium dose	High dose
Beclomethasone, 42 or 84 µg/puff	168–504 ug; 4–12 puffs of 42 µg; 2–6 puffs of 84 µg	504–840 µg; 12–20 puffs of 42 µg; 6–10 puffs of 84 µg	>840 µg; >20 puffs of 42 µg; >10 puffs of 84 µg
Budesonide DPI, 200 µg/puff	200–400 µg, 1–2 puffs	400–600 µg, 2–3 puffs	>600 µg, >3 puffs
Flunisolide, 250 µg/puff	500–1,000 µg; 2–4 puffs	1,000–2,000 µg; 4–8 puffs	>2,000 µg, >8 puffs
Fluticasone metered-dose inhaler: 44, 110, 220 µg/puff; DPI: 50, 100, 250 µg/dose	88–264 µg; 2–6 puffs of 44 µg; 2 puffs of 110 µg; 88–264 µg (2–6 puffs of 50 µg)	264–660 µg, 2–6 puffs of 110 µg, 264–660 µg (3–6 puffs of 100 µg)	>660 µg, >6 puffs of 100 µg; >3 puffs of 220 µg; >660 µg (6 puffs of 100 or 2 of 250 µg)
Triamcinolone, 100 µg	400–1,000 µg (4–10 puffs)	1,000–2,000 µg (10–20 puffs)	>2,000 µg (>20 puffs)

Note: All bid drugs.
Source: NIH Expert Panel 2. Guidelines for the diagnosis and management of asthma. NIH Guidelines Publication #97-4051, August 1997.

PULMONARY EMBOLISM (PE)   *(Am J Respir Crit Care Med 159:1, 1999; JAMA 263:2753, 1990; N Engl J Med 339:93, 1998)*

Fast Facts
- 500,000 cases of PE each year
- 50,000 deaths per year (10%)
- Only 30% of fatal PE diagnosed premortem

Symptoms
- Dyspnea (61–73%)
- Pleuritic pain (54–66%)
- Cough (37%)
- Syncope (in large PE)
- Hemoptysis (13–18%)

Signs
- Tachypnea (70–73%)
- Rales (51%)
- Tachycardia (30%)
- S_4 (24%)
- P_2 (23%)
- Accessory muscles (21%)
- Jugular venous pressure elevation (12%)
- Chest wall pain (10%)

Diagnosis
- Chest x-ray (usually normal or pleural effusion)
    - Watermark's sign: focal oligemia
    - Hampton's hump: peripheral wedge
    - Palla's sign: large right descending pulmonary artery
- $\dot{V}/\dot{Q}$ scan
- Lower-extremity Dopplers (up to 50% negative with PE)
- Pulmonary angiogram
- Spiral CT (angiogram protocol)
- Echocardiogram
- ECG usually shows sinus tachycardia, wide S in I, Q and T wave inversion in III ($S_1Q_3T_3$), acute RBBB, right axis deviation, T wave inversion also in V_1–V_4, ST depression in II
- D-Dimer (latex positive >500)
- $\dot{V}/\dot{Q}$ scan: PIOPED data for frequency of PE *(JAMA 263:2753, 1990)* given clinical suspicion (c-prob) and $\dot{V}/\dot{Q}$ scan results

	c-prob 80–100%	c-prob 20–79%	c-prob 0–20%	All prob
$\dot{V}/\dot{Q}$ high prob	96%	88%	56%	87%
$\dot{V}/\dot{Q}$ intermediate	66%	28%	16%	30%
$\dot{V}/\dot{Q}$ low prob	40%	16%	4%	14%*
Near normal	0%	6%	2%	4%

*McMaster data ≈ 30% PE for low prob $\dot{V}/\dot{Q}$ scan alone.
Source: *JAMA* 263:2753, 1990. Copyright 1990, American Medical Association.

continued

PULMONARY

- Spiral CT vs. V̇/Q̇ (*Radiology* 208:201, 1998; *Ann Emerg Med* 33:520, 1999)
  Spiral CT: 87% sensitive/95% specific (not reliable in subsegmental vessels)
- V̇/Q̇ scan: 65% sensitive/94% specific

Management

- Heparin IV (consider LMW heparin in stable patients)
- Oxygen
- Thrombolysis: reduced mortality in people with RV dilation/hypokinesis or acute tricuspid regurgitation up to 14 days post-PE (*Circulation* 96:88)
- Consider inferior vena cava catheter (Greenfield) filter if PE occurred while on therapeutic anticoagulation
- Consider hypercoagulable workup if appropriate

HEPARIN SLIDING SCALE   (*Ann Intern Med* 119:874, 1993; Stanford Medical Center Hematology/Anticoagulation Guidelines)

- Heparin (by weight) nomogram: bolus 80 units/kg IV, then 15 units/kg/hour IV gtt
- Empirically: bolus 5,000 units IV, then 1,000 units/hour
- √Partial thromboplastin time at baseline and q6h; titrate to 1.5–2.0 times control

Stanford Protocol

Activated partial thromboplastin time	Action	Rate change	Recheck
<40	Bolus 5,000 U	↑200 units/hour	6 hours
40–54	—	↑100 units/hour	6 hours
55–95	—	—	Next A.M.
96–120	Hold 30 min	↓100 units/hour	6 hours
>120	Hold 1 hour	↓200 units/hour	6 hours

HEMOPTYSIS (*J Crit Illness* 11:446, 1996; *Chest* 97:469, 1990)

Definition
- Massive hemoptysis: ≥100–600 ml/24 hours

History and Physical Examination
- Prior lung, cardiac, renal, GI pathology or disease; prior hemoptysis
- Bleeding disorders or use of NSAIDs, anticoagulants
- Tobacco use
- Infectious symptoms or rash
- Travel history
- Family history of hemoptysis or brain aneurysms (telangiectasia)

Physical Signs
- Telangiectasias
- Skin rash (SLE, vasculitis, fat embolism, endocarditis)
- Splinter hemorrhages, needle tracks (endocarditis)
- Clubbing
- Pulmonary hypertension (tricuspid regurgitation, pulmonary insufficiency, loud P_2)
- Cardiac murmurs (mitral stenosis, CHD, pulmonary hypertension)
- Lower-extremity deep venous thrombosis

Etiology
- Airway diseases: most common (bronchitis, bronchiectasis, neoplasms, foreign body)
- Vascular (PE, arteriovenous malformation, mitral stenosis or left ventricular failure, perforation of artery with pulmonary artery catheter)
- Bronchial arteries (systemic pressure from the aorta, subclavian, intercostal arteries) are more common etiologies than pulmonary arteries (low pressure)
- Parenchymal diseases (infection, inflammatory or autoimmune disease, coagulopathy)
- Cryptogenic: in ≤30% no cause found

Diagnostic Tests
- **Bronchoscopy** (bronchi is most common source, then pulmonary, systemic): early while the patient is bleeding provides highest yield.
- **Arteriography** after bronchoscopy
- **Chest CT** helps with diagnosis: bronchiectasis, lung abscess, mass lesion, arteri-ovenous malformation, fungus, tuberculosis
- **Tagged RBC scan** not very useful

Initial Management
- Monitor in ICU setting and consult pulmonary and thoracic surgery
- Oxygen
- Suction
- May need packed red blood cells, fluids
- If bleeding site is known, place patient in lateral decubitus position (bleeding side down)
- If bleeding continues and oxygenation compromised→intubate (double lumen if possible)

PULMONARY

PLEURAL EFFUSION (*Clin Chest Med* 19:407, 1998; *Am Rev Respir Dis* 148:813, 1993)

Diagnosis

- Chest x-ray (posteroanterior and lateral)
  - Blunting of costophrenic angle (lateral) 25–50 cc; posteroanterior >150-cc effusion
- **Always** take lateral decubitus film
  - Check if free flowing (tap if >10 mm)
  - Check for underlying pleural thickening, pulmonary infiltrate, evidence of CHF
- Thoracentesis

Pleural Fluid Analysis

- Cell count with differential
- Protein, glucose, lactate dehydrogenase (LDH)
- *pH, if potentially parapneumonic versus abscess (collect in ABG syringe and keep closed to avoid change in P_{CO_2} and pH)
- Culture (Gram's stain, bacterial, acid-fast bacilli)
- Cytology (requires large volume)
- Consider cholesterol, amylase, triglycerides, antinuclear antibodies
- ?Pleural biopsy

Transudate	Exudate
Criteria	**Criteria**
Light's criteria	Fails criteria for transudate
LDH fluid/serum ratio <0.6	Check pH: <7.2→chest tube
Protein ratio <0.5	<7.3→tuberculosis
New criteria	>7.3→cancer
LDH ≤200 IU	**Differential diagnosis**
Cholesterol <45 mg/dl	Bloody: Hct >1% or RBC >100,000 (tumor, thrombus/infarction, trauma)
pH >7.4	Chylous: triglycerides >110 mg/dl→tumor (lymphoma), thrombus (superior vena cava), trauma (surgical), lymphangiomatosis
Specific gravity <1.016	
Total protein <3 g/100 ml	
WBC <1,000; RBC <10,000/mm³	↑Amylase →pancreatitis, tumor (salivary), esophageal perforation (pH <6, glucose ≤60 mg/dl)
Differential diagnosis	↑Eosinophil→Churg-Strauss, paragonimiasis (glucose <60), drug, parasite, asbestosis
CHF (right >left, pH 7.35–7.45)	
Ascites (fluid protein >2.5)	↑Polymorphonuclear lymphocytes→empyema (>50,000), pneumonia (glucose <60 mg/dl), pancreatitis, PE, rheumatoid arthritis, subphrenic abscess, inflammation
Nephrotic syndrome	
PE	
Hypothyroidism	Lymphocytes >50%→malignancy, tuberculosis (↑antinuclear antibodies→SLE)
Constrictive pericarditis	
Peritoneal dialysis	Variable: Meig's syndrome (ovarian fibroma), Dressler's syndrome, asbestosis

Unclear Etiologies of Pleural Effusion

- Glucose <60: rule out rheumatoid arthritis
  (fluid rheumatoid factor >1:320, multinucleated macrophage, background
  necrotic debris, subcutaneous nodes)
- Pleural biopsy to rule out tuberculosis (granuloma) and malignancy (cytology ×
  3→80%)
  If negative, check PPD
  Treat for tuberculosis
  Recheck x-ray/PPD/thoracentesis for LDH in 6 weeks if initial PPD negative
  Acid-fast bacilli positive in 20–30%, even if initial PPD negative
- $\dot{V}/\dot{Q}$ scan to rule out PE

Management of Parapneumonic Effusions

Class 1: Parapneumonic: <10 mm, no loculation	No tap
Class 2: Typical parapneumonic: glucose >40, pH >7.2, culture and Gram's stain negative	Antibiotics
Class 3: Borderline complicated: pH 7.0–7.2, LDH >1,000 mg/dl or glucose >40, culture and Gram's stain negative	Serial taps, antibiotics
Class 4: Simple complicated: pH <7.4, glucose <40, Gram's stain or culture positive, no pus or loculation	Chest tube, antibiotics
Class 5: Complex complicated: pH <7.0, glucose <40, Gram's stain or culture positive, multi-loculated	Chest tube or local lytics, rarely decortication
Class 6: Simple empyema: pus, single locule or free	Chest tube/decortication
Class 7: Complex empyema: pus, multiple locules	CT scan plus lytics, decortication

Source: Reproduced with permission from RW Light. A new classification of parapneumonic effusions and empyema. *Chest* 108:299, 1995.

PULMONARY

PULMONARY FUNCTION TESTING (N Engl J Med 331:25, 1994; Am Rev Respir Dis 144:1202, 1991)

Terminology

	Definition	Obstructive	Restrictive
FVC	Maximum air expelled in forced expiration	Normal/↓	↓
FEV_1	Forced expiratory volume in 1 second	↓↓	Normal/↓
FEV_1/FVC	FEV_1/VC × 100%	↓↓	Normal/↑
RV	Volume remaining after maximum expiration	Normal/↑	↓
TLC	Total lung capacity	Normal/↑	↓

FVC = forced vital capacity; FEV_1 = forced expiratory volume in 1 second; RV = residual volume; TLC = total lung capacity.

- FEF 25–75 more useful than FEV_1/FVC with early airflow obstruction
- TLC = VC + RV = functional residual capacity (FRC) + inspiratory capacity (IC)
- **Bronchodilator response:** improvement in FEV_1/FVC >10% or FEF 25–75 >25%; 15–25% considered good; ≥25% considered excellent
- DL_{CO} (diffusing capacity)
  Increases in ↑hemoglobin, ↑pulmonary blood volume (CHF), hemorrhage
  Decreases in interstitial lung disease, emphysema, vascular disease

Grading of Severity (in 60- to 70-kg person)

- Obstructive (↓flow)
- Restrictive (↓TLC)

Severity	FEV_1 (liters)	FVC	TLC	DL_{CO}	Limitation
Mild	>3	65–79%	75–80%	60–75%	Severe exercise
Moderate	2–3	50–64%	55–75%	50–60%	Rapid walking
Severe	0.5–1.0	<50%	<50%	<40%	Walking <1 block
Very severe	<0.5	—	—	—	Room bound

Differential Diagnosis of Pulmonary Disease

Disease	Air flow FEV_1/FVC	TLC	VC	Air trap	DL_{CO}	ABG
Emphysema	↓	↑	↓	++	↓	N/↓PO_2
Chronic bronchitis	↓	N/↑	N/↓	+	N/↓	↓PO_2
Asthma	↓	N/↑	N/↓	+	N/↑	N/↓PO_2
Interstitial lung disease	N	↓	↓	↓	↓	↓PO_2
Obesity	N/↓	N/↓	N/↓	—	N	↓PO_2

3. Renal

URINALYSIS

	Properties	Interpretation
Specific gravity (SG)	SG 1.030 ~ uOsm 120 SG 1.018 ~ uOsm 750 SG 1.003 ~ uOsm 40	↓SG in free water loss or ↓reabsorption ↑SG in ↓mineralocorticoids, ↓effective circulation
pH	Normal pH 4.5–8	If >7, consider urea splitters (*Proteus, Pseudomonas, Klebsiella*), UTI or renal tubular acidosis, acetazolamide, ↓aldosterone
Protein	Globin, Tamm-Horsfall protein	See Proteinuria—Differential Diagnosis
Leukocyte esterase/ nitrite	Neutrophilic granules released in urine/bacteria reduce nitrate	UTI
Glucose	Glucose oxidase test	Positive in diabetes mellitus, Cushing's syndrome, hyperthyroidism, pheochromocytoma
Ketones	Acetoacetic acid only	Starvation vs. ketoacidosis
Bilirubin	Conjugated bilirubin (direct)	Negative in hemolysis, ↑in biliary obstruction
Urobilinogen	↑Bilirubin production	↑In hemolysis and hepatic diseases, CHF
WBC	Urine eos (Hansel stain)	Acute interstitial nephritis, UTI, glomerulonephritis, urethritis
Heme/RBC	RBC/myoglobin/free Hgb	Renal (glomeruli/tubules/collecting) vs. postrenal
Epithelial	Usually indicates contaminants	Oval fat bodies/fatty cast→nephrotic syndrome
Casts	Tamm-Horsfall protein secreted by renal tubules in matrices	RBC cast→glomerular disease WBC cast→inflammation (acute interstitial nephritis, glomerulonephritis, pyelonephritis) Tubular cast→acute tubular nephritis Hyaline cast→concentrated Waxy cast→chronic renal failure (stasis) Granular cast→"muddy brown" acute tubular nephritis Pigmented cast (hemoglobin, myoglobin, bilirubin)
Crystals	Formed in acid urine	Amorphous urates (Ca^{+2}, Mg^{+2}, Na^+, K^+) Crystalline urates (Na^+, K^+, NH_4) Uric acid (hexagonal) Ca oxalate (diamond, envelope)
	Formed in alkaline urine	Amorphous phosphate (Ca^{+2} pyroPO_4, Mg^{+2}) Struvite (rectangle) $CaCO_3$ (dumbbell) NH_4 biurate
	Miscellaneous	Contrast (plate) Sulfa (haystack) Cystine (cross)

RENALChinese

PROTEINURIA (N Engl J Med 338:1202, 1998; Mayo Clin Proc 69:1154, 1994)

Definition
- 24-hour urine collection for protein
  - Normal: <150 mg/day
  - Low-grade proteinuria: 1–2 g/day
  - Nephrotic range: 3.5 g/day
  - *or*
- Urine protein-to-creatinine ratio
  - Normal = 0.1
  - Nephrotic range: >3

Microalbuminuria
- Albumin/creatinine: >30 mg/g
  - *or*
- 24-hour urine protein: 30–300 mg
  - *or*
- Timed collection: >20 µg/minute

Differential Diagnosis by Pathophysiology
- Overflow of normal or abnormal protein: myeloma, Bence-Jones
- ↑Glomerular permeability of protein: glomerulonephritis (2–3 g/day)
- ↓Reabsorption of protein: tubulointerstitial disease (<2 g/day)
- Alterations in renal hemodynamics: fever, exercise, orthostatic proteinuria, seizure

NEPHROTIC SYNDROME (N Engl J Med 338:1202, 1998)

Definition
- Urine protein >3.5 g/day, hypoalbuminemia, hyperlipidemia

Adult Incidence
- Minimal change (10–15%)
- Focal segmental glomerular sclerosis (15–25%)
- Membranous (25–35%)
- Membranoproliferative glomerulonephritis (5%)

HEMATURIA (JAMA 263:2475, 1990)

Definition
- ≥3–5 RBCs/hpf in a urine specimen
- Positive dipstick also caused by ascorbic acid, myoglobin

Differential Diagnosis
- Urologic: neoplasm, nephrolithiasis, polycystic kidney disease, UTI
- Hematologic: coagulopathies, sickle-cell disease
- Glomerular: IgA nephropathy, hereditary glomerulonephritis (with proteinuria/deformed RBCs)

SPECIAL URINE TESTS
Wood's Lamp Test
• Positive for ethylene glycol, porphyria

Urine Protein Electrophoresis (uPEP)
• Qualitative analysis, paraprotein (e.g., myeloma)

Endocrine Tests
• 5-HIAA → carcinoid
• Melanin → melanoma
• Vanillylmandelic acid (VMA)/catechols → pheochromocytoma
• Ketosteroids → Cushing's

Urine Urea Nitrogen (uUN) for Nutritional Status
• N balance (g) = [Protein intake(g)/6.25] – [uUN + 4]
   →goal: positive 4–6 g/day
• If uUN >30 g/day, use factor of 6 instead of 6.25 in equation

Screening Tests
• Uric acid (uricosuria >750 mg/day)
• Myoglobin (positive with dipstick + heme but no RBC→rhabdomyolysis)
• Hemosiderin (positive if hemolysis)
• Amylase (2-hour collection, ↑in mumps and pancreatitis)
• Pregnancy (β-hCG)
• Calcium (>150 mg/day if calciuria)

RENAL

URINE ELECTROLYTES AND FUNCTIONAL TESTS AND WHEN TO USE THEM

Parameter	Indication	Remarks
Sodium	Assessment of volume status	<15 mmol/liter in low effective intravascular volume. Limited by changes in diuretic dose, hypoaldosteronism, and renal salt wasting
	Diagnosis of hyponatremia	Reflects level of ADH activity
	Diagnosis of acute renal failure	<15 mmol/liter in prerenal states; higher in acute tubular necrosis
	Dietary compliance in patients with hypertension	Adequate adherence: <100 mEq/day
	Evaluation of calcium and uric acid excretion in stone formers	Na^+ excretion 75–100 mEq/day excludes volume depletion
Chloride	Similar to that for Na excretion	Na^+ and Cl^- excretion vary in parallel
		May use urine Cl^- in patients with higher than expected urine Na^+
	Diagnosis of metabolic alkalosis	"Saline-responsive" metabolic alkalosis, <15 mmol/liter
		"Saline-resistant" metabolic alkalosis, >15 mmol/liter
Potassium	Diagnosis of hypokalemia	<20 mmol/liter suggests extrarenal losses
		>20 mmol/liter implies urinary losses
Osmolality	Diagnosis of hyponatremia	<100 mOsm/kg→excess water
		Very high osmolality→volume depletion or SIADH
	Diagnosis of hypernatremia	600–800 mOsm/kg→extrarenal water loss or Na intake in excess of water
		uOsm<pOsm→ inadequate ADH or resistance
	Diagnosis of acute renal failure	High uOsm excludes acute tubular necrosis
pH	Diagnosis of renal tubular acidosis	>5.3 in metabolic acidosis suggests renal tubular acidosis
	Efficacy of treatment in metabolic alkalosis	<6 in metabolic alkalosis suggests need for volume replacement
	Efficacy of treatment of uric acid stone disease	Target pH: 6.0–6.5

Source: Reproduced with permission from BD Rose. *Clinical Physiology of Acid-Base and Electrolyte Disorders* (4th ed). New York: McGraw-Hill, 1994

FUNCTIONAL TESTS AND WHEN TO USE THEM

Fractional Excretion of Sodium (FENa)

Differentiation between prerenal and renal failure:
- Value <1% is highly sensitive and specific for prerenal etiology
- May be <1% for NSAIDs, ACE inhibitors, IV contrast use, amphotericin B, rhabdomyolysis, vasculitis

$$FENa = \frac{Excreted\ Na^+}{Filtered\ Na^+} = \frac{UNa \times SCr}{UCr \times SNa^+}$$

Urine Net Charge

Differential diagnosis of nongap metabolic acidosis:
- Ammonium excretion increases in attempt to excrete acid
- Urine net charge provides index of ammonium excretion
- A net negative charge means ammonium excretion >80 mmol/day (e.g., diarrhea)
- A net positive charge means deficient ammonium excretion (e.g., renal tubular acidosis)

Calculated Creatinine Clearance

$$CrCl = \frac{UCr \times Uvol}{SCr} \times Time \approx \frac{(140 - age) \times wt\ (kg)}{SCr \times 72} \quad [female \times 0.85]$$

Blood Urea Nitrogen (BUN) to Creatinine Ratio

- ↑BUN/Cr (>10:1): ↑Urea input: ↑protein, GI bleed, hemolysis, sepsis/catabolic state
  ↓Circulating volume: ↓volume, CHF, cirrhosis/ascites, nephrosis
- ↓BUN/Cr (<10:1): ↓Urea input: starvation, liver disease; ↑Cr production: rhabdomyolysis
  ↑Circulating volume: SIADH, iatrogenic, chronic renal failure with dialysis

RENAL

RENAL IMAGING TECHNIQUES AND WHEN TO USE THEM

Renal Ultrasonography
- Role: Accurately measures renal size; detects obstruction and stones >5 mm
- Differentiates between solid and cystic structures >3 cm
- Advantages: May be done at any level of renal function; noninvasive
- Renovascular disease: Duplex ultrasonography has sensitivity >90%

Intravenous Pyelogram (IVP)
- Role: To evaluate nonglomerular hematuria, UTI, and voiding disorders
- Complications: Radiocontrast nephrotoxicity
- Renovascular disease: Not sensitive or specific

Computed Tomography
- Role: Noncontrast study used for renal stone investigation, suspected hemorrhage
- Role: Contrast study allows better definition of renal masses
- Advantages: Allows for identification of mass and staging

Radionuclide Scintigraphy
- Role: Used to assess renal perfusion, comparing left and right
- Renovascular disease: 75% sensitivity, ↑92% with captopril challenge

Renal Arteriography
- Role: Used to assess renal artery disease
- Complications: Atheroembolic and contrast-mediated acute renal failure

Renal Biopsy
- Role: For diagnosis of glomerular diseases and unusual cases of renal failure
- Contraindications: Uncontrolled hypertensions, infection, bleeding disorder, cystic kidney
- Complications: Gross hematuria (1/10), transfusion (1/100), nephrectomy (1/1,000)

HYPERNATREMIA *(Lancet 352:220, 1998)*

Symptoms
- Nausea/vomiting, anorexia, headache, agitation, confusion, seizure, coma

Evaluation
- First rule out pseudohypernatremia: ↓lipids, ↓glucose, ↓protein, lab error

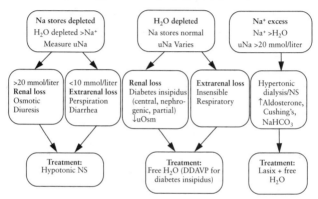

Na stores depleted H_2O depleted >Na⁺ Measure uNa		H_2O depleted Na stores normal uNa Varies		Na⁺ excess Na⁺ >H_2O uNa >20 mmol/liter
>20 mmol/liter **Renal loss** Osmotic Diuresis	<10 mmol/liter **Extrarenal loss** Perspiration Diarrhea	**Renal loss** Diabetes insipidus (central, nephro- genic, partial) ↓uOsm	**Extrarenal loss** Insensible Respiratory	Hypertonic dialysis/NS ↑Aldosterone, Cushing's, $NaHCO_3$
Treatment: Hypotonic NS		**Treatment:** Free H_2O (DDAVP for diabetes insipidus)		**Treatment:** Lasix + free H_2O

Therapy
- Determine free water deficit

Estimated free H_2O deficit:
   (Male) 0.6 × lean wt (kg) × (measured Na⁺/140 – 1)
   (Female) 0.5 × lean wt (kg) × (measured Na⁺/140 – 1)

- Replace 50% of deficit over 24 hours, remaining 50% over 48–72 hours (≤0.5 mEq/liter/hour)

RENAL

HYPONATREMIA   *(Lancet 352:220, 1998)*

Symptoms
- Headache, nausea/vomiting, ileus, lethargy, disorientation, cramps, seizure, coma

Evaluation
- Assess extracellular volume (ECV) by orthostasis, edema, mucous membrane, turgor, BUN/Cr, HCO_3, uNa
- Rule out pseudohyponatremia (pOsm <280: ↑lipids, ↑protein; pOsm >295: ↑glucose)

> Corrected Na^+ = measured Na^+ + (glucose − 100) × 1.6 (i.e., Na^+ ↓1.6 mEq per ↑100 mg/dl glucose)

- Proceed with algorithm

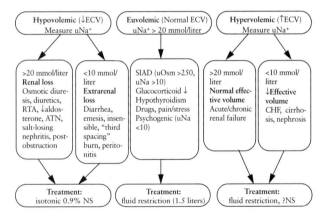

Hypovolemic (↓ECV) Measure uNa⁺		Euvolemic (Normal ECV) uNa⁺ > 20 mmol/liter	Hypervolemic (↑ECV) Measure uNa⁺	
>20 mmol/liter **Renal loss** Osmotic diuresis, diuretics, RTA, ↓aldosterone, ATN, salt-losing nephritis, postobstruction	<10 mmol/liter **Extrarenal loss** Diarrhea, emesis, insensible, "third spacing" burn, peritonitis	SIAD (uOsm >250, uNa >10) Glucocorticoid ↓ Hypothyroidism Drugs, pain/stress Psychogenic (uNa <10)	>20 mmol/liter **Normal effective volume** Acute/chronic renal failure	<10 mmol/liter **↓Effective volume** CHF, cirrhosis, nephrosis
Treatment: isotonic 0.9% NS		Treatment: fluid restriction (1.5 liters)	Treatment: fluid restriction, ?NS	

Therapy for Acute, Symptomatic Hyponatremia

- Calculate fluid/Na+ replacement

1. Total Na deficit (TSD)	(Men) 0.6 × lean wt (kg) × (desired Na+ − measured Na+) (Women) 0.5 × lean wt × (desired Na+ − measured Na+)[a]
2. Desired correction rate	Rapid: 1.5 mEq/liter/hour (emergent, symptomatic)[b] Standard: 0.5 mEq/liter/hour (<12 mEq/liter/day)
3. Desired CF	0.9% NS (154 mEq/liter, 0.15 mEq/cc) – hypovolemia 3% NS (514 mEq/liter, 0.5 mEq/cc) – euvolemia/hyper- volemia
4. Establish correction duration (CD)	(desired Na − measured Na+) ÷ correction rate
5. Actual correction rate	(TSD ÷ CD) ÷ CF Na+ content (mEq/cc) [cc/hour]

TSD = total sodium deficit; CF = correction fluid; CD = correction duration.
[a]TBW = total body weight = lean weight × 0.6 (men), or lean weight × 0.5 (women).
[b]Plasma Na can be raised at initial rate of 1.5–2.0 mEq/liter/hour for first 3–4 hours during severe hyponatremia, especially in premenopausal women.

- Correction parameters:
    <2.0 mEq/liter/hour correction rate, <25 mEq/liter absolute increase over 48 hours
    Correct only to 120–130 mEq/liter in 48 hours
- Correct remainder by water restriction/0.9 NS
- Closely monitor electrolytes (q2–3h) and complications (central pontine myelinolysis—neurologic examination)

RENAL

SYNDROME OF INAPPROPRIATE ANTIDIURESIS (SIAD)

(Am J Med 42:790, 1967)

Essential
- Decreased effective osmolality of the extracellular fluid (pOsm <275 mOsm/kg H_2O)
- Inappropriate urinary concentration (uOsm >100 mOsm/kg H_2O) with normal renal function at some level of hypo-osmolality
- Clinical euvolemia
- Elevated urinary sodium excretion while on a normal salt/water intake
- Absence of other potential causes of euvolemic hypo-osmolality:
  - Hypothyroidism
  - Hypocorticalism (Addison's disease or pituitary ACTH insufficiency)
  - Diuretic use

Supplementary
- Abnormal water load test:
  - Inability to excrete at least 90% of a 20-ml/kg water load in 4 hours *and/or* failure to dilute uOsm to <100 mOsm/kg H_2O
- Plasma aqueous vasopressin (AVP) level inappropriately elevated relative to plasma osmolality
- No significant correction of plasma [Na^+] with volume expansion but improvement after fluid restriction

Common Etiologies of Syndrome of Inappropriate Antidiuresis

Tumors
- Pulmonary/mediastinal (bronchogenic carcinoma, mesothelioma, thymoma)
- Non-chest (pancreatic, ureteral/prostate, uterine, nasopharyngeal cancer, leukemia)

Central Nervous System Disorders
- Mass lesions (tumors, brain abscess, subdural hematoma)
- Inflammatory disease (encephalitis, meningitis, lupus)
- Degenerative/demyelinative disease (Guillain-Barré syndrome, spinal cord lesions)
- Subarachnoid hemorrhage, head trauma, psychosis, delirium tremens

Drug Induced
- Stimulate AVP release (nicotine, phenothiazines, tricyclic antidepressants, selective serotonin reuptake inhibitors)
- Direct renal effects (desmopressin, oxytocin, prostaglandin synthesis inhibitors)
- Chlorpropamide, clofibrate, carbamazepine, cyclophosphamide, vincristine

Pulmonary
- Infection (TB, aspergillosis, pneumonia, empyema)
- Mechanical/ventilatory (acute respiratory failure, COPD, mechanical ventilation)

HYPERKALEMIA *(Lancet 352:135, 1998; J Am Soc Nephrol 9:1535, 1982)*

Symptoms and Signs
- ↓Deep tendon reflex (DTR), paresthesia, paralysis, confusion, respiratory failure, arrhythmia

ECG findings	K⁺ Level (mEq/liter)
Peaked Ts	>5.5
PR increase, lost P	>6.5
QRS widening, ST changes	>7.0
PSVT, ventricular tachycardia/fibrillation, asystole	Any level

Evaluation
- Rule out pseudohyperkalemia: hemolysis, WBC >100,000, platelet count >1 × 10^9, tourniquet, lab error
- Rule out redistribution: ↓insulin, acidosis, beta blocker, digoxin toxicity, hyperkalemic periodic paralysis

Corrections: K⁺ ↑0.6 mEq/liter per ↓0.1 in pH, or ↑10 mOsm

- Proceed with algorithm

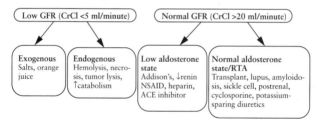

continued

RENAL

Treatment (in Suggested Order)

Mechanism	Therapy	Dose	Time of action/remarks
Antagonism of membrane action	CaCl/gluconate	1 amp (1 g) IV over 3 mins	Minutes, but very brief effect
Increased K entry into cells	Glucose and insulin	D50 2 amps with regular insulin, 10 units IV	30–60 mins, lasting several hours
	NaHCO₃	1 amp IV (44 mEq) over 5 mins	30–60 mins, lasting several hours. Best with other agents
	Albuterol nebulizers (if shortness of breath or respiratory distress)	10–20 mg by nebulizer	Within 30 mins
Removal of excess potassium	Lasix		Hypoaldosteronism, CHF, potassium secretory defect
	Kayexalate	1 g/kg PO/PR q6–12h	Hours
	Hemodialysis		Last resort

HYPOKALEMIA (*Lancet* 352:135, 1998; *N Engl J Med* 339:451, 1998; *J Am Soc Nephrol* 8:1179, 1997)

Symptoms

• Weakness, tetany, ileus, paresthesia, arrhythmias (<2.5 mEq)

Evaluation

• Rule out pseudohypokalemia: WBC >100,000 after storage at room temperature, lab error
• Rule out redistribution: ↑insulin, alkalosis, β agonist, hypokalemic periodic paralysis
• ECG changes
    T inversion, U waves, ↑QT, wide QRS, ST↓ (digoxin toxic)
    Ectopy, paroxysmal supraventricular tachycardia/atrial fibrillation
• Estimated total body potassium deficit: ~200–400 mEq per ↓1 mEq
    Estimates: 100 mEq (K$^+$ 3.0–3.5), 200 mEq (K$^+$ 2.5–2.9), 300–400 mEq (K$^+$ 2.0–2.4)
• For etiology proceed with algorithm:

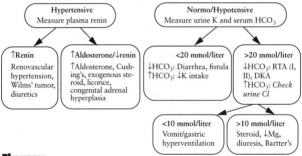

Therapy

• Opt for oral therapy if possible
• Scale: For each K ↓0.1 mEq ≤5.0, give 2 mEq IV or 3 mEq PO (preferred) KCl (standing sliding scales can be a problem)
• Maximum infusion rate
    ≤10 mEq/hour in peripheral IV
    ≤20 mEq/hour in central line
    May add 1% lidocaine to bag to decrease pain
• Replete magnesium

RENAL

HYPERCALCEMIA   (*Lancet* 352:306, 1998; *N Engl J Med* 326:1196, 1992)

Symptoms
- "Stones, bones, groans, and psychic overtones"
- Nausea/vomiting, constipation, hypertension, acute renal failure, nephrolithiasis

Evaluation
- Repeat lab, correct for albumin
- Rule out pseudohypercalcemia: ↑albumin, lab error

> Corrected Ca^{+2} = measured Ca^{+2} + 0.8 × (4 − albumin) [i.e., Ca^{+2} ↓0.8 mg/dl per ↓1 g/dl albumin]

- Review patient's history and medication list
- Check parathyroid hormone (PTH), identify PO_4, alkaline phosphatase, ±1,25-OH_2 vitamin D
- If malignancy suspected, check PTH-related protein
- PTH tests:
  Radioimmunoassay: mid-region (44–68), carboxyhemoglobin (69–84)
  Immunoradiometric assay: ↑sensitivity
- Diagnostic algorithm:

High PTH	Normal/low PTH

Primary hyperpara-
thyroidism (<12
mg/dl) (adenoma,
MEN I/IIa)
Renal failure
(acute/chronic)
Familial hypocal-
ciuria (↓uCa)
Lithium

Acute: Rule out malignancy, check PTHrP

Chronic: Measure vitamin D

	1,25-OH_2D	AlkPhos	uCa	PTHrP
Squamous cell cancer	↓	↑	↑	↑↑
Metastases/myeloma/thyroid/Paget's	↓	↑	↑	0
Vitamin D toxicity	↑	↓	↑	0
Lymphoma/granulo-matous disease	↑	↑	↑	0
Milk-alkali, Addison's disease	N	N	N	0
Thiazides	N	N	↓	0

Therapy

Drug	Onset	Duration	Comments	Toxicities
Furosemide (Lasix), 20–40 IV q2h + NS	Hours	Infusion	Avoid in Cr >1.3 mg/dl	Check electrolytes, CHF
Pamidronate, 90 mg IV	1–2 days	10–14 days	Potent	Fever, ↓PO_4, ↓Mg
Prednisone, 40 mg PO qd	Days	Weeks	Antitumor, ↓GI absorption	Malignancy-related
Phosphate, 20–30 mg/kg IV q12h	Hours	Infusion	Potent, ↑extravascular	Ectopic Ca^{+2}
Calcitonin, 4 IU/kg SQ q12h	Hours	2–3 days	↓1–3 mg/dl in 6–8 hrs	Tachyphylaxis
Mithramycin, 25 μg/kg IV qd	12 hrs	3–7 days	Antitumor	↓Platelets, acute rena failure, acute heart failure
Dialysis	Hours	≤48 hrs	In renal failure	Needs setup

- Indications for admissions: dehydration, Ca^{+2} >14 mg/dl, altered mental status, severe symptoms
- Indications for parathyroid surgery: Ca^{+2} >11.4 mg/dl, ↓CrCl, urine Ca^{+2} >400 mg/day, ↓bone mass, nephrolithiasis

RENAL

HYPOCALCEMIA   (*Lancet* 352:306, 1998)

Symptoms
- Neuromuscular irritability (Chvostek's: CN 7; Trousseau's: median nerve), tetany, paresthesia, seizure, hyperreflexia
- Bronchospasm
- ECG findings: $\uparrow$QT interval
- Lenticular cataracts
- Lethargy

Evaluation
- Rule out pseudohypocalcemia: Check albumin, ionized Ca^{+2}, Mg^{+2}/PO_4

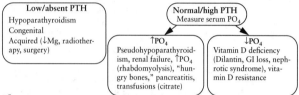

Low/absent PTH
Hypoparathyroidism
Congenital
Acquired ($\downarrow$Mg, radiotherapy, surgery)

Normal/high PTH
Measure serum PO_4

$\uparrow PO_4$
Pseudohypoparathyroidism, renal failure, $\uparrow PO_4$ (rhabdomyolysis), "hungry bones," pancreatitis, transfusions (citrate)

$\downarrow PO_4$
Vitamin D deficiency (Dilantin, GI loss, nephrotic syndrome), vitamin D resistance

Therapy
For severe hypocalcemia (<7.5 mg/dl) use IV calcium:
- Ca^{+2} gluconate (1 amp = 100 mg = 90 mg elemental Ca^{+2}/10 ml in 100 cc D_5W)
- Load 200 mg IV over 10 minutes, then 50–150 mg/hour IV $\approx$ $\uparrow$Ca 2–3 mg/dl for 15 mg/kg infusion
- Then check calcium q4–6h

For chronic hypocalcemia:
- Oral $CaCO_3$, 1–2 g/day (Tums-EX, 250 mg; Rolaids, 220 mg; OsCal, 500 mg)
- Vitamin D
- Ensure that magnesium is replete

HYPERPHOSPHATEMIA (*Lancet* 352:391, 1998; *Nephrol Dialysis Transplant* 14:2085, 1999)

Symptoms
- Related to $\downarrow Ca^{+2}$ due to Ca^{+2}-PO_4^- complexes
- Tetany, spasms, $\downarrow BP$, lethargy, organ dysfunction

Solubility product = $[Ca] \times [PO_4] \geq 60 \rightarrow$ deposition

Evaluation
- Rule out pseudohyperphosphatemia: multiple myeloma
- Determine patient's glomerular filtration rate (GFR)
  - **Low GFR (<30):** renal insufficiency ($\downarrow PO_4$ excretion, rarely $PO_4 > 10$)
  - **Normal/high GFR (≥ 30 ml/minute/m²):**
    - $\uparrow$**Renal absorption:** $\downarrow PTH$, $\uparrow$growth hormone, $\uparrow$thyroid, tumoral calcinosis, diphosphonates, $\downarrow ECV$
    - $\uparrow$**Phosphate loading:** exogenous, endogenous (rhabdomyolysis, necrosis, tumor lysis)
    - **Transcellular shifts:** catabolic states, infection, acidosis

Therapy
- Low PO_4 diet; $CaCO_3$; calcium acetate (PhosLo); dialysis; ?acetazolamide, 15 mg/kg PO q4h

HYPOPHOSPHATEMIA

Symptoms
- Myopathy ($\downarrow ATP$), obtundation, osteomalacia, RBC/WBC/platelet dysfunction, rhabdomyolysis, CHF

Evaluation
- Rule out redistribution: glucose/DKA, alkalosis, EtOH, $\uparrow$catecholamine state, $\uparrow Ca^{+2}/\downarrow Mg^{+2}$
- Evaluate for $\downarrow$dietary intake: starvation, TPN
- For further evaluation check urine phosphorus level

Hyperphosphaturia ($U_{PO_4} > 5$–10 mg/dl)   **Hypophosphaturia** ($U_{PO_4} < 5$–10 mg/dl)

Renal losses

GI losses: malabsorption, diarrhea (EtOH) phosphate binders

Measure urine lytes   *Measure serum Ca^{+2}*
Renal tubular defects $\uparrow Ca$: primary $\uparrow PTH$
(Wilson's, Fanconi's,   N/$\downarrow Ca^{+2}$: secondary
metal tox, SLE, RTA) $\uparrow PTH \downarrow VitD$ (EtOH)

Therapy	IV replacement		PO replacement	
Dosage	**Na-Phos,** IV 0.25– 0.5 mmol/kg (q4h)	**K-Phos,** IV 0.25– 0.5 mmol/ kg (q4h)	**Neutra-Phos** K/Na (1.25 mg), 2 tablets PO tid	**Phospho-Soda,** 5 ml PO tid
PO_4	93 mg (3 mmol)/ml	93 mg (3 mmol)/ml	250 mg (8 mmol)/tablet	129 mg (mmol)/ml
Other	Na^+, 4 mEq/ml	K^+, 4.4 mEq/ml	K^+/Na^+, 7.125 mEq/tablet	Na^+, 4.8 mEq/ml

RENAL

HYPERMAGNESEMIA (*J Am Soc Nephrol* 10:1616, 1999; *Lancet* 352:391, 1998)

Symptoms
- Manifesting as weakness or paralysis, confusion
- ECG changes: ↑PR, ↑QRS, ↑T

Cause
- Almost always related to renal insufficiency

Therapy
- $CaCl_2$ at 100 mg (4.5 mmol)/minute as antagonist, dialysis (usually in renal failure)

HYPOMAGNESEMIA

Symptoms
- Weakness, muscle cramps, tremor, + Babinski, hypertension
- Arrhythmia/ventricular tachycardia
- ECG changes: prolonged QT and ST segments
- Hypokalemia, hypocalcemia

Causes
- ↓Absorption: diarrhea, laxatives, EtOH, TPN, small-bowel bypass
- ↑Loss: DKA, diuretics, diarrhea, ↑aldosterone, Bartter's syndrome, ↑calciuria, renal wasting
- Unexplained: ↑PTH, vitamin D therapy, amphotericin B, aminoglycosides, cisplatin

Therapy

Options
- Mg gluconate, 500 mg PO (2.5 mEq)
- MgO_2, 140 mg PO (7 mEq)
- $MgSO_4$, 1 amp IV (8 mEq/1 g)

Magnesium Scale (Cr ≤1.2 mg/dl) for IV Replacement
- 2 amp (Mg 1.3–1.5 mg/dl)
- 3 amp (1.0–1.2 mg/dl)
- 4 amp (0.7–0.9 mg/dl)
- 6 amp (0.4–0.6 mg/dl)

ACID-BASE PRIMER (*West J Med* 155:146, 1991; *Semin Nephrol* 18:83, 1998)

1. Primary→pH: Determine **acidemia** (pH <7.38) versus **alkalemia** (pH >7.42)

2. Secondary→PaCO$_2$ (normal 38–42) and HCO$_3$ (normal 22–26)

	pH	PaCO$_2$	HCO$_3$	Go to
Respiratory acidosis	↓	↑	↑	Step 3
Respiratory alkalosis	↑	↓	↓	Step 3
Metabolic acidosis	↓	↓	↓	Step 4
Metabolic alkalosis	↑	↑	↑	Step 4

3. Primary respiratory: Determine **metabolic compensation** (acute versus chronic) (±4)

Secondary metabolic compensation		Respiratory acidosis		Respiratory alkalosis	
		(PaCO$_2$ ↑10 mm Hg)		(PaCO$_2$ ↓10 mm Hg)	
		Acute	Chronic	Acute	Chronic
	HCO$_3$	↑1 mEq	↑3 mEq	↓2 mEq	↓5 mEq
	pH	↓0.08	↓0.03	↑0.07	↑0.02

Calculated ΔpH In respiratory acidosis	(acute) $0.08 \times \dfrac{\Delta PaCO_2}{10}$	(chronic) $0.03 \times \dfrac{\Delta PaCO_2}{10}$

- Differences between measured and calculated values represent degree of chronicity (% mixture between acute and chronic)

4. Primary metabolic: Compare measured with calculated **respiratory compensation**

Secondary respiratory compensation	Metabolic acidosis	Metabolic alkalosis
	(HCO$_3$ ↓1 mg/dl)	(HCO$_3$ ↑1 mg/dl)
	PaCO$_2$ ↓1.25 mm Hg	PaCO$_2$ ↑0.75 mm Hg

Calculated PaCO$_2$	(acute)(1.5 × HCO$_3$) + 8(±2)	(chronic)(0.7 × HCO$_3$) + 20(±1.5)

Difference between measured and calculated values suggests a **secondary disorder:**
- If measured PaCO$_2$ > calculated PaCO$_2$→underlying respiratory acidosis
- If measured PaCO$_2$ < calculated PaCO$_2$→underlying respiratory alkalosis

5. Tertiary→Determine concomitant tertiary metabolic acidosis

    Anion gap = [Na − (Cl + HCO$_3$)]   [Normal = 12 ± 2]
        •Anion gap >20 have metabolic acidosis regardless

    Delta-delta = [(anion gap − 12) + HCO$_3$]   [Normal = 24 ± 1]
        •Underlying metabolic alkalosis if >30
        •Underlying nonanion gap metabolic acidosis if <23

    Urine anion gap = [UNa + UK − UCl]   [Normal <0 in pH <5.5]
        •Renal tubular acidosis if urine anion gap >0 and pH >5.5
        •GI loss if urine anion gap <0 and pH >5.5

RENAL

EVALUATION OF METABOLIC ACIDOSIS

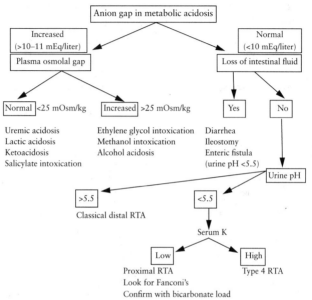

RTA = renal tubular acidosis.
Source: Reproduced with permission from American College of Physicians, MKSAP 11, Nephrology, p. 705.

Differential Diagnosis

- Anion gap (**MUDPILES**): **m**ethanol, **u**remia, **D**KA, **p**araldehyde, **i**schemia, **l**actic acidosis, **e**thylene glycol, **s**alicylates
- Nonanion gap (**HARD UP**): **h**yperalimentation, **a**cetazolamide, **r**enal tubular acidosis, **d**iarrhea/GI losses, **u**reterosigmoidostomy, **p**ancreatic fistula. Others include ↓aldosterone, ↑K⁺/Ca⁺²/Mg⁺², myeloma, lithium

RENAL TUBULAR ACIDOSIS (*Arch Intern Med* 156:1629, 1996; *Semin Nephrol* 18:317, 1998)

	Hypokalemic distal (type I)	Proximal (type II)	Type IV
Prevalence	Rare	Rare	Very common
Plasma K	Low	Low	High
Plasma HCO_3	<10 mEq	14–20 mEq	>15 mEq
Urine pH	>5.3 (NH_4Cl)	<5.3 (threshold)	<5.3
Urine NH_4	Low	Normal	Low
Diagnosis	↓K^+, response to $NaHCO_3/NH_4Cl$	Response to $NaHCO_3$	Check plasma aldosterone
Defect	↓H^+ pump; ↓acid secretion distally, intact tubules	↓Proximal HCO_3 transport	↓NH_3, ↓aldosterone effect, ↓renin
Treatment	HCO_3, 1–2 mEq/kg/day	Diuretics, HCO_3 10–15 mEq/kg/day	Diuretics, HCO_3 1–3 mEq/kg/day
Complications	Nephrocalcinosis	Osteomalacia	None
Example	Amphotericin, cirrhosis	Acetazolamide, myeloma	Diabetes, chronic renal failure

RENAL

EVALUATION OF METABOLIC ALKALOSIS (*Lancet* 352:474, 1998;
N Engl J Med 338:107, 1998; *J Am Soc Nephrol* 8:1462, 1997)

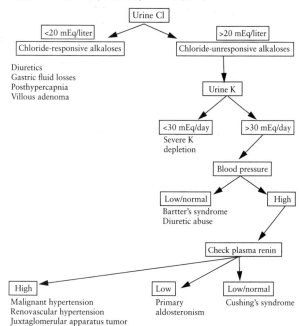

Source: Reproduced with permission from American College of Physicians, MKSAP 11, Nephrology, p. 707.

Differential Diagnosis

- Saline responsive (UcCl <20): volume depletion (vomiting, nasogastric drainage, diuretics)
- Saline unresponsive: Bartter's syndrome, $\downarrow K^+$, refeeding (normotensive); aldosteronism, adrenal deficiency, exogenous mineralocorticoid use (hypertension)

ACUTE RENAL FAILURE   (*Lancet* 346:1533, 1995; *N Engl J Med* 334:1448, 1996; *N Engl J Med* 338:571, 1998)

Fast Facts
- 2–5% of inpatients develop renal failure; 2–55% of cases are iatrogenic
- Renal failure increases mortality by 15-fold (risk: age, hypertension, Cr >1.7)

Definition
- Oliguria = urine output <400–500 ml/day

Evaluation

Condition	Dipstick	Sediment	BUN/Cr	uNa	uOsm	FENa
Prerenal	Trace or no pro-teinuria	A few hyaline casts possible	>20:1	<20	>500	<1
Renal	—	—	<20:1	>40	<350	>1
Ischemia	Mild/moderate proteinuria	Pigmented granu-lar casts	—	—	<350	>1
Nephro-toxins	Mild/moderate proteinuria	Pigmented granu-lar casts	—	—	<350	>1
Acute inter-stitial nephritis	Mild/moderate proteinuria; hemoglobin; leukocytes	White cells and white cell casts; eosinophils and eosinophil casts; red cells	—	—	<350	>1
Acute glo-merulo-nephritis	Moderate/severe proteinuria; hemoglobin	Red cells and red cell casts: red cells can be dys-morphic	—	—	>500	<1
Postrenal	Trace or no pro-teinuria; can have hemoglo-bin, leukocytes	Crystals, red cells, and white cells possible	Variable	>40	<350	>1

Therapy
Maintain renal perfusion: most effective prophylactic strategy.
- Fluid management can be dicey; follow examination intake and output, weight, and perhaps invasive monitoring

Preventive and supportive measures:
- Discontinue nephrotoxins, renal dosing for all medications
- Monitor and avoid K^+/Mg^{+2}/PO_4^{-3}, maintain renal diet, and watch acidosis
- Monitor and treat anemia, bleeding disorders
- Leading causes of death in renal failure are infectious complications

Converting oliguric to nonoliguric renal failure with diuretics (evidence is paltry).
Increasing urine volume with diuretics, if possible, makes patients easier to manage.

continued **87**

RENAL

Indications for Dialysis (AEIOU)

- Metabolic acidosis: unresponsive to bicarbonate therapy
- Electrolytes: refractory hyperkalemia, with ECG changes unresponsive to therapy
- Intoxications: methanol, ethylene glycol, lithium, ASA
- Volume overload: with pulmonary edema
- Uremia: pericarditis, encephalopthy, seizures, bleeding, enteropathy

DRUGS ASSOCIATED WITH RENAL FAILURE (N Engl J Med 334:1448, 1996; N Engl J Med 338:571, 1998)

Mechanism	Drug
Reduction in renal perfusion through alteration of intrarenal hemodynamics	NSAIDs, ACE inhibitors, cyclosporine, tacrolimus, radiocontrast agents, amphotericin B, interleukin-2
Direct tubular toxicity	Aminoglycosides, radiocontrast agents, cisplatin, cyclosporine, tacrolimus, amphotericin B, methotrexate, foscarnet, pentamidine, organic solvents, heavy metals, IVIG
Heme pigment–induced tubular toxicity	Cocaine, ethanol, lovastatin
Intratubular obstruction by precipitation of the agent or its metabolites or by-products	Acyclovir, sulfonamides, ethylene glycol, chemotherapeutic agents, methotrexate
Allergic interstitial nephritis	Penicillins, cephalosporins, sulfonamides, rifampin, ciprofloxacin, NSAIDs, thiazide diuretics, furosemide, cimetidine, phenytoin, allopurinol
Hemolytic-uremic syndrome	Cyclosporine, tacrolimus, mitomycin, cocaine, quinine, conjugated estrogens

Source: Reprinted with permission from N Engl J Med 334:1451, 1996. Copyright © 1996, Massachusetts Medical Society. All rights reserved.

HEPATORENAL SYNDROME *(Hepatology* 23:164,1996; *J Am Soc Nephrol* 10:1833, 1999)

Diagnostic Criteria

- Renal insufficiency (Cr >1.5 mg/dl/CrCl <40 mg/minute) despite 1.5 liters plasma expander in liver failure
- Rule out shock, hypovolemia, proteinuria <500 mg/day, no neurotoxin
- Additional criteria: urinary volume <500 ml/day, uNa <10 mEq/liter, uOsm >pOsm, uRBC <50/hpf, pNa <130

RHABDOMYOLYSIS AND PIGMENT NEPHROPATHY
(Medicine 61:141, 1982)

Risks

- Dehydration, hyperosmolality, acidosis, $\downarrow K^+$

Symptoms

- Extremity pain and weakness, contractures, fever, malaise, abdominal pain, mental status changes, cardiac arrest

Causes

- Trauma, hypothermia, drug/EtOH overdose, infection, seizure, diabetes, heat shock

Diagnosis

- $\uparrow$Muscle enzymes: CK (may be >100K), both MM and MB released
- Myoglobin in urine (heme + dipstick but no blood seen, no color change in urine)
- Renal failure and electrolyte abnormalities ($\uparrow K^+$, $\uparrow PO_4^{-3}$, $\downarrow Ca^{+2}$)
- $\uparrow$Uric acid; metabolic acidosis also may be seen

Therapy

- Mainstay: IV fluids (0.9% NS), HCO_3 to keep urine pH >8
- Lasix/mannitol if oliguric (uNa <25 reflects intact tubules)
- Dialysis, kayexalate/sorbitol for $\uparrow K^+$
- Calcium acetate prn for $\uparrow PO_4^{-3}$
- Compartment syndrome may develop after fluid resuscitation

RENAL

CHRONIC RENAL FAILURE (*Lancet* 338:423, 1991)

Causes
- Diabetes mellitus and hypertension make up 60% of cases
- Chronic glomerulonephritis: 15%
- Interstitial nephritis, polycystic kidney disease, obstructive uropathy

Therapy
Find Reversible Factors
- Volume depletion
- Congestive heart failure
- Urinary tract obstruction
- Accelerated hypertension
- Drugs
- Contrast media
- Ischemic renal disease

Slow Progression
- Control of BP to <120/75: **ACE inhibitor may have selective advantage**
- Protein-restricted diet: Variable results from clinical trials; need renal dietician
- Blood sugar control in diabetics: Proven benefit in type I but applies to type II

Treating Complications
- Hypertension and volume status: dietary restriction, BP medications, and loop diuretics
- Hyperkalemia: Limit K^+ intake; careful use of NSAIDs, ACE inhibitors, beta blockers, digoxin
- Bone disease: Phosphate binder—calcium acetate (PhosLo), 667 mg PO tid with meals; $CaCO_3$, 1,250 mg PO tid for bones/acidosis
- Anemia: Folate, 1 mg PO qd; $FeSO_4$, 325 mg PO tid; if needed, epoetin α (Epogen) start at 2,000–4,000 units/week (up to 10,000 units)
- Dietary considerations: Renal diet (low Na^+/K^+/PO_4^{-3}), dialysis vitamin supplement (Nephrocaps), 1 tablet PO qd

End-Stage Renal Disease (*J Am Soc Nephrol* 10:872, 1999; *Lancet* 353:737, 1999; *Lancet* 353:823, 1999)
- Dialysis versus transplant: clear survival advantage with cadaveric transplant
- For nondiabetic dialysis when CrCl <0.16 ml/second, diabetics CrCl 0.16–0.25 ml/second
- Peritoneal dialysis: Option for patients who want control; catheter placed 2 weeks before
- Hemodialysis: AV fistula or catheter required weeks to months in advance

NEPHROLITHIASIS (*Lancet* 351:1797, 1998; *J Am Soc Nephrol* 9:917, 1998; *Semin Nephrol* 19:381, 1999)

Fast Facts

- Peak incidence at ages 20–50 years
- Ratio of occurrence in men to that in women is 4:1
- Calcium stones account for 80% of stones; others are uric acid, struvite, and cystine
- Recurrence is common: 10% per year and 75% per lifetime
- Risk factors for recurrence:

Middle-aged white male	Family history of renal stones
Renal tubular acidosis	Chronic bowel disease
Uric acid stones	

  Extrarenal manifestations of stone-related abnormality (gout, bone loss)
- Stones pass spontaneously 80% of the time; stones >8 mm only pass 10% of the time
- Complications: renal failure if obstruction unrelieved >7 days

Prediction Rule for Nephrolithiasis

- Patients with abdominal and flank pain should have a urinalysis
- If prior history of stones and hematuria is present, then evaluation may stop
- If no prior history of stones and hematuria is present, then proceed with x-ray examination of kidneys, ureter, and bladder (KUB)
- Patient with flank pain, hematuria, and positive KUB has almost 100% chance of stone
- If KUB is negative, proceed with CT scan or IVP

Therapy for Acute Nephrolithiasis

- Hydration and pain medications (ketorolac/NSAIDs or narcotics) adequate for <5-mm stone
- Strain urine
- Hospitalize for dehydration, prolonged pain, suspected infection, stone in solitary kidney
- Consult urology for pain >72 hours, obstruction, concurrent infection
- Treatment of obstruction:

  Percutaneous nephrostomy with stent
  Percutaneous nephrolithotomy
  Ureteroscopic stone removal (best method if stone at ureteropelvic junction)
  Extracorporeal shock wave lithotripsy (treatment of choice in 85% of cases)
  Open surgical removal

Management After First Stone

- Check serum calcium if radiopaque stones and serum uric acid if radiolucent
- Encourage fluid intake >2 liters/day
- KUB or ultrasound at 1 year and, if negative, every 3–5 years thereafter

Management After Recurrent Stones

- Screen for hypercalcemia and hyperuricemia
- Send 24-hour urine collection for urine volume, excretion of calcium, uric acid, citrate, oxalate, creatinine, pH, and sodium. May need two collections of urine.

4. Gastroenterology

BEDSIDE DIAGNOSIS: ABDOMINAL PAIN
Differential Diagnosis of Abdominal Pain by Location
(Reproduced with permission from F. Ferri. *Practical Guide to the Care of the Medical Patient*. St. Louis: Mosby–Year Book, 1991)

Right Upper Quadrant
Biliary: calculi, infection, inflammation, neoplasm
Hepatic: hepatitis, abscess, hepatic congestion, neoplasm, trauma
Gastric: peptic ulcer disease, pyloric stenosis, neoplasm, alcoholic gastritis, hiatal hernia
Pancreatic: pancreatitis, neoplasm, stone
Renal: calculi, pyelonephritis, neoplasm
Pulmonary: pneumonia, pulmonary infarction
Intestinal: retrocecal appendicitis, intestinal obstruction, high fecal impaction

Epigastric
Gastric: peptic ulcer disease, gastric outlet obstruction, gastric ulcer
Duodenal: peptic ulcer disease, duodenitis
Biliary: cholecystitis, cholangitis
Hepatic: hepatitis
Pancreatic: pancreatitis
Intestinal: high small-bowel obstruction, early appendicitis
Cardiac: angina, MI, pericarditis
Pulmonary: pneumonia, pleurisy, pneumothorax
Subphrenic abscess

Left Upper Quadrant
Gastric: peptic ulcer disease, gastritis, pyloric stenosis, hiatal hernia
Pancreatic: pancreatitis, neoplasm, stone
Cardiac: MI, angina
Splenic: splenomegaly, ruptured spleen, splenic abscess, infarction
Renal: calculi, pyelonephritis, neoplasm
Pulmonary: pneumonia, pulmonary infarction
Vascular: ruptured aortic aneurysm
Cutaneous: herpes zoster
Trauma
Intestinal: high fecal impaction, perforated colon

Right Lower Quadrant
Intestinal: acute appendicitis, regional enteritis, incarcerated hernia, cecal diverticulitis, intestinal obstruction, perforated ulcer, perforated cecum, Meckel's diverticulum
Reproductive: ectopic pregnancy, ovarian cyst, torsion of cyst, salpingitis, tubo-ovarian abscess, mittelschmerz, endometriosis, seminal vesiculitis
Renal: renal and ureteral calculi, neoplasm, pyelonephritis
Vascular: leaking aortic aneurysm
Psoas abscess
Trauma
Cholecystitis

Periumbilical
Intestinal: small-bowel obstruction or gangrene, early appendicitis
Vascular: mesenteric thrombosis, dissecting aortic aneurysm
Pancreatic: pancreatitis
Metabolic: uremia, diabetic ketoacidosis
Trauma

Left Lower Quadrant
Intestinal: diverticulitis, intestinal obstruction, perforated ulcer, inflammatory bowel disease, perforated descending colon, inguinal hernia, neoplasm, appendicitis
Reproductive: ectopic pregnancy, ovarian cyst, torsion of cyst, salpingitis, tubo-ovarian abscess, mittelschmerz, endometriosis, seminal vesiculitis
Renal: renal and ureteral calculi, neoplasm, pyelonephritis
Vascular: leaking aortic aneurysm
Psoas abscess
Trauma

GASTROINTESTINAL ENDOSCOPY (A. Fauci et al. [eds]. *Harrison's*
Principles of Internal Medicine [14th ed]. New York: McGraw-Hill, 1997)

Procedure	Indications	Complications	Preparation
Esophago-gastroduo-denoscopy (EGD)	Evaluation for upper GI bleed, dysphagia, gastroesophageal reflux, peptic ulcer disease, upper GI cancer; placement of percutaneous endoscopic gastrostomy tube; palliation of esophageal cancer	1 in 500 patients have complications; 1 in 10,000 patients die (cardiopulmonary complications and perforation most common)	NPO × 8 hours
Endoscopic retrograde cholangiography	Unclear persistent jaundice despite negative ultrasound, CT, HIDA scan; biliary pain; postoperative cholangitis; changes in results of liver function tests	Asymptomatic increase in amylase in 40–75%; transient symptomatic pancreatitis in 1–7%; mortality of 0.2%	NPO × 8 hours
Endoscopic retrograde pancreatography	Recent or chronic pancreatitis; rule out pancreatic cancer; painless steatorrhea	Same as above	Same as above
Therapeutic ERCP	Removal of stones from pancreatic or biliary tree; placement of stents over strictures	Same as above	Same as above
Colonoscopy	Polyp evaluation; follow-up on abnormal barium enema findings; narrowing on x-ray; chronic GI bleeding; inflammatory bowel disease; as part of routine colon cancer screening	Bleeding or perforation in 0.5–1.3%; mortality of 0.02%	Clear liquid diet × 2 days; GoLYTELY, 4 liters over 3 hours in the afternoon of the day before; NPO × 8 hours

GASTROENTEROLOGY

GASTROINTESTINAL FUNCTIONAL TESTS
Best Choices in Liver Function Tests

Disorder		Best tests
Acute hepatitis		ALT, AST
Chronic hepatitis		ALT, AST
Cholestasis		Bilirubin, ALP, GGT
Cirrhosis	Biliary	ALP, bilirubin
	Nonbiliary	Early: GGT, AST Advanced: albumin, GGT, AST, bilirubin
Tumor metastasis		GGT, ALP

Some Causes of Hyperbilirubinemia

Unconju-gated	Increased production	Hemolysis
	Decreased uptake	Gilbert's syndrome
	Decreased conjugation	Prematurity/newborn, Gilbert's, Crigler-Najjar syndrome
Conju-gated	Decreased secretion	Dubin-Johnson syndrome; Rotor syndrome
	Hepatocellular disease	Hepatitis, cirrhosis
	Intrahepatic cholestasis	Sclerosing cholangitis, primary biliary cirrhosis, drugs
	Extrahepatic cholestasis	Stone, neoplasm, stricture

Urinary Bilirubin and Urobilinogen

	Bilirubin	Urobilinogen
Healthy	Absent	Trace
Hemolytic disease	Absent	Increased
Gilbert's syndrome	Absent	Normal
Hepatocellular disease	Present	Early: increased Late: decreased
Cholestasis	Present	Decreased

Typical Plasma Aminotransferase Changes in Liver Disease

Disease	Frequency of abnormality (%)	Level (× upper reference limit)	Relative activity
Viral hepatitis (acute)	100	>10	ALT >AST
Chronic hepatitis	<90	5–10	ALT >AST
Cirrhosis	<50	<5	AST >ALT
Hepatic metastases	<50	<5	AST >ALT
Cholestatic jaundice	>90	<10	ALT >AST

All tables on this page reproduced with permission from SB Rosaki, JS Dooley. Liver function profiles and their interpretation. *Br J Hosp Med* 51:181, 1994.

GASTROINTESTINAL BLEEDING: ACUTE MANAGEMENT

(*JAMA* 278:2151, 1997)

Fast Fact

• Mortality rate for GI bleed: 5–14%

Management

Stabilize patient hemodynamically!

Initial Assessment

• Check for hypovolemia, orthostatics; initiate cardiac monitoring
• Obtain access (16-gauge IVs × 2), send blood for Hgb/Hct, coagulation, type, and cross

Volume Resuscitation

• Saline [transfuse blood, platelets, fresh-frozen plasma (if indicated)]
• With large saline infusion or large-volume transfusion, consider replacing calcium, fresh-frozen plasma,
  cryoprecipitate as these factors may be diluted

Additional Orders

• Hgb/Hct q2–6h
• Hold NSAIDs, anticoagulants (unless indicated), sucralfate, antacids, iron, food
• H$_2$-blocker IV: Pepcid, 20 mg IV bid
• Exclude underlying anemia

General Evaluation

• Nasogastric lavage to determine upper GI source (check bilirubin by dipstick)

Differential Diagnosis

Upper GI bleed	Lower GI bleed
Gastritis/esophagitis/duodenitis	Upper GI bleed
Peptic ulcer disease	Hemorrhoid
Mallory-Weiss tear	Diverticulosis/diverticulitis
Variceal bleed	Arteriovenous malformation
Arteriovenous malformation	Neoplasm
	Inflammatory (inflammatory bowel disease, infection)

continued

GASTROENTEROLOGY

Further Evaluation of Upper GI Bleed

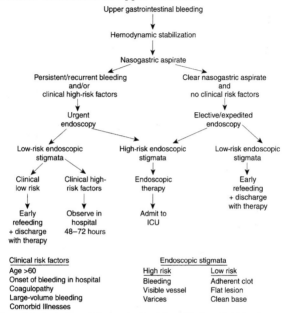

Upper gastrointestinal bleeding

Hemodynamic stabilization

Nasogastric aspirate

Persistent/recurrent bleeding and/or clinical high-risk factors → Urgent endoscopy

Clear nasogastric aspirate and no clinical risk factors → Elective/expedited endoscopy

Low-risk endoscopic stigmata

High-risk endoscopic stigmata → Endoscopic therapy → Admit to ICU

Low-risk endoscopic stigmata → Early refeeding + discharge with therapy

Clinical low risk → Early refeeding + discharge with therapy

Clinical high-risk factors → Observe in hospital 48–72 hours

Clinical risk factors
Age >60
Onset of bleeding in hospital
Coagulopathy
Large-volume bleeding
Comorbid Illnesses

Endoscopic stigmata	
High risk	Low risk
Bleeding	Adherent clot
Visible vessel	Flat lesion
Varices	Clean base

Source: Reproduced with permission from American College of Physicians, MKSAP 11, Gastroenterology and Hepatology, p. 1030.

Further Evaluation of Lower GI Bleed

- Initial test: Colonoscopy after rapid colonic purge
- If vigorous bleeding:
  ^{99m}Technetium-RBC angiography: detects 1 ml/minute active bleeding
  RBC scan: detects 0.5 ml/minute active bleeding
- Melena requires >50-ml bleed
- Hemoccult positive >20-ml bleed (false positives: high peroxidases—e.g., red meat, raw fruits and vegetables, vitamin C)

GASTROENTEROLOGY

NAUSEA AND VOMITING
Differential Diagnosis
- CNS disorders
- Gastrointestinal irritation: gastroenteritis
- Obstruction
- Medication: chemotherapy
- Pregnancy
- Systemic diseases

Evaluation
- Consider upper GI bleed
- Check KUB
- Check electrolytes/consider arterial blood gas
- Upper GI series/small-bowel follow-through
- EGD-manometry

Management
- General: NPO, nasogastric tube, treat underlying disease (obstruction/CNS/infection)

Drug	Dosage	Indications
Centrally acting anti-emetic: ondansetron (Zofran)	8 mg IVP, then 9 mg PO tid (0.15 mg/kg IV q4h × 3)	Chemotherapy-induced
Corticosteroid: dexa-methasone (Decadron)	10 mg IV q6h (check glucose)	Chemotherapy-induced
Dopamine antagonists:		Severe nausea and vomiting. Side effects include sedation, hypotension, and parkinsonism; helpful in all types except motion sickness or inner ear disturbance
Prochlorperazine (Compazine)	10 mg PO/IM/IV q6h or 25 mg PR q12h	
Promethazine (Phenergan)	25 mg PO/PR/IM/IV tid	
Metoclopramide (Reglan)	1–3 mg/kg/day (10–20 mg) q4–6h	
Antihistamine: diphenhydramine (Benadryl)	25–50 mg PO/IV q4–6h	Motion sickness/inner ear disturbance, pregnancy, uremia, postoperative nausea and vomiting
Sedative: Lorazepam (Ativan)	0.5–2.0 mg PO/IV q4–6h	Psychogenic and anticipatory

GASTROENTEROLOGY

ACUTE DIARRHEA

Fast Fact
- Almost all acute diarrhea is self-limited, so identification of organism is rarely needed

Definition
- Abnormal increase in daily stool weight (>200 g/day) or frequency

Dichotomies to Consider
- Infectious versus noninfectious: history of travel, sexual exposure, food exposure, hospitalization, medications (especially antibiotics), systemic illness (e.g., diabetes mellitus)
- Acute versus chronic; acute usually related to infection or drugs
- Inflammatory versus noninflammatory
- Bloody versus nonbloody
- Large bowel (frequent, small bowel movements) versus small bowel (infrequent voluminous bowel movements)

Evaluation
- First check stool fecal leukocytes to rule out inflammatory diarrhea, then tailor evaluation
- If inflammatory diarrhea is suspected (toxic appearance, outbreaks, blood/mucus, >10 bowel movements/day, lasting >4–5 days, on antibiotics, ↓immune/underlying illness, changed electrolytes)→bacterial culture (*Shigella, Salmonella, Yersinia, Campylobacter*)
- If history of antibiotic use→√*Clostridium difficile* toxin
- If history of suspected raw meat ingestion, outbreak, bloody stools→alert microcyte laboratory for specific serotyping for enterohemorrhagic *E. coli*
- *Aeromonas, Cryptosporidium, Vibrio*→specific cultivation should be ordered
- *Giardia*→ELISA for antigen
- If diarrhea >10 days, send ova and parasites × 3
- Sigmoidoscopy or colonoscopy may be necessary if symptoms >10 days

Management
- Rest, with fluid and electrolyte replacement
- Initial absorbents:
    Attapulgite (Kaopectate), 60–120 ml PO q3–4h
    Bismuth subsalicylate (Pepto-Bismol), 30 ml PO q6h
- Opioids (antiperistaltic): may precipitate toxic megacolon in invasive colitis
    Loperamide HCl (Imodium), 2–4mg PO qid
    Diphenoxylate HCl (Lomotil), 5 mg PO qid
    Paregoric, 4–8 ml PO qid (max 32 ml qd)
- Antidiarrheals may be given with antibiotics for traveler's diarrhea

CLOSTRIDIUM DIFFICILE COLITIS (*Am J Gastroenterol* 92:739, 1997)

Tests for *Clostridium Difficile*

Test	Remarks
Endoscopy with biopsy	Diagnostic when pseudomembranes are seen
	Best and most rapid method
Tissue culture tests for toxin B	"Gold standard" lab test
	Negative result does not rule out *C. difficile*
ELISA for toxin A and B	Rapidly performed and inexpensive
	Sensitivity 70–95%; specificity is better
Latex agglutination	Also rapidly performed and inexpensive
	Detects glutamate dehydrogenase
	As sensitive as ELISA but not as specific
Stool culture	Problem is some people are carriers

Practice Guidelines for Diagnosis (Reprinted with permission from the American College of Gastroenterology, *Am J Gastroenterol* 92:739, 1997)

1. Suspect in anyone with diarrhea
   - who has received antibiotics within the previous 2 months and
   - whose diarrhea began 72 hours or more after hospitalization
2. If suspected, send a single stool specimen for *C. difficile* and its toxin
3. If test is negative and symptoms persist, send one or two additional specimens
4. Endoscopy is reserved for
   - when rapid diagnosis is needed and test results are delayed
   - when test is not highly sensitive
   - when patient has ileus and stool is not available
   - when other colonic diseases are in the differential

Practice Guidelines for Treatment (Reprinted with permission from the American College of Gastroenterology, *Am J Gastroenterol* 92:739, 1997)

1. Antibiotics should be discontinued if possible
2. Nonspecific supportive therapy
3. Oral metronidazole is preferred
   Oral: 250–500 mg qid or 500–750 mg tid for 7–10 days
   IV: 500–750 mg IV tid or qid
4. If suspicion is high but test result not available, may treat
5. Vancomycin should be reserved for
   - patients who have failed a course of metronidazole
   - organism resistant to metronidazole
   - patient unable to tolerate metronidazole or allergic to it, or patient taking ethanol-containing solutions
   - patient is pregnant or a child <10 years old

continued

- patient is critically ill because of associated diarrhea or colitis
- any evidence that *Staphylococcus aureus* might be a cause of diarrhea

Vancomycin: 125 mg qid for 7–10 days or 500 mg qid

Management of Relapses (Reprinted with permission from the American College of Gastroenterology, *Am J Gastroenterol* 92:739, 1997)

1. Reconfirm diagnosis, usually relapse, not resistance
2. Decrease diarrhea-inducing medications; give supportive care
3. If diagnosis reconfirmed, give standard course of metronidazole or vancomycin PO as recommended
4. Avoid antibiotics if possible for the next 2 months
5. For repeated episodes:
   - Oral metronidazole or vancomycin
   - Specific therapy with above drugs for 1–2 months every other day, every week, or with taper, or therapy with cholestyramine or colestipol
   - Oral vancomycin with rifampin
   - Oral yogurt, *Lactobacillus* preparations
   - *Saccharomyces boulardii* (500 mg PO bid) × 1 month (for immunocompetent patients, may begin 4 days before antibiotics course completed)
   - IVIG for immunodeficiency

CONSTIPATION

Fast Facts

- "Constipation" means many things to many people
- Medical definition: <2 bowel movements/week or excessive difficulty straining at defecation

Evaluation

- Check stool for occult blood, CBC, electrolytes, thyroid function tests, calcium
- Check medication list: opiates, aluminum, iron, calcium channel blockers, anticholinergics, anticonvulsants

Management

Chronic Constipation

- Dietary modifications: fiber
- Docusate sodium (Colace), 250 mg PO bid (softener, large sodium load)
- Psyllium (Metamucil), 7 g PO tid (bulk)

Acute Constipation

- Rule of thumb: Begin with "afterload" before "preload" or "inotropy":

Afterload	Preload	Inotropy
Bisacodyl (Dulcolax) tablets, 10–15 mg PO/suppository 10 mg PR qd	Milk of magnesia, 30 ml PO qhs (not in impacted patients)	Magnesium citrate, 18 g/10 oz PO qd (**not in patients with renal failure**)
Bisacodyl (Fleets) enema, 500 ml PO until clear (alternatives: soap suds, tap water, mineral oil)		Senna, 25–50 mg PO qd
		Misoprostol, 0.2 mg PO qid

- Alternatives:
  Lactulose, 30 ml PO q6–8h
  Sorbitol, 25 ml of 75% solution PO tid
  GoLYTELY, up to 4 liters over 3 hours (chilled)
  Disimpaction

GASTROENTEROLOGY

PANCREATITIS (N Engl J Med 330:1198, 1994)

Etiology
- Gallstones (45%)
- Alcohol (35%)
- Idiopathic (10%)
- Drugs, trauma, infection (virus, TB)
- Hypertriglyceridemia, hypercalcemia
- Cancer

Evaluation
- Serum markers: amylase (peaks at 20–30 hours); lipase (peaks at 24 hours)
- Ranson's prognostic criteria (number of criteria predictive of mortality):

Admission criteria	Initial 48 hours criteria	Mortality
Age >55 years	Drop in Hct >10%	<3 criteria→1%
WBC >16,000/µl	BUN increase >5 mg/dl	3–4→15%
Glucose >200 mg/dl	Ca^{+2} <8 mg/dl	5–6→40%
LDH >350 IU/liter	PaO$_2$ <60 mm Hg	>7→100%
AST >250 IU/liter	Base deficit >4 mg/dl	
	Fluid sequestered >6 liters	

- Abdominal CT: Pancreatic protocol (*Radiology*, 174:331, 1990): assess pancreatic necrosis

Stage	Description	Mortality
A	Normal appearance	Minimal
B	Enlargement of pancreas	Minimal
C	Peripancreatic inflammation	Minimal
D	Single, ill-defined fluid collection (phlegmon)	30–50% infection rate, need CT-guided aspiration for diagnosis; 8% mortality
E	≥2 poorly defined fluid collections or gas in or adjacent to pancreas	30–50% infection rate, need CT-guided aspiration for diagnosis; 17% mortality

Management
- Hydration with normal saline, "bowel rest" with NPO, TPN via central line, pain control [meperidine HCl (Demerol)], frequent laboratory draws for Hct, calcium, glucose, renal function, LDH; rule out infection, hold antibiotics

Complications
- Sepsis is most common cause of death (70–80%)
- Phlegmon: may become infected leading to abscess (10%)
- Pseudocyst: complicated by pain, rupture (mortality 14%), hemorrhage (60%), abscess
- Pancreatic ascites
- Abscess (100% mortality if undrained)

CIRRHOSIS AND CHRONIC HEPATITIS
Child's Criteria for Cirrhosis

Criteria	A (minimal)	B (moderate)	C (advanced)
Bilirubin	<2 mg/dl	2–3 mg/dl	>3 mg/dl
Albumin	>3.5 mg/dl	3–3.5 mg/dl	<3 mg/dl
Ascites	None	Easily controlled	Poor control
Mental status changes/ encephalopathy	None	Minimal	Advanced/coma
Nutrition	Excellent	Good	Poor/wasting
Mortality (30 days)	<2%	20%	50%

Ascites   (*Arch Intern Med* 146:2259, 1986; *Arch Intern Med* 117:215, 1966; *N Engl J Med* 330:337, 1994)

Fast Facts
- 50% of patients with cirrhosis develop ascites within 10 years
- 50% of patients with cirrhotic ascites live 2 years

Physical Examination
- Shifting dullness (88% sensitivity, 56% specificity)
- Fluid wave (53% sensitivity, 90% specificity)
- Abdominal distention (72% sensitivity, 65% specificity)
- Bulging flanks (72% sensitivity, 70% specificity)

Diagnostic Studies
Ultrasound
- Minimal detection 100 ml; rule out hepatoma; portal vein thrombosis
- May require ultrasound-guided paracentesis if small volume of fluid

Paracentesis
- Indicated in new-onset ascites
- Therapeutic due to distention, pulmonary compromise
- Deterioration after hospital admission or hypotension
- Send fluid for CBC/differential, ascitic fluid albumin (with simultaneous serum albumin), culture, total protein
- Optional: glucose, LDH, amylase, Gram's stain; unusual: acid-fast bacilli, cytology
- Serum-ascites albumin gradient = serum albumin – ascitic albumin

Wide (>1.1)	Narrow (<1.1)
Chronic liver disease	Peritoneal cancer
Hepatic metastasis	Peritoneal inflammation
Veno-occlusive disease	TB, fungal
Budd-Chiari	Serositis
Cardiac failure	Viscus leak: pancreatic, bilious, chylous, ureteric
Spontaneous bacterial peritonitis	Nephrotic syndrome
Myxedema	Protein-losing enteropathy
	Idiopathic

GASTROENTEROLOGY

Management
- **Bed rest** (50% resolution of ascites)
- **Low-sodium diet,** 44–88 mEq/day (2 g), fluid restriction (if ↓Na$^+$)
- **Paracentesis** for shortness of breath, tense ascites, early satiety
- **Diuretics:** Start furosemide (Lasix) (40 mg/day) and spironolactone (Aldactone) (100 mg/day)
- If without weight loss and/or urinary sodium <20 mEq/day ↑furosemide by 40 mg and ↑spironolactone by 100 mg (repeat until 160 mg/day furosemide and 400 mg/day spironolactone)
- Stop diuretics in patients with renal dysfunction, hepatic encephalopathy, or no weight loss despite maximum dosing
- Consider **shunt/**transjugular intrahepatic porta-systemic shunt/transplant if there is no adequate response despite maximum diuretics

Hepatic Encephalopathy

Fast Facts
- Ammonia is the most readily identified toxin, but ammonia level is not correlative with symptoms
- Brought on by alkalosis, potassium deficiency, sedating drugs, systemic infection, hypovolemia, GI bleed, hepatocellular carcinoma (HCC)

Management
- Treat underlying problem: infection/sepsis/GI bleed workup; consider evaluation for HCC
- Monitor coagulants and liver function tests; low-protein diet
- Hold hepatotoxins, sedatives, diuretics
- Correct uremia, abnormal electrolytes/glucose; treat alcohol withdrawal
- Lactulose, 30–50 ml q2–6h until diarrhea, then titrate to 2–4 soft stools qd (comatose: 300 ml in 700 ml normal saline retention enemas for 30 minutes q4h)
- Neomycin, 1–2 g PO qid, ?metronidazole

Spontaneous Bacterial Peritonitis (SBP) *(Clin Infect Dis* 24:1035, 1997)

Fast Fact

- In patients with cirrhosis, onset is insidious, with fever, hepatic encephalopathy, possible tenderness, hypoactive bowel sounds, vomiting

Diagnosis

- Bedside paracentesis and inoculation of blood culture bottles with ascitic fluid at the bedside
- Typical findings: WBC >500, PMN >250, and protein <1 g/dl (if clinically indicated)
- Bacteremia in 75% with aerobic SBP, rare with anaerobic; also check fungal, acid-fast bacilli

Etiologic Agents

- *E. coli*
- *Klebsiella*
- *Streptococcus pneumoniae*

Management

Empiric

- Cefotaxime, 2 g q8–12h × 5 days
- Clinical improvement should occur in 24–48 hours

Prophylaxis

For high-risk patients, protein <1 g/dl

- Ciprofloxacin, 750 mg/week
- Trimethoprim/sulfamethoxazole: 1 double-strength tablet 5×/week

GASTROENTEROLOGY

ACUTE HEPATITIS
Hepatitis B

Interpretation	HbsAg	Anti-HBs	Anti-HBc	HBeAg	Anti-HBe
Acute HBV	+	−	IgM	+	−
Chronic HBV (active viral replication)	+	−	IgG	+	−
Chronic HBV (low viral replication)	+	−	IgG	−	+
Chronic HBV (heterotypic anti-HBs)	+	+	IgG	±	±
Recovery from HBV (immunity)	−	+	IgG	−	±
Vaccination (immunity)	−	+	−	−	−
False-positive/ remote HBV	−	−	IgG	−	−

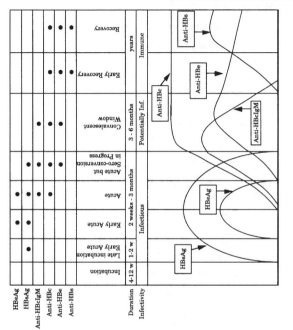

Courtesy of Abbott Laboratories

GASTROENTEROLOGY

Hepatitis C *(Clin Infect Dis* 20:1361, 1995)

Transmission (Most Common to Least Common)
- Unidentified route
- Parenteral transmission
- Sexual transmission
- Needle-stick

Symptoms
- Incubation: 6–7 weeks
- 20–30% have symptoms
- Most common symptom: jaundice (50%)
- Leading indication for liver transplantation is ultrasonography

Time Course
- Chronic hepatitis (10 years)
- Cirrhosis 20–30% (21 years)
- ↑Risk of hepatocellular carcinoma (29 years)

Diagnosis
- HCV antibody: initial screen
- HCV RNA if antibody positive
  ↑ALT in chronic hepatitis
  Normal ALT in carrier
- HCV antibody positive but HCV RNA negative = prior acute HCV
- Liver biopsy for those considering therapy with interferon (IFN)

Treatment: IFN-α and Ribavarin *(N Engl J Med* 339:1485, 1998)

- ≤75 kg: IFN-α 3 million IU three times/week SQ, and ribavirin, 400 mg PO every morning, 600 mg PO every evening; >75 kg: IFN-α 3 million IU three times/week SQ, and ribavirin 600 mg PO bid; goal is 24–48 weeks of therapy (improved virologic: 31–38% vs. 13%; biochemical: 26–34% vs. 5–12%; and histologic: 57–61% vs. 41–44% response over treatment with IFN alone).
- Pregnancy absolutely contraindicated during use and for 6 months after treatment.
- Reversible hemolytic anemia increased with ribavirin use; check Hgb at weeks and 4 and as clinically indicated during treatment; if Hgb <10, discontinue or reduce dose (reduction leads to 1–1.5 g/dl increase in Hgb)
- Careful screening of all possible patients; can exacerbate depression

FULMINANT HEPATIC FAILURE

Definition

- Liver failure without history of liver disease and leading to encephalopathy within 8 weeks of diagnosis. Transaminitis/hyperbilirubinemia/coagulopathy.

Etiology

- Viral: 75% cases [HBV (many with D) = 50% >non-A, non-B >HAV >HCV], HSV, mononucleosis, cytomegalovirus
- Toxin: Bacterial, cereolysin (*Bacillus cereus*), aflatoxin, mushroom
- Drugs: Acetaminophen, carbon tetrachloride, halothane, phenytoin, AZT, keto-conazole, gold, valproate, isoniazid
- Autoimmune (anti–smooth muscle antibody)
- Neoplastic
- Genetic: Wilson's disease (Kayser-Fleischer rings, 24-hour urine copper, serum ceruloplasmin); α_1-antitrypsin deficiency (pulmonary); hemochromatosis (iron)
- Other: Primary biliary cirrhosis (antimitochondrial antibody), veno-occlusive disease, Budd-Chiari syndrome, Reye's syndrome

Evaluation

- Splenomegaly, intravascular hemolysis, AST >ALT, low-alkaline phosphatase: bilirubin ratio, CNS

Management

Encephalopathy

- Prognosis is poor if onset of encephalopathy within 7 days of hyperbilirubinemia
- Reduce protein in diet, lactulose (not known to be effective but can be tried)

Cerebral Edema

- Most common cause of death in fulminant hepatic failure
- Occurs in >75% of patients with grade 4 encephalopathy
- Hypertension, hyperventilation, abnormal pupillary reflexes, rigidity, decerebrate
- Treat by decreased tactile stimulation, raise head of bed, avoid hypotension, hypoxia, hypercarbia
- Treat with mannitol, hyperventilation, intubation

Renal Failure

- Early with acetaminophen overdose, later with other etiologies

Metabolic Disorders

- Hypoglycemia: D10 drip
- Acidosis (especially in acetaminophen)

Coagulopathy

- Usually GI bleed; prophylax with H_2-blocker
- Transfuse fresh-frozen plasma if needed

Sepsis

- Common with bacterial and fungal fulminant hepatic failure (80% in patients with coma)
- Treat fevers empirically

5. Hematology

PERIPHERAL BLOOD SMEAR

Red cell variant	Major clinical associations
Acanthocyte	Abetalipoproteinemia, alcoholic cirrhosis (with hemolysis)
Basophilic stippling	Lead poisoning, thalassemia, hemolysis, myelodysplastic syndrome
Blister cells	Disseminated intravascular coagulation, microangiopathic hemolytic anemia, hemolysis, sickle cell, drug-induced hemolysis
Burr cell	Uremia, gastric ulcer/cancer, renal disease
Elliptocyte	Normal (few), hereditary elliptocytosis, iron-deficiency anemia
Heinz bodies	Drug-induced oxidative hemolysis
Howell-Jolly bodies	Hemolytic anemias, hyposplenism, megaloblastic anemia, thalassemia
Macro-ovalocyte	Megaloblastic anemia, myeloproliferative disease, MDS
Nucleated RBCs, reticulocytes	Increased erythropoiesis
Poikilocyte (teardrop)	Myelophthisic states
Pappenheimer bodies (siderocytes)	Sideroblastic anemia, lead poisoning, thalassemia
Parasites	Malaria, *Bartonella*
Rouleaux of RBCs	Increased plasma protein
Schistocytes	Disseminated intravascular coagulation, microangiopathic hemolytic anemia, hemolysis, cardiac valve replacement, severe burns, uremia
Sickle cell	Sickle cell disease and variants
Spherocyte	Hereditary spherocytosis, immune and other hemolytic anemias
Stomatocyte	Hereditary stomatocytosis, alcoholism
Target cell	Hemoglobinopathies, iron deficiency, liver disease

RED BLOOD CELL INDICES

Hemoglobin (Hgb)

- Determined by converting Hgb→methemoglobin→cyanmethemoglobin
- Sources of error: variation in volume, insoluble abnormal hemoglobins
- Normal (g/dl): males (14–18), females (12–16)

Hematocrit (Hct) (Packed Cell Volume)

- Determined by centrifugation of blood in heparinized capillary tube
- Can be electronically calculated with mean cell volume (MCV) and RBC count
- Sources of error: variation in volume, inadequate mixing or centrifugation
- Normal (%): males (0.41–0.51), females (0.37–0.47)
- Hct ≈ Hgb × 3

Red Blood Cell Count

- Determined by electronic particle counting
- Normal ($\times 10^{12}$/liter): males (4.4–6.0), females (4.2–5.5)

Mean Corpuscular Volume (MCV)

- Essential for classification of anemia
- (Hct × 1,000) ÷ RBC count
- Normal (femtoliters/cell): 82–101

Red Cell Distribution Width (RDW)

- In combination with MCV can help distinguish between iron deficiency and anemia of chronic disease
- (Standard deviation of RBC size) ÷ MCV
- Normal (%): 11.5–14.5

Mean Cell Hemoglobin (MCH)

- May be used in distinguishing between anemias, but limited value
- (Hgb × 10) ÷ RBC count
- Normal (pg/cell): 27–34

Mean Cell Hemoglobin Concentration (MCHC)

- Used to test lab quality control
- Hgb ÷ Hct
- Normal (g/dl): 31.5–36.0

Reticulocyte Count

- Indicator of bone marrow erythroid activity
- Normal: 0.5–1.5%; not accurate in anemia, so use index

Reticulocyte Index

$$\text{Reticulocyte index} = \text{Reticulocyte count} \times \frac{\text{Hct (measured)}}{45\% \text{ (normal Hct)}} \quad \text{(normal} <2)$$

HEMATOLOGY

HEMATOLOGY COAGULATION TESTS

Prothrombin Time (PT)
- Tests extrinsic/common pathway
- Add calcium + tissue factor + phospholipid to platelet-poor plasma

Partial Thromboplastin Time (PTT)
- Tests intrinsic/common pathway
- Add partial thromboplastin, an inactivating agent, and calcium chloride to plasma

Thrombin Time (TT)
- Tests common pathway (conversion of fibrinogen→fibrin affected by heparin)
- Add thrombin to plasma (fibrinogen) forms fibrin

Reptilase Time (RT)
- Also tests common pathway but test not affected by heparin
- ↑Thrombin time and normal RT = heparin present

Mixing Study
- Used in evaluation of prolonged coagulation times
- Add normal plasma to patient's plasma (50:50)
- If problem corrects→factor deficiency (VIII, IX, XI, VII, high molecular weight kinogen)
- Otherwise, √ for inhibitor:
    Specific versus antiphospholipids/lupus anticoagulant
    Prolonged Russell viper venom time (X→Xa): indicates lupus anticoagulant

Bleeding Time
- Primarily indicates problem with platelet function and vascular function
- Blood-letting technique (earlobe/finger): √ time to stop bleeding
- Very operator dependent

COAGULATION CASCADE [Reproduced with permission from DC Dale, DD Federman (eds). *Scientific American Medicine*. VI. Disorders of Hemostasis and Coagulation. New York: Scientific American, 1996.]

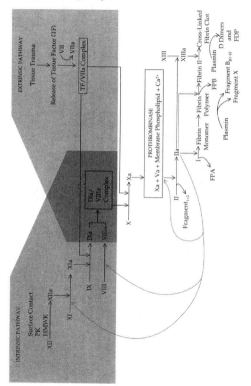

HEMATOLOGY

HEPARIN SLIDING SCALE   (*Ann Intern Med* 119:874, 1993; Stanford Medical Center Hematology/Anticoagulation Guidelines)

- Heparin (by weight) nomogram: bolus 80 units/kg IV, then 15 units/kg/hour IV gtt
- Empirically: bolus 5,000 units IV, then 1,000 units/hour; √ partial thromboplastin time in 6 hours to titrate

Stanford Protocol

Activated partial thromboplastin time	Action	Rate change	Recheck
<40	Bolus 5,000 U	↑200 units/hour	6 hours
40–54	—	↑100 units/hour	6 hours
55–95	—	—	Next A.M.
96–120	Hold 30 minutes	↓100 units/hour	6 hours
>120	Hold 1 hour	↓200 units/hour	6 hours

LOW-MOLECULAR-WEIGHT HEPARIN (LMWH)[a]   (*Chest* 115:1419, 1999)

Indication	Dose	Duration
Hip replacement surgery	Enox, 30 mg q12h or 40 mg qd	First dose 12–24 hrs postop if no significant bleeding; treat 7–10 days
Extended hip prophylaxis	Enox, 40 mg qd	For an additional 3 wks after above
Knee replacement surgery	Enox, 30 mg q12h; or ardeparin, 50 U/kg q12h	(As with hip replacement)
General surgery	Enox, 40 mg qd; or dalteparin, 2,500 U qd; or dalteparin 5,000 U qd	First dose 2 hrs preop; second dose after 24 hrs if no significant bleeding; treat 7–10 days
Unstable angina/non–Q wave MI	Enox, 1 mg/kg q12h (plus ASA)	Treat for a minimum of 2 days, until clinically stable (2–8 days usually); if cathetered, leave sheath in place 6–8 hrs and do not give enox for 6–8 hrs post–sheath removal
DVT	Enox, 1 mg/kg q12h (while starting warfarin[b])	Continue treatment until stable, appropriate INR reached; usually 3–5 days overlap (in some patients hospitalization unnecessary)
DVT ± PE	Enox, 1 mg/kg q12h; or enox, 1.5 mg/kg q24h (while starting warfarin[b])	q24h regimen approved by FDA only for inpatients

Enox = enoxaparin.
[a]FDA approval for LMWH is only for subcutaneous administration.
[b]See warfarin algorithm (p. 116).

Considerations in Using LMHW

Outpatient Treatment

In patients without significant comorbidity or hemodynamic instability:

• No need to check PTT or anti–factor Xa level except as below
• Start warfarin the evening of first dose of LMWH

Inpatient Treatment

• Consider inpatient use, or standard IV heparin in patient with significant comorbidities
• Comorbid conditions or poor support system may affect ability to care for self and administer treatment
• Comorbid conditions may complicate treatment: Enoxaparin clearance decreased with renal failure; monitor anti-Xa levels (therapeutic level 0.5–1.2) if Cr >2; morbid obesity: initial dose as usual but adjust per anti-Xa levels
• Consider conversion to outpatient LMWH use when patient is stabilized; remember to initiate patient teaching re: injection.
• Decreased incidence of heparin-induced thrombocytopenia vs. unfractionated heparin, but may cross-react
• Safety in pregnancy not fully established, but off-label use common

HEMATOLOGY

WARFARIN (Stanford Medical Center Hematology/Anticoagulation Guidelines)

Warfarin Sodium (Coumadin) Dosing Algorithm

(for patients with a target INR of 2–3)[a,b] (*Ann Intern Med* 126:133, 1997; *Ann Intern Med* 127:332, 1997)

Day	INR	Warfarin sodium dosage
1		5 mg
2	<1.5	5
	1.5–1.9	2.5
	2.0–2.5	1.0–2.5
	>2.5	0
3	<1.5	5–10
	1.5–1.9	2.5–5.0
	2.0–2.5	0–2.5
	2.5–3.0	0–2.5
	>3.0	0
4	<1.5	10
	1.5–1.9	5.0–7.5
	2.0–3.0	0–5.0
	>3.0	0
5	<1.5	10
	1.5–1.9	7.5–10
	2–3	0–5
	>3	0
6	<1.5	7.5–12.5
	1.5–1.9	5–10
	2–3	0–7.5
	>3.0	0

[a]After day 4, check PT/INR at least once a week, and adjust warfarin sodium to maintain INR 2–3 until stable.
[b]Only indication for anticoagulation beyond 2–3 is mechanical prosthetic valve (2.5–3.5).
Source: Reproduced with permission from W Camahan, J Bracikowski. Warfarin: less may be better. *Ann Intern Med* 127:332, 1997.

Reversal of Warfarin Sodium with Vitamin K and Fresh Frozen Plasma (*Ann Intern Med* 126:959, 1997)

INR 5.0–10.0 and No Significant Bleeding

- Hold warfarin for 1–2 days and give vitamin K, 2.5 mg PO (96% had INR brought down <5 without further resistance to anticoagulation within 24–48 hours)

Fresh Frozen Plasma (FFP)

- Plasma volume approximately 40 ml/kg
  1 ml of plasma has ≈ 1%/kg unit of factor activity
  Formula for FFP needed (ml) = % activity desired (in decimal form) × (wt in kg × 40)
- Patient with an INR of 2 has approximately 15% of total activity
- Goal for reversal: ≈ 50–60% total activity
- Thus, in a 70-kg patient: plasma volume = 2,800 ml with goal of increasing activity from 15% to 50% = 0.35 × 2,800 = 960 ml of FFP needed

Drugs That Can Augment or Interfere with the Effects of Warfarin

May potentiate (strong evidence)	May potentiate (some evidence)	May inhibit
Trimethoprim-sulfamethoxazole	Ciprofloxacin	Nafcillin sodium
Erythromycin	Itraconazole	Rifampin
Isoniazid	Tetracycline hydrochloride	Griseofulvin
Fluconazole	Quinidine	Cholestyramine
Miconazole nitrate	Simvastatin	Barbiturates
Metronidazole	Acetylsalicylic acid	Carbamazepine
Amiodarone	Acetaminophen	Chlordiazepoxide
Propafenone hydrochloride	Tamoxifen	Sucralfate
Propranolol	Influenza vaccines	Enteral feeds with high vitamin K content
Phenylbutazone		
Piroxicam		
Cimetidine		
Omeprazole		

HEMATOLOGY

HYPERCOAGULABLE STATES
Evaluation
- Start evaluation before anticoagulation
  Evaluation may be tailored to suspicion
- If on heparin, do not send antithrombin III or lupus anticoagulant screen
- If on warfarin sodium, do not send protein C or S

Hypercoagulable state	Screening test	Prevalence
Natural anticoagulants		
Protein C deficiency	Protein C activity	2%
Protein S deficiency	Protein S activity	2%
Activated protein C resistant (factor V Leiden)	Factor V Leiden DNA assay	20%
Antithrombin deficiency	Antithrombin III activity	3–5%
Prothrombin gene mutation 20210		
Fibrinolysis	Suspect if euglobulin lysis time abnormal	5–15%
Plasminogen deficiency	Plasminogen activity	
Poor tissue plasminogen activator release		
Excessive plasminogen activator inhibitor	Plasminogen activator inhibitor activity	
Dysfibrinogenemia		
Antiphospholipid-antibodies		10–20%
Lupus anticoagulant	Activated partial thromboplastin time, Russell viper venom	
Anticardiolipin antibody	Anticardiolipin antibody titers	
Hyperhomocysteinemia	Serum homocysteine	
	Methionine load	
Malignancy/myeloproliferation disorder	Age-appropriate cancer screening	
Systemic disorders		
Nephrotic syndrome	Urinalysis, 24-hour urinary protein excretion	
Vasculitis	ESR, vasculitis workup	

EVALUATION OF A BLEEDING PATIENT

Basic Screening Lab Tests

- CBC
- Peripheral smear
- Prothrombin time
- Activated partial thromboplastin time
- Thrombin time

Prolonged Thrombin Time

- Heparin
- Hypo/dysfibrinogenemia
- Heparin-like inhibitor
- Fibrin split products (e.g., DIC)
- Paraprotein myeloma
- Thrombin antibody
- Rule out heparin effect: √ RT; ↑PTT, ↑TT and normal RT = heparin effect
- Rule out DIC: √ fibrinogen and D-dimer
- Consider immunologic fibrinogen level
- Consider mixing study to rule out inhibitor

Prolonged Prothrombin Time, Normal Thrombin Time

- Liver disease
- Warfarin sodium
- Early vitamin K deficiency
- Factor VII deficiency

Prolonged Partial Thromboplastin Time, Normal Thrombin Time, Normal Prothrombin Time

- VIII deficiency (hemophilia A or von Willebrand's)
- IX deficiency (hemophilia B)
- Von Willebrand's disease
- Acquired inhibitor of VIII (bleeding)
- Lupus anticoagulant (no bleeding)
- Other deficiencies of XI, XII, prekallikrein, or HMWK
- √ mixing study; if no correction, acquired inhibitor or lupus anticoagulant

Prolonged Prothrombin Time and Prolonged Partial Thromboplastin Time

- Dysfibrinogenemias
- Vitamin K deficiency
- Lupus anticoagulants
- Massive transfusion
- Warfarin sodium
- Moderate to severe liver disease
- Disseminated intravascular coagulation
- Factors X, V, II deficiency
- Plasmapheresis without fresh frozen plasma replacement

Normal Thrombin Time, Prothrombin Time, Partial Thromboplastin Time, Decreased Platelet Count

- Disseminated intravascular coagulation
- Drug-induced thrombocytopenia
- Aplastic anemia
- Check peripheral smear; consider bone marrow biopsy

HEMATOLOGY

ANEMIAS

Categorization by Erythrocyte Size and Reticulocyte Response

Reticulocytes	Low MCV (<83 fl)	Normal MCV (83–97 fl)	High MCV (>97 fl)
Elevated (>100 k/µl)	Thalassemia major; chronic intravascular hemolytic anemia (**paroxysmal nocturnal hemoglobinuria**); severe fragmentation hemolysis	Hemolytic anemia (intravascular and extravascular)	Hemolytic anemia (intravascular and extravascular)
Decreased or normal (<100 k/µl)	Iron-deficiency anemia; β-thalassemia minor; α-thalassemia; HbE; anemia of chronic disease; **hyperthyroidism**; sideroblastic anemia (hereditary)	Anemia of renal failure; **aplastic anemia**; anemia of chronic disease; **hyperthyroidism** and hypothyroidism; hypopituitarism; hypoadrenalism; hypogonadism; sideroblastic anemia (acquired); **myelodysplastic syndrome (MDS)**; pure red cell aplasia; **leukemia**; infiltrative disease of bone marrow; increased splenic pooling	Megaloblastic anemia; aplastic anemia; hypothyroidism; MDS; pure red cell aplasia; leukemia

Bold type = disorders in which low leukocyte count and low platelet count may coexist.
Source: Reproduced with permission from American College of Physicians, MKSAP 11: Hematology, p. 1097.

Iron Studies and Microcytic Anemias (*Am Fam Physician* 59:851, 1999)

Type	Serum iron	Total iron-binding capacity	Ferritin	Red blood cell distribution width
Iron deficiency	↓	↑	↓	↑
Anemia of chronic disease	↓	↓/Normal	↑/Normal	Normal
Thalassemia	Normal/↑	Normal	Normal/↑	Normal/↑
Sideroblastic/MDS	↑	Normal/↓	Normal/↑	Normal

ETIOLOGIES OF THROMBOCYTOPENIA

Decreased marrow production	Increased platelet destruction
Aplastic anemia	Connective tissue diseases
Congenital	Disseminated intravascular coagulation
Drugs	Drugs
Infections	Infections
Ineffective thrombocytopoiesis (e.g., folate or vitamin B_{12} deficiency, MDS)	Hypersplenism
	Idiopathic thrombocytopenic purpura
Marrow replacement (myelofibrosis, myelophthisic process)	Lymphomas and other malignancies
	Mechanical (e.g., artificial heart valve)
Radiation	Paroxysmal nocturnal hemoglobinuria
Toxins (e.g., alcohol)	Thrombotic thrombocytopenic purpura
	Post-transfusion purpura
Others: dilutional	

Source: Reprinted with permission from K Goldstein, N Abramson. Efficient diagnosis of thrombocytopenia. *Am Fam Physician* 53:916, 1996.

PANCYTOPENIA

Causes of pancytopenia	Changes in the CBC and blood smear
Impaired production	
Disorders of precursors	
Aplastic anemia	MCV may be high
MDS	MCV may be high; occasional blasts
Aleukemic leukemia	Occasional blasts
Idiopathic myelofibrosis	Leukoerythroblastosis
Infiltrative disease of bone marrow	
Cancer	Leukoerythroblastosis occasionally
Lymphoma	
Multiple myeloma	
Infection, granuloma	Leukoerythroblastosis occasionally
Exogenous factors	
Drugs or toxins	
Cobalamin or folate deficiency	High MCV, hypersegmented neutrophils
Viral infection	
Increased destruction	
Autoimmune	Reticulocytosis, anisocytosis, spherocytosis; MCV and MPV may be high
Hemophagocytic syndrome	
Paroxysmal nocturnal hemoglobinuria	Reticulocytosis; MCV may be low or high
Splenic pooling	

Source: Reproduced with permission from American College of Physicians, MKSAP 11: Hematology, p. 1419.

HEMATOLOGY

TRANSFUSIONS   (N Engl J Med 340:438, 1999)

Fast Facts

- For each 10 packed red blood cells, consider replacing fresh frozen plasma and platelets
- Replete calcium secondary to precipitation with acetate or citrate with packed red blood cells
- Risks: hemolysis, 1/250,000 to 1/2,000,000 units; HBV, 1/30,000 to 1/250,000; HCV, 1:30,000 to 1/150,000; HIV, 1/200,000 to 1/2,000,000; HTLV (I or II), 1/250,000 to 1/2,000,000.

Indications*

Packed Red Blood Cells (PRBCs)

- Hgb <9 g/dl or Hct <27% in uncompromised cardiovascular function
- Hgb <10 g/dl or Hct <30% in cardiac/septic patient

Platelets (plt)

- <5,000–10,000/mm^3 if not actively bleeding
- Prophylactically for platelet count <20,000/mm^3
- <50,000/mm^3 in bleeding/preprocedure
- <100,000/mm^3 in bleeding/procedure in high-risk site (e.g., CNS, eye) or platelet dysfunction (contraindicated in thrombotic thrombocytopenic purpura, hemolytic-uremic syndrome; relatively contraindicated in idiopathic thrombocytopenic purpura, disseminated intravascular coagulation, heparin-induced thrombocytopenia)

Cryoprecipitate (cryo)

- Bleeding/preprocedure in patient with hemophilia A, von Willebrand's disease, dysfibrinogenemia, uremia, or fibinogen <100 mg/dl

Fresh Frozen Plasma (FFP)

- Factors II, V, X, XI, XIII; protein C and/or protein S deficiency; other deficiencies INR >6–8 (INR >1.1 with bleeding or invasive procedures); thrombotic thrombocytopenic purpura and hemolytic-uremic syndrome; warfarin sodium reversal

*Reprinted with permission from Stanford University Transfusion Service guidelines.

TRANSFUSION REACTIONS (Hematol Oncol Clin North Am 9:187, 1995; J Postgrad Med 98:159, 1995)

Transfusion reaction	Etiology	Frequency (units PRBC)	Onset	Symptoms	Diagnosis	Treatment
Acute hemolytic	Incompatibility of blood groups causing acute hemolysis through complement; 83% due to ABO incompatibility	1/25,000	Early in transfusion period	Fever and chills, nausea, flushing, shortness of breath, oliguria, hypotension, hemoglobinemia, hemoglobinuria, DIC	Coombs, direct antiglobulin testing, Hgb/Hct, haptoglobin, total/direct bilirubin, LDH, renal function, coagulation	Stop transfusion; fluids and low-dose dopamine prn; treat DIC
Delayed hemolytic	Gradual immunologic destruction of sensitized donor cells, either primary immunization or secondary amnestic response with at least one antibody (i.e., Rh, Kidd, Duffy, Kell)	1/1,600	5–10 days for amnestic; several weeks for primary	Drop in post-transfusion Hct, fever and chills, mild jaundice	Coombs, direct antiglobulin testing, Hgb/Hct, total/direct bilirubin, LDH, renal function, coagulation	No treatment for mild; treat anemia prn; avoid future exposure
Febrile non-hemolytic	Antibodies to donor HLA antigens or granulocyte-specific antibodies	1/100	<2 hrs of transfusion completion	↑In temp of ≥1°C; sometimes chills, nausea and vomiting, headache, back pain	Coombs, direct antiglobulin testing, Hgb/Hct	Discontinue; rule out acute hemolytic reaction; acetaminophen for fever; hydrocortisone (100 mg); Demerol for chills; use leuko-poor/washed RBCs
Allergic	Recipient antibodies to donor plasma proteins	Urticaria: 1/1,000; anaphylaxis: 1/20,000 to 1/300,000	Early in transfusion period	Urticaria, itch, headache, nausea and vomiting, shortness of breath, wheeze, anxiety, ↓BP, no fever	If anaphylactic, consider test for IgA deficiency	If mild, discontinue; give diphenhydramine and may resume; if anaphylaxis, discontinue, give epinephrine, steroids; wash next blood and avoid FFP
Acute lung injury	Unclear	1/10,000	2–4 hrs after	PE, respiratory failure	Chest x-ray	Stop transfusion; oxygen/ventilator support; consider diuretics, steroids

PRBC = packed red blood cells; LDH = lactate dehydrogenase; DIC = disseminated intravascular coagulation; FFP = fresh frozen plasma; PE = pulmonary edema.

HEMATOLOGY

THROMBOTIC THROMBOCYTOPENIC PURPURA (TTP)/ HEMOLYTIC UREMIC SYNDROME (HUS)   (*Lancet* 343:398, 1994; *N Engl J Med* 325:393, 1991)

TTP and HUS are now thought to be a continuum of disease.

TTP
- Classically defined as fever, fluctuating neurologic changes (twitch, coma, seizure, ataxia), renal failure, microangiopathic hemolytic anemia, thrombocytopenia
- Causes include infection, malignancy, pregnancy, drugs
- TTP is the term preferred in adults in whom neurologic symptoms predominate

HUS
- Marked by acute renal insufficiency, microangiopathic hemolytic anemia, and thrombocytopenia
- Renal biopsy shows vasculopathy with septicemia; can also have evidence of DIC and hematologic complications
- Causes include infection (especially diarrheal [*E. coli* 0157-H7, *Shigella*, HIV]), idiopathic, familial, drugs, malignancy, pregnancy, SLE
- HUS is the term preferred in children in whom renal failure predominates.
- Treat the underlying cause

Diagnosis
- Classic signs and symptoms with suggestive laboratory results
- Test for hemolysis (anemia, ↓haptoglobin, ↑indirect bilirubin, ↑LDH), ↓platelets; coags often normal (PT/PTT) unless concurrent DIC

Treatment
- Supportive: correct volume deficits with normal saline or blood products (RBCs, FFP as needed; platelets may worsen prognosis and ischemia); monitor renal function (consider hydration, diuresis, dialysis); treat hypertensive complications
- Plasma exchange with FFP for 5 days or for 2 days after the platelet count normalizes and symptoms resolve
- For TTP, improved outcome seen with steroids (methylprednisolone, 200 mg IV qd); consider antiplatelet therapy (ASA)
- In chronic relapsing situations, consider splenectomy and immunosuppression

DISSEMINATED INTRAVASCULAR COAGULATION (DIC)

(N Engl J Med 341:586, 1999)

- Consumptive coagulopathy
- Suspect in critically ill patients or those with predisposing conditions with bleeding and clotting abnormalities
- Predisposing conditions: sepsis, trauma, liver disease, malignancy (especially acute promyelocytic leukemia), toxin, TTP-HUS

Diagnosis

- Lab values in a patient with predisposing condition
- ↑PT/PTT, ↓fibrinogen (may be normal early or elevated as an acute phase reactant), ↓platelets (<100,000), ↑D-dimers (fibrin degradation products), ↓AT III

Treatment

- Treat the underlying cause
- Supportive:
    FFP to correct ↑PT/PTT if patient is bleeding or preprocedure
    Cryoprecipitate if fibrinogen <100
    Platelets if <20,000 and bleeding
    Heparin is controversial; consider low dose (300–500 U/hr IV)
    Consider AT III replacement in severe cases

6. Oncology

EVALUATION OF THE CANCER PATIENT
Fast Facts
- First priority is to define the extent of disease and prognosis.
- Biopsy for grading and staging: **Tissue is the issue.**

Physical Performance Scales
- Major determinant in treatment outcome, with Karnofsky status <70 having a poorer diagnosis

Physical condition	Karnofsky scale	Zubrod scale (ECOG)
No complaints or evidence of illness	100	0
Normal activities, minor symptoms	90	1 (symptoms)
Some symptoms on exertion	80	
Self-care, unable to engage in normal activity or do active work	70	2 (symptoms, <50% time in bed)
Occasional assistance, mostly self-care	60	
Considerable assistance, frequent medical care	50	3 (in bed >50% time)
Handicapped, specialized nursing	40	
Severely disabled, admission indicated	30	4 (bedridden, hospital)
Very ill, active supportive treatment	20	
Moribund	10	
Dead	0	

Mouth Care
- Stanford mouthwash (tetracycline + nystatin + hydrocortisone + chlorpheniramine), swish and swallow qid
- Thrush: **Prophylaxis:** nystatin suspension 5–10 ml swish and swallow qid; clotrimazole (Mycelex) troches, 10 mg, 5 × per day; **treatment:** fluconazole, 100 mg PO qd
- Herpes simplex: Acyclovir, 800 mg PO, 5 × per day
- Xerostomia: Viscous lidocaine 1% or dyclonine 1%, 5–10 ml swish and swallow q2–4 h

Growth Factors
- G-CSF (filgrastim), 5 µg/kg SC/IV qd (round to ampule size, 240, 300, 480 µg)
- GM-CSF (sargramostim), 250 µg/m^2 SC qd
- Erythropoietin (epoetin alfa), 50–100 units/kg SC three times per week
- Thrombopoietin (experimental): Rarely used

Clotted Hickman Catheter Protocol
- Urokinase 5,000 units each lumen × 30 minutes, then aspirate; repeat with 10,000 if unsuccessful

126

TUMOR MARKERS

Tumor marker	Cancer	Non-neoplastic conditions
β-hCG	Gestational trophoblastic disease, gonadal germ cell tumor	Pregnancy
Calcitonin	Medullary thyroid cancer	
Catecholamines	Pheochromocytoma	
α-Fetoprotein	Hepatocellular carcinoma, gonadal germ cell tumor	Cirrhosis, hepatitis
Carcinoembryonic antigen	Adenocarcinomas (colon, pancreas, lung, breast, ovary)	Pancreatitis, hepatitis, smoking, inflammatory bowel
Prostatic acid phosphatase, prostate-specific antigen	Prostate cancer	Prostatitis, prostatic hypertrophy
Neuron-specific enolase	Small-cell lung carcinoma, neuroblastoma	
Monoclonal immunoglobulin, β_2-microglobulin	Myeloma	Infection, monoclonal gammopathy of undetermined significance
CA-125	Ovarian cancer, lymphoma	Menstruation, peritonitis, pregnancy
CA 19-9	Colon, pancreatic, breast cancer	Pancreatitis, ulcerative colitis
CD30	Hodgkin's disease, anaplastic large-cell lymphoma	
CD25	Hairy cell leukemia, adult T-cell leukemia/lymphoma	
HER-2/neu	Breast cancer (poor prognosis)	

Source: Reprinted with permission from Longo DL. Approach to the Patient with Cancer. In AS Fauci et al. (eds), *Harrison's Principles of Internal Medicine* (14th ed). New York: McGraw-Hill, 1998;497.

METASTASIS

	Thyroid	Lung	Breast	Stomach	Colon	Pancreas	Biliary	Kidney	Bladder	Prostate	Testis	Sarcoma	Uterus/cervix	Melanoma	Lymphoma
Brain	1+	3+	2+	1+	1+	1+	—	1+	—	—	—	1+	—	2+	1+
Lung	1+	1+	3+	1+	1+	1+	1+	2+	1+	1+	2+	—	1+	2+	—
Pleura	—	2+	3+	—	1+	—	—	—	—	—	—	—	—	1+	2+
Liver	1+	1+	2+	2+	3+	2+	3+	1+	—	—	—	—	2+	2+	1+
Bone	2+	2+	3+	1+	1+	—	—	1+	2+	3+	—	1+	1+	1+	—

Reprinted with permission from M von Planta (ed). *Memorix Innere Medizin* (4th ed). © Chapman & Hall, Weinheim 1996; Hippokrates Verlag Stuttgart 1999.

SIDE EFFECTS OF CHEMOTHERAPY

Class	Generic name	Abbreviations	Elimination L Liver / K Kidney	Toxicity Leuco-cytes	Platelets	Nausea/ vomiting	Hair loss	Other organs
Alkylating agents	Busulphan	BSF/BUS	L	++	++	+		Pulmonary fibrosis
	BCNU (carmustine)	BCNU	L	+++	+++	++	+	Pulmonary fibrosis
	CCNU (lomustine)	CCNU	L	+++	+++	++		
	Chlorambucil	CLB		(+)	(+)	+		
	Cisplatin	CDDP	L/K	(+)	(+)	+++	++	Nephro-/ototoxic
	Carboplatin	CBCDA		+++	+++	++	++	
	Cyclophosphamide	CMP/CTX	L	++	++	++	++	Cystitis
	Melphalan	MEL	L	++	+++	+		
	Thiotepa	TTP		+++	+++	+	+	
Antimeta-bolites	Cytarabine	ARA-C	L	+	+	++	++	Diarrhoea, stomatitis
	Fluorouracil	FU	L	++	+	+		
	Mercaptopurine	MP	L	+	+	+		Hepatotoxic
	Methotrexate	MTX	K	++	+	+		Mouth ulcers, neuro-/hepatotoxic
	Thioguanine	TG	L	++	++	+		
Alkaloids	Vinblastine	VLB	L	++	++	(+)	(+)	
	Vincristine	VCR	L	(+)	(+)		++	Neurotoxic, paralytic ileus
	Vindesine	VDS						
	Etoposide	VP 16	L/K	+	-	++	++	Neurotoxic
Antibiotics	Actinomycin	AC	L/K	++	++	++	++	Stomatitis
	Bleomycin	BLM	K	(+)	(+)	(+)	(+)	Pulmonary fibrosis
	Doxorubicin	ADM	L	+++	+++	+++	+++	Cardiotoxic
	Mitozandrone	MIT	L	++	+++	++		Cardiotoxic
	Mitomycin	MM	L	++	++	++	(+)	Nephro-/neurotoxic
Others	Asparaginase	ASP	L	+	+	+		Pancreatitis, allergy
	Dacarbazine	DIC	L	+++	++	+++		Pseudo-influenza
	Estramustine	EMP						
	Hydroxyurea	HUR		++	++	++		
	Procarbazine	PCZ	L	++	++	++		Neurotoxic

Source: Reprinted with permission from M von Planta (ed). *Memorix Innere Medizin* (4th ed). © Chapman & Hall, Weinheim 1996; Hippokrates Verlag Stuttgart 1999.

RECOMMENDED ANTIEMETICS   (S Horning. *Chemotherapy Manual*. Stanford University Medical Center, 1995)

For Highly Emetogenic Agents

- Ondansetron, 32 mg IV, with dexamethasone, 10–20 mg IV, 30 minutes before chemotherapy qd **or**
- Granisetron, 10 µg/kg IV, with dexamethasone, 10–20 mg IV, 30 minutes before chemotherapy **or**
- Ondansetron, 0.15 mg/kg IV, with dexamethasone 10–20 mg IV, 30 minutes before chemotherapy followed by ondansetron, 0.15 mg/kg q4h, for a total of three doses on each day drug is administered. With 12- to 24-hour infusion regimens, dose q6h and continue for two doses after infusion containing the agent is ended **or**
- Ondansetron, 8 mg IV, with dexamethasone, 10–20 mg IV, 30 minutes before chemotherapy followed by ondansetron, 1 mg/hour IV continuous for minimum 24 hours **or**
- Metoclopramide, 2–3 mg/kg IV, with dexamethasone, 10–20 mg IV, and diphenhydramine, 50 mg IV, 30 minutes before chemotherapy followed by metoclopramide, 2 mg/kg IV q2h, for total of three doses. Diphenhydramine, 50 mg IV q4h prn for restlessness or acute dystonic reaction

For Moderately Emetogenic Agents

- Metoclopramide, 1 mg/kg IV, with dexamethasone, 10–20 mg PO/IV, and diphenhydramine, 50 mg IV, 30 minutes before chemotherapy, followed by metoclopramide, 1 mg/kg q2h for total of three doses. Diphenhydramine, 50 mg IV q4h prn for restlessness or acute dystonic reaction **or**
- Ondansetron, 8–10 mg IV, with dexamethasone, 10–20 mg IV, 30 minutes before chemotherapy followed by ondansetron, 8 mg PO q4h × two doses

Delayed Nausea

Metoclopramide, 0.5 mg/kg PO qid × 2 days, with dexamethasone, 8 mg PO bid × 2 days, then 4 mg PO bid × 2 days. Diphenhydramine, 50 mg PO/IV q4h prn for restlessness or dystonic reaction (especially for cyclophosphamide, cisplatin, doxorubicin ≥40 mg/m2, and carboplatin). Metoclopramide with dexamethasone is more effective than ondansetron in this setting.

Ondansetron (Zofran)
Granisetron (Kytril)
Metoclopramide (Reglan)
Diphenhydramine (Benadryl)
Dexamethasone (Decadron)

Note: High-dose ondansetron and granisetron should be administered in slow IVP; low doses should be administered over 5 minutes.

ONCOLOGY

ONCOLOGIC EMERGENCIES
Tumor Lysis Syndrome   (*Semin Nephrol* 13:273, 1993)
- Massive tumor cell death from rapidly growing tumors (e.g., lymphoma) or chemo
- Diagnosis: $\uparrow$Uric acid, $\uparrow PO_4^{-3}$, $\uparrow K^+$, $\downarrow Ca^{+2}$ (arrhythmia), acute renal failure
- Treatment: allopurinol, 300 mg PO qd, $NaHCO_3$/acetazolamide, IV fluids, correct electrolytes, dialysis

Neutropenic Fever   (*N Engl J Med* 328:1323, 1993; *Clin Infect Dis* 25:551, 1997)
- Neutropenia = <500 PMNs and/or bands/mm. Fever = once >38.5°C or three times >38°C in 24 hours
- Diagnosis: pan-culture (blood, urine, sputum, wound, chest x-ray) 85% source from endogenous flora
- Treatment: **monotherapy:** ceftazidime, 2 g IV q8h, or imipenem, 10 mg/kg q6–8h; **two-drug:** gentamicin, 5 mg/kg IV qd, plus ticarcillin/clavulanic acid, 3.1 g IV q6h, **or** piper-acillin/tazobactam, 4.5 g IV q6h; **for line infection** add vancomycin, 1 g IV q12h; add: vancomycin (48–72 hours) and amphotericin B (4–7 days) if no improvement

Spinal Cord Compression   (*N Engl J Med* 327:614, 1992; *Ann Intern Med* 131:37, 1999)
- Symptoms: >95% with progressive central or radicular back pain (sensory → motor → saddle anesthesia, bowel/bladder dysfunction, lumbosacral dermatomal paresthesia)
- Diagnosis: plain film, MRI (?vertebral collapse, osteolytic lesion, pedicle erosion, mass)
- Treatment: STAT radiology-oncology (for emergent radiotherapy) and neuro-surgical consultation; dexamethasone, 10-mg IV load, then 4 mg IV q6h (controversial use of high dose, 100 mg IV)

Superior Vena Cava Syndrome   (*Arch Intern Med* 153:384, 1993)
- Symptoms: headache, visual changes, changed mental status, pleural effusion, head/neck edema, venous engorgement, dyspnea, cough, chest pain, dysphagia, $\downarrow$cardiac output (squamous/small-cell carcinoma, lymphoma)
- Diagnosis: Chest x-ray with distended azygos, mediastinal mass; chest CT with engorged vessels
- Treatment: elevate head, O_2, dexamethasone, 6–10 mg IV q6h, STAT radiology-oncology consultation for radiotherapy, consider possible localized thrombolytic infusion as last resort

Pericardial Effusion and Tamponade   (*JAMA* 272:59, 1994)
- Encasement of the heart by tumor, malignant effusion, or pericarditis → $\downarrow$diastolic filling
- Symptoms: Beck's triad ($\downarrow$BP, $\downarrow$heart sounds, $\uparrow$jugular venous distention), cyanosis, $\uparrow$heart rate, $\uparrow$jugular venous distention, pulsus paradoxus, hepatomegaly, friction rub, dyspnea, chest pain, cough, epigastric pain, hiccups
- Diagnosis: STAT echo (diastolic RV collapse), chest x-ray with globular heart, non-specific ST-T wave changes, low voltage in ECG, electrical alternans
- Treatment: echocardiographically guided pericardiocentesis, $\sqrt{}$fluid cytology

CANCER STATISTICS

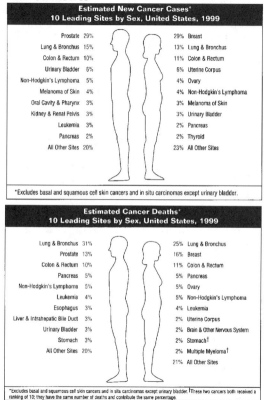

Estimated New Cancer Cases*
10 Leading Sites by Sex, United States, 1999

Prostate 29%	29% Breast
Lung & Bronchus 15%	13% Lung & Bronchus
Colon & Rectum 10%	11% Colon & Rectum
Urinary Bladder 6%	6% Uterine Corpus
Non-Hodgkin's Lymphoma 5%	4% Ovary
Melanoma of Skin 4%	4% Non-Hodgkin's Lymphoma
Oral Cavity & Pharynx 3%	3% Melanoma of Skin
Kidney & Renal Pelvis 3%	3% Urinary Bladder
Leukemia 3%	2% Pancreas
Pancreas 2%	2% Thyroid
All Other Sites 20%	23% All Other Sites

*Excludes basal and squamous cell skin cancers and in situ carcinomas except urinary bladder.

Estimated Cancer Deaths*
10 Leading Sites by Sex, United States, 1999

Lung & Bronchus 31%	25% Lung & Bronchus
Prostate 13%	16% Breast
Colon & Rectum 10%	11% Colon & Rectum
Pancreas 5%	5% Pancreas
Non-Hodgkin's Lymphoma 5%	5% Ovary
Leukemia 4%	5% Non-Hodgkin's Lymphoma
Esophagus 3%	4% Leukemia
Liver & Intrahepatic Bile Duct 3%	2% Uterine Corpus
Urinary Bladder 3%	2% Brain & Other Nervous System
Stomach 3%	2% Stomach†
All Other Sites 20%	2% Multiple Myeloma†
	21% All Other Sites

*Excludes basal and squamous cell skin cancers and in situ carcinomas except urinary bladder. †These two cancers both received a ranking of 10; they have the same number of deaths and contribute the same percentage.

Source: Reproduced with permission from SH Landis, et al. Cancer statistics 1999. *CA* 49:8, 1999.

ONCOLOGY

LH Sobin, CH Wittekind, eds. *TNM Classification of Malignant Tumors*, 5th ed. New York: Wiley, 1997.

NON–SMALL CELL LUNG CANCER: TNM CLASSIFICATION

Primary tumor (T)

T0	No evidence of primary tumor
TX	Positive cytology only or primary tumor cannot be assessed
Tis	Carcinoma in situ
T1	≤3 cm
T2	At least one of the following: • >3 cm in size • Involvement of mainstem bronchus ≥2 cm from the carina • Invasion of visceral pleura • Associated with atelectasis extending to the hilum but not involving the entire lung • Associated with atelectasis/pneumonitis extending to the hilum not involving the entire lung
T3	At least one of the following: • Extension to parietal pleura, chest wall, diaphragm, mediastinal pleura • <2 cm from but not involving the carina • Atelectasis or associated with atelectasis/pneumonitis of the entire lung
T4	Invasion of mediastinal structures, vertebral body, or carina or malignant pleural effusion

Nodal involvement (N)

NX	Regional nodes not assessed
N0	No nodal metastases
N1	Peribronchial/ipsilateral hilar nodes
N2	Ipsilateral mediastinal nodes
N3	Contralateral mediastinal or hilar nodes, or ipsilateral or contralateral supraclavicular nodes

Distant metastasis (M)

MX	Not assessed
M0	No distant metastases
M1	Distant metastases

Staging

Occult	TX, N0, M0
Stage 0	Tis, N0, M0
Stage I	T1, N0, M0
	T2, N0, M0
Stage II	T1, N1, M0
	T2, N1, M0
Stage IIIA	T1, N2, M0
Stage IIIB	Any T, N3, M0
	T4, Any N, M0
Stage IV	Any T, Any N, M1

Source: American Joint Committee on Cancer. *Manual for Staging Cancer*, 4th ed. Philadelphia: Lippincott, 1992.

BREAST CANCER: TNM CLASSIFICATION

Primary tumor (T)

T0	No evidence of primary tumor
Tis	Paget's disease of the nipple with no demonstrable tumor, in situ carcinoma
T1	Tumor ≤2 cm in greatest dimension
	T1a ≤0.5 cm
	T1b >0.5–1.0 cm
	T1c >1–2 cm
T2	Tumor >2 cm, ≤5 cm in greatest dimension
T3	Tumor >5 cm in greatest dimension
T4	Tumor of any size with direct extension to chest wall or skin
	a) Fixation to chest wall
	b) Edema (including peau d'orange), ulceration of the skin, skin nodules confined to the same breast
	c) Both of the above
	d) Inflammatory carcinoma

Nodal involvement (N)

N0	No regional lymph node involvement
N1	Metastasis to movable ipsilateral axillary nodes
N2	Metastasis to ipsilateral axillary node(s) fixed to one another or to other structures
N3	Metastasis to ipsilateral internal mammary lymph node(s)

Distant metastasis (M)

M0	No (known) distant metastasis
M1	Distant metastasis (include supraclavicular nodes)

continued

BREAST CANCER: *continued*

Staging

Stage 0	Tis
Stage I	T1, N0, M0
Stage IIA	T0, N1, M0
	T1, N1, M0
	T2, N0, M0
Stage IIB	T2, N1, M0
	T3, N0, M0
Stage IIIA	T0, N2, M0
	T1, N2, M0
	T2, N2, M0
	T3, N1, M0
	T3, N2, M0
Stage IIIB	Any T, N3, M0
	T4, any N, M0
Stage IV	Any T, any N, M1

		Standard management	
		Premenopausal	Postmenopausal
Node −	ER +	Tamoxifen; consider CT	Tamoxifen or observation
	ER −	Chemotherapy	Chemotherapy
Node +	ER +	Chemotherapy	Tamoxifen ± chemotherapy
	ER −	Chemotherapy	Chemotherapy
Metastatic ER and/or indolent disease		Tamoxifen (nonresponders proceed to chemotherapy)	Tamoxifen (nonresponders proceed to chemotherapy)
ER − or liver or pulmonary compromise		Chemotherapy	Chemotherapy

ER = estrogen receptor.
Source: American Joint Committee on Cancer. *Manual for Staging Cancer*, 4th ed. Philadelphia: Lippincott, 1992.

COLORECTAL CANCER: TNM CLASSIFICATION

Primary tumor (T)

TX	Primary tumor cannot be assessed
T0	No evidence of primary tumor
Tis	Carcinoma in situ; intraepithelial or invasion of lamina propria
T1	Tumor invades submucosa
T2	Tumor invades muscularis propria
T3	Tumor invades through muscularis propria into subserosa, or into non-peritonealized pericolic or perirectal tissues
T4	Tumor perforates the visceral peritoneum or directly invades other organs or structures

Nodal involvement (N)

NX	Regional lymph nodes cannot be assessed
N0	No regional lymph node metastasis
N1	Metastasis in 1–3 pericolic or perirectal lymph nodes
N2	Metastasis in 4 or more pericolic or perirectal lymph nodes
N3	Metastasis in any lymph node along the course of a named vascular trunk

Distant metastasis (M)

MX	Presence of distant metastasis cannot be assessed
M0	No (known) distant metastasis
M1	Distant metastasis present

Staging

Stage 0	Tis, N0, M0
Stage I	T1, N0, M0
	T2, N0, M0
Stage II	T3, N0, M0
	T4, N0, M0
Stage III	Any T, N1, M0
	Any T, N2–3, M0
Stage IV	Any T, any N, M1

Dukes' Staging System

A	T1, N0, M0
	T2, N0, M0
B	T3, N0, M0
	T4, N0, M0
C	T (any), N1, M0
	T (any), N2, M0
C2	T (any), N3, M0
D	T (any), N (any), M1

Source: American Joint Committee on Cancer. *Manual for Staging Cancer*, 4th ed. Philadelphia: Lippincott, 1992.

ONCOLOGY
PROSTATE CANCER: TNM CLASSIFICATION

Primary tumor (T)

TX	Primary tumor cannot be assessed
T0	No evidence of primary tumor
T1	Clinically inapparent tumor not palpable or visible by imaging
T1a	Tumor incidental histologic finding in ≤5% of tissue resected
T1b	Tumor incidental histologic finding in >5% of tissue resected
T1c	Tumor identified by needle biopsy (e.g., because of elevated prostate-specific antigen level)
T2	Palpable tumor confined within prostate[a]
T2a	Tumor involves half of a lobe or less
T2b	Tumor involves more than half of a lobe, but not both lobes
T3	Tumor extends through the prostatic capsule[b]
T3a	Unilateral extracapsular extension
T3b	Bilateral extracapsular extension
T3c	Tumor invades seminal vesicle(s)
T4	Tumor fixed or invades adjacent structures other than seminal vesicles
T4a	Tumor invades external sphincter and/or bladder neck and/or rectum
T4b	Tumor invades levator muscles and/or is fixed to pelvic wall

Nodal involvement (N)

NX	Regional lymph nodes cannot be assessed
N0	No regional lymph node metastasis
N1	Metastasis in a single lymph node ≤2 cm in greatest dimension
N2	Metastasis in a single lymph node >2 cm and ≤5 cm in greatest dimension, or multiple lymph nodes, none >5 cm in greatest dimension
N3	Metastasis in a lymph node >5 cm in greatest dimension

Distant metastasis (M)

MX	Presence of distant metastasis cannot be assessed
M0	No (known) distant metastasis
M1	Distant metastasis[c]
M1a	Nonregional lymph nodes
M1b	Bone
M1c	Other sites

Staging

Stage I	T1a or b, T2a; N0, M0
Stage II	T2b, N0, M0
Stage III	T3a or b, N0, M0
	Any T, N1, M0
Stage IV	T4, N0, M0
	Any T, N2 or 3, M0
	Any T, any N, M1

Jewett staging

Stage A1	T1a, N0, M0
Stage A2	T1b or Gleason >4, N0, M0
Stage B1	T2a (≤1.5 cm), N0, M0
Stage B2	T2b (>1.5 cm or 1 or 2 lobes), N0, M0
Stage C1	T3, N0, M0
Stage C2	T4, N0, M0
Stage D1	Any T ≤3 pelvic lymph nodes
Stage D2	Any T >3 pelvic lymph nodes, M0
	Any T, any N, M1

[a]Tumor found in one or both lobes by needle biopsy, but not palpable or visible by imaging is classified as T1c.
[b]Invasion into the prostate apex or into (but not beyond) the prostatic capsule is not classified as T3, but as T2.
[c]When more than one site of metastasis is present, the most advanced category (M1c) is used.
Source: American Joint Committee on Cancer. *Manual for Staging Cancer*, 4th ed. Philadelphia: Lippincott, 1992.

Pathologic Scoring of Prostate Cancer

The Gleason sum is based on the glandular pattern of the sample at low magnification. It is the sum of two scores (primary = pattern of the largest section of the specimen; secondary = pattern of the second largest area). It is usually reported as (primary score 1–5) + (secondary score 1–5), but may be reported as a sum [i.e., Gleason sum (2 + 2) or 4].

7. Infectious Disease

STANFORD ADULT PARENTERAL ANTIMICROBIAL DOSING
GUIDELINES (Information reprinted courtesy of R Lafayette, M.D., Department of
Nephrology, Stanford Health Services.)

Drug	CrCl >50 ml/min	CrCl 10–50 ml/min[b]	CrCl <10 ml/min[b]
Acyclovir			
HSV infection	5 mg/kg/dose q8h	5 mg/kg/dose q12–24h	2.5 mg/kg/dose q24h[c]
HSV encephalitis/herpes zoster	10 mg/kg/dose q8h	10 mg/kg/dose q12–24h	5 mg/kg/dose q24h[c]
Amikacin	>80 ml/min: 7.5–8.0 mg/kg q8h 60–80 ml/min: 4–5 mg/kg q8h	40–60 ml/min: 4–5 mg/kg q12h 20–40 ml/min: 6 mg/kg q12–24h	10–20 ml/min: 6 mg/kg q24–48h <10 ml/min: 4–6 mg/kg q48–72h
Amphotericin B[d]	0.3–1.0 mg/kg/day	No change	No change
Ampicillin	1–2 g q4–6h (max 8 g/day)	1.0–1.5 g q6h	1 g q8–12h[c]
Ampicillin/sulbactam	1.5–3.0 g q6–8h	1.5–3.0 g q6–8h	1.5–3.0 g q12–24h
Azithromycin IV	500 mg q24h × 2 doses, then 250–500 mg q24h	No change	No change[e]
Aztreonam	1–2 g q6–8h (max 8 g/d)	1–2 g q8h	500 mg q8h[c]
Cefazolin	1–2 g q8h	0.5–1.5 g q12h	0.5–1.0 g q24h[c]
Cefotaxime[f]	1–2 g q8h	1–2 g q8–12h	0.5–1.0 g q12h[c,e]
Cefotetan	1–2 g q12h	1–2 g q12h	1–2 g q24h
Ceftazidime	1–2 g q8h	1–2 g q12–24h	0.5 g q24h[c]
Ceftriaxone	1–2 g q24h (2 g q12h in meningitis)	1–2 g q24h	1 g q24h[c]
Cefuroxime	0.75–1.50 g q8h	0.75–1.50 mg q12–24h	0.75–1.50 g q24h[c]
Ciprofloxacin (IV)[g]	200–400 mg q8–12h	30–50 ml/min: no change 10–30 ml/min: 200 q12h	200 mg q24h[c]
Clarithromycin*	250–500 mg q12h	250–500 mg q12h	250–500 mg q24h[e]

138

Drug	CrCl >50 ml/min	CrCl 10–50 ml/min[b]	CrCl <10 ml/min[b]
Clindamycin	600–900 mg q8h	No change	No change[e]
Doxycycline	100 mg q12h	No change	No change
Erythromycin[h]	500–1,000 mg q6h	No change	No change[e]
Ethambutol HCl	15–25 mg/kg qd	7.5–10.0 mg/kg qd	5 mg/kg qd[c]
Fluconazole	100–400 mg q24h	50–200 mg q24h	50–100 mg q24h[i]
Flucytosine (PO)[j]	12.5–37.5 mg/kg/dose q6h	25–50 ml/min: 12.5–37.5 mg/kg q12h 10–25 ml/min: 12.5–37.5 mg/kg q24h	12.5–25.0 mg/kg q24h
Ganciclovir	>80 ml/min: 5 mg/kg/dose q12h <80 ml/min: 2.5 mg/kg/dose q12h	1.25–2.50 mg/kg q12–24h	1.25 mg/kg q24h[k]
Gentamicin[l]	>80 ml/min: 1.5–1.8 mg/kg q8h 60–80 ml/min: 1.2–1.6 mg/kg q8h	40–60 ml/min: 1.2–1.6 mg/kg q12h 20–40 ml/min: 1.5 mg/kg q12–24h	10–20 ml/min: 1.5 mg/kg q24–48h <10 ml/min: 1.0–1.5 mg/kg q48–72h
Imipenem[m]	500 mg to 1 g q6h (max 4 g/day)	500–750 mg q8h	250–500 mg q12h[c]
Isoniazid*	300 mg qd	No change	No change[e]
Itraconazole	200 mg q12–24h	No change	No change[e]
Ketoconazole*	200–400 mg qd	No change	No change
Levofloxacin	500 mg q24h	250 mg q24h	250 mg q48h
Meropenem	1 g q8h	500 mg q12h	500 mg q24h
Metronidazole[n]	500 mg q8h	500 mg q8–12h	500 mg q12h[c,e]
Nafcillin	1–2 g q4h	No change	No change
Nitrofurantoin*[o]	50–100 mg q6h	Avoid	Avoid[e]
Penicillin G[p]	2–3 million units q4h	1–2 MU q4–6h	1 MU q6h[c]
Pentamidine	3–4 mg/kg q24h	No change	No change[e]
Piperacillin	3–4 g q6h	3–4 g q6h	2–3 g q8h[c]
Piperacillin/tazobactam	>40 ml/min Life-threatening = 4.5 g q6h Moderate = 4.5 g q8h	20–40 ml/min Life-threatening = 4.5 g q8h Moderate = 4.5 g q12h	<20 ml/min Life-threatening = 4.5 g q12h[a] Moderate = 3.375 g q12h[a]
Pyrazinamide*	15–30 mg/kg q24h (usually in 2–4 doses, commonly 500 mg tid; max 2 g/day)	No change	12–20 mg/kg q24h[e]

INFECTIOUS DISEASE

Drug	CrCl >50 ml/min	CrCl 10–50 ml/min[b]	CrCl <10 ml/min[b]
Rifampin	600 mg qd	No change	No change[e]
Ticarcillin/clavulanate	3.1 g q4–6h	2.07–3.10 g q6–8h	2.07 g q12h[c]
Tobramycin	See gentamicin	See gentamicin	See gentamicin
Trimethoprim-sulfamethoxazole (TMP/SMX)[q]	Systemic GNR infections: 10 mg TMP/kg/day divided q6–12h	5.0–7.5 mg TMP/kg/day divided q12–24h	2.5–5.0 mg TMP/kg q24h[c,e]
Vancomycin[r]	>60 ml/min: 10–15 mg/kg q12h 40–60 ml/min: 10–15 mg/kg q12–24h	20–40 ml/min: 10–15 mg/kg q24–48h 10–20 ml/min: 10–15 mg/kg q48–72h	10–15 mg/kg q4–7d

CrCl = creatinine clearance.

*All drugs are PO only, except for isoniazid (PO/IM) and ketoconazole (PO/topical).

[a] Doses recommended for systemic infections commonly treated with this agent.

[b] For patients with minimal renal function or those with end-stage renal disease (ESRD). For information about the dosing of antimicrobial agents in the setting of hemodialysis or hepatic failure, contact your pharmacist.

[c] Dose after hemodialysis.

[d] Dosage reductions in renal disease are not necessary. However, because of the nephrotoxic potential of the drug, reducing or holding the drug in the setting of a rising creatinine may be warranted.

[e] Dose adjust or use caution in patients with hepatic dysfunction.

[f] Cefotaxime dosing recommendations in ESRD are based on pharmacokinetic data for the parent compound. Accumulation of the active metabolite (desacetyl-cefotaxime) may also occur in renal failure.

[g] The use of q12h dosing intervals is recommended in ESRD due to the variability in the half-life data observed in anephric patients.

[h] Erythromycin dosing does not require adjustment for renal disease, but an increased risk of ototoxicity has been associated with IV doses >2 g/day in patients with renal insufficiency.

[i] 200 mg fluconazole after hemodialysis.

[j] Steady-state serum 5-flucytosine (5-FC) level measurements are difficult to obtain. However, they may be useful in guiding dosing of 5-FC in anuria. Bone marrow suppression has been associated with 2-hour postdose 5-FC peaks of >100 mg/liter.

[k] Ganciclovir 1.25 mg/kg three times a week after hemodialysis.

[l] Gentamicin/tobramycin dosing should be guided by serum level measurements (peaks 30 minutes after the end of IV infusion and trough <30 minutes before the next dose). The dosage ranges suggested are those used in the treatment of gram-negative infection and are meant to provide peaks of 5–8 mg/liter and troughs of <2 mg/liter.

[m] Imipenem dosages must be adjusted in patients with decreased renal function to reduce the potential for seizures.

[n] Metronidazole metabolites accumulate in renal failure. To minimize the potential for toxicity, q12h dosing intervals are recommended.

[o] Nitrofurantoin metabolites accumulate in renal insufficiency and are toxic.

[p] Dosages for penicillin are based on penicillin (PCN) (MU/day) = CrCl (ml/min)/7.0 + 3.2. For end-stage hepatic disease with concomitant ESRD, the maximum recommended dose is PCN (MU/day) = CrCl (ml/min)/7.0 + 1.5.

[q] See page 163 for PCP dosing for HIV patients.

[r] Vancomycin dosing should be guided by serum level measurements in settings such as osteomyelitis, endocarditis, CNS infections, and dialysis. Trough levels (<30 minutes before next dose) should be 5–15 mg/liter and peak (1 hour after completion of infusion) should be 25–35 mg/liter. Ototoxicity has been associated with peak levels >50 mg/liter.

VANCOMYCIN AND AMINOGLYCOSIDE MONITORING

Vancomycin Dosing (Information reprinted courtesy of R Lafayette, M.D., Department of Nephrology, Stanford Health Services.)

Creatinine clearance (ml/min)	Dose	Interval
90–120	15 mg/kg	q12h
60–89	10 mg/kg	q12h
40–59	15 mg/kg	q24h
20–39	15 mg/kg	q48h
<20	15 mg/kg	See pharmacy

- Round dose to nearest 250-mg increment.
- Dose is based on ideal body weight.

Peak Levels Rarely Indicated
Target trough = 5–15 µg/ml
Target peak = 25–35 µg/ml

When to Obtain Serum Troughs
- Coadministration of nephrotoxic medications
- Patients who have unstable renal function
- Patients on dialysis
- Life-threatening infections
- Patients with meningitis, endocarditis, osteomyelitis
- Treating organisms with high minimal inhibitory concentration (MIC)

Aminoglycoside Dosing
Standard Gentamicin and Tobramycin Dosing

CrCl (ml/min)	Dose*	Interval
>70	1.5–1.7 mg/kg	q8h
40–70	1.5–2.0 mg/kg	q12h
20–40	1.5 mg/kg	q12h
10–20	1.5 mg/kg	q24h
<10	1.0–1.5 mg/kg	q48h

*Round to nearest 20 mg.

- Check peak and trough levels after the third dose.
- Goal peak level for bacteremia is 6 µg/ml; for pneumonia, 8 µg/ml.
- Goal trough level is <1 µg/ml to minimize toxicity.

INFECTIOUS DISEASE

SINGLE DAILY AMINOGLYCOSIDE DOSING (Infect Dis Clin Pract 5:12, 1996; AAC 39:650, 1995; Eur J Clin Microbiol Infect Dis 14:1029, 1995; Ann Intern Med 124:717, 1996)

Fast Facts

- Dependent on the postantibiotic effect; continued bacterial growth suppression when serum concentration is below MIC. Usually lasts 2–4 hours.
- Trend toward less renal toxicity.
- 33% reduction in ototoxicity.

Indications for use	Limited data	Not recommended for use
Uncomplicated gram-negative infections	Burn victims	Bacteremic with *Pseudomonas*
Abdominal wound infections	Obesity	Cystic fibrosis
Pelvic inflammatory infections	Elderly	Pregnancy or postpartum <6 wks
Urinary tract infections	Pediatrics	Endocarditis
	Critically ill	Meningitis
	Neutropenic	
	Renal disease	
	Organ transplant	

Creatinine clearance (ml/min)	Gentamicin dose	Interval
>90	7 mg/kg	q24h
50–89	5 mg/kg	q24h
30–49	2.5–3.5 mg/kg	q24h
<30 or dialysis	Call pharmacy	Call pharmacy

Gentamicin dose	Desired 8-hour level (μg/ml)
7 mg/kg q24h	2–5
5 mg/kg q24h	2–5
2.5–3.5 mg/kg q24h	2.5–5.0

Adjusting Gentamicin Dosing

Gentamicin has linear pharmacokinetics. Any adjustment in the dose will change the measured peak by the same amount (i.e., for a dose of 80 mg and peak of 4 μg/ml, a change in the dose to 120 mg will increase the peak to 6 μg/ml). [Note: It actually is more complicated because the measured peak is not the true peak (peaks are usually measured 30 minutes to 1 hour postinfusion), and the actual peak also will reflect that the infusion is not instantaneous but spread over a span of time. However, the above guidelines work well in practice. For more accurate adjustments in dosing, consult a pharmacist.]

FEVER AND RASH DIFFERENTIAL DIAGNOSIS [Modified from AS Fauci et al. (eds). *Harrison's Principles of Internal Medicine* [14th ed]. New York: McGraw-Hill, 1998.]

Centrally Distributed Maculopapular Eruptions

- Measles (paramyxovirus)
- German measles (togavirus)
- Fifth disease (erythema infectiosum)
- Roseola (exanthem subitum, HHV-6)
- Primary HIV
- Infectious mononucleosis
- Exanthematous drug eruptions
- Endemic typhus (*Rickettsia typhi*)
- Scrub typhus (*Rickettsia tsutsugamushi*)
- Rickettsial spotted fevers

- Ehrlichiosis
- Leptospirosis
- Lyme disease
- Typhoid fever
- Rat-bite fever (Sodoku; *Spirillum minus*)
- Relapsing fever (*Borrelia* species)
- Erythema marginatum (rheumatic fever)
- SLE
- Adult-onset Still's disease

Peripheral Eruptions

- Chronic meningococcemia
- Rocky Mountain spotted fever (*Rickettsia rickettsii*)
- Secondary syphilis
- Atypical measles

- Hand-foot-and-mouth disease
- Erythema multiforme
- Rat-bite fever (Haverhill fever; *Spirillum minus*)
- Bacterial endocarditis

Confluent Desquamative Erythema

- Scarlet fever (group A streptococcus)
- Kawasaki disease
- Staphylococcal scalded-skin syndrome
- Toxic epidermal necrolysis

- Staphylococcal TSS (*Staphylococcus aureus*)
- Streptococcal TSS (group A streptococcus)
- Exfoliative erythroderma syndrome

Vesiculobullous Eruptions

- Hand-foot-and-mouth syndrome
- Staphylococcal scalded-skin syndrome
- Toxic epidermal necrolysis
- Varicella

- Rickettsial pox (*Rickettsia akari*)
- Disseminated *Vibrio vulnificus* infection
- Ecthyma gangrenosum (*Pseudomonas aeruginosa*, gram-negative, and fungi)

continued

INFECTIOUS DISEASE

Urticarial Eruptions

- Urticarial vasculitis (serum sickness, connective tissue disease, infection, idiopathic causes)

Nodular Eruptions

- Disseminated infection (fungi)
- Erythema nodosum (infection, drugs, sarcoidosis, idiopathic)

- Sweet's syndrome (acute febrile neutrophilic dermatosis; *Yersinia* infection, lymphoproliferative disorders, idiopathic)

Purpuric Eruptions

- Rocky Mountain spotted fever
- Endocarditis
- Epidemic typhus
- Acute meningococcemia
- Purpura fulminans (severe DIC)

- Chronic meningococcemia
- Disseminated gonococcal infection
- Enteroviral petechial rash
- Viral hemorrhagic fever (arboviruses and arenaviruses)
- Thrombotic thrombocytopenic purpura

FEVER OF UNKNOWN ORIGIN (*Clin Infect Dis* 24:291, 1997)

Definitions

Classic Fever of Unknown Origin (FUO)
- Fever ≥3 weeks
- Three outpatient visits or 3 hospital days without elucidation of cause

Nosocomial Fever of Unknown Origin
- Hospitalization, no acute infection on admission
- No source in 3 days of hospitalization

Neutropenic Fever of Unknown Origin
- ANC ≤500/µl or expected to reach that level in 1–2 days
- No source in 3 days of hospitalization (2 days of culture incubation)

HIV-Associated Fever of Unknown Origin
- Confirmed HIV positive
- No source in 3 days of hospitalization or 4 weeks as outpatient

Differential Diagnosis of Classic Fever of Unknown Origin [Modified from AS Fauci, JB Martin, E Braunwald, et al. (eds). *Harrison's Principles of Internal Medicine*, 14th ed. New York: McGraw-Hill, 1998.]

Localized Pyogenic Infections
- Appendicitis
- Cholangitis
- Cholecystitis
- Dental abscess
- Diverticulitis/abscess
- Liver abscess
- Perinephric/interrenal abscess
- PID
- Prostatic abscess
- Sinusitis

Intravascular Infections
- Bacterial aortitis
- Bacterial endocarditis

Systemic Bacterial Infections
- Bartonellosis
- Brucellosis
- *Campylobacter* infection
- Cat-scratch disease
- Gonococcemia
- Legionnaire's disease
- Leptospirosis
- Listeriosis
- Lyme disease
- Rat-bite fever
- Relapsing fever
- Salmonellosis
- Syphilis
- Tularemia
- Typhoid fever
- Vibriosis
- *Yersinia* infection

continued

INFECTIOUS DISEASE

Mycobacterial Infection
- TB and atypical

Fungal Infections
- Aspergillosis
- Blastomycosis
- Candidiasis
- Coccidioidomycosis
- Cryptococcosis
- Histoplasmosis
- Mucormycosis

Other Bacterial Infections
- Actinomycosis
- Ehrlichiosis
- Murine typhus
- Nocardiosis
- Q fever
- Rickettsia
- Rocky Mountain spotted fever
- Whipple's disease

Viral Infections
- Coxsackievirus group B
- CMV
- Dengue
- Epstein-Barr virus
- Hepatitis A, B, C, D, and E
- HIV

Parasitic Infections
- Amebiasis
- Babesiasis
- Chagas' disease
- Leishmaniasis
- Malaria
- PCP
- Strongyloidiasis
- Toxocariasis
- Toxoplasmosis
- Trichinosis

Malignant Neoplasms
- Colon
- Hepatoma
- Hodgkin's lymphoma
- Leukemia
- Non-Hodgkin's lymphoma
- Renal cell carcinoma

Benign Neoplasms
- Atrial myxoma

Collagen Vascular Diseases
- Adult Still's disease
- Behçet's disease
- Erythema multiforme
- Erythema nodosum
- Giant cell arteritis
- Mixed connective-tissue disease
- Polyarteritis nodosa
- Relapsing polychondritis
- SLE
- Takayasu's arteritis
- Wegener's granulomatosis

Drugs

- Antiarrhythmics (quinidine, procainamide)
- Antiepileptics
- Antihistamines
- Antihypertensives (hydralazine, methyldopa)
- Antimicrobials
- Antithyroid drugs
- Iodides
- NSAIDs

Other Miscellaneous

- Aortic dissection
- Gout
- Hematomas
- Hemolytic diseases
- Laennec's cirrhosis
- Post-myocardial infarction
- Recurrent pulmonary emboli
- Subacute thyroiditis
- Tissue infarction/necrosis

Inherited and Metabolic Disease

- Adrenal insufficiency
- Familial Mediterranean fever

Thermoregulatory Disorders

Central

- Brain tumor
- Cerebrovascular accident
- Encephalitis
- Hypothalamic dysfunction

Peripheral

- Factitious fever
- Hyperthyroidism
- Pheochromocytoma

INFECTIOUS DISEASE

SEVERE SOFT-TISSUE INFECTIONS
Necrotizing Infections of the Soft Tissues*

Type	Usual etiologic agents	Predisposing causes	Clinical manifestations
Meleney's synergistic gangrene	*S. aureus*, microaerophilic streptococci	Surgery	Slowly expanding ulceration confined to superficial fascia
Clostridial cellulitis	*Clostridium perfringens*	Local trauma or surgery	Gas in skin, fascia spared, little systemic toxicity
Nonclostridial anaerobic cellulitis	Mixed aerobes and anaerobes	Diabetes mellitus	Gas in tissues
Gas gangrene	Clostridial species (*C. perfringens*, *C. histolyticum*, or *C. septicum*)	Trauma, crush injuries, epinephrine injections, spontaneous cases related to cancer, neutropenia, cancer chemotherapy	Myonecrosis, gas formation, evident systemic toxicity, shock
Necrotizing fasciitis type 1	Mixed anaerobes, gram-negative aerobic bacilli, enterococci	Surgery, diabetes mellitus, peripheral vascular disease	Destruction of fat and fascia, skin may be spared, involvement of perineal area in Fournier's gangrene
Necrotizing fasciitis type 2	Group A *streptococcus*	Penetrating injuries, surgical procedures, varicella, burns, minor cuts, trauma	Systemic toxicity, severe local pain, rapidly extending necrosis of subcutaneous tissues and skin, gangrene, shock, multiorgan failure

*All necrotizing infections are surgical emergencies until proved otherwise.

Source: Reprinted with permission from *N Engl J Med* 334:240, 1996. Copyright © 1996 Massachusetts Medical Society. All rights reserved.

ENDOCARDITIS *(Am J Med 96:200, 1994)*

Diagnosis: Duke's Clinical Criteria

Two major, one major and three minor, or five minor criteria make definitive diagnosis.

Major Criteria

Positive blood culture:	Either typical microorganism from two separate blood cultures, persistently positive blood cultures from cultures drawn >12 hrs apart, or three out of three or majority of ≥4 cultures
Positive echo-cardiogram:	Vegetation, abscess, new partial dehiscence of prosthetic valve, new valvular regurgitation

Minor Criteria

Fever:	≥38.0°C
Vascular phenomena:	Arterial emboli, septic pulmonary infarcts, mycotic aneurysm, intracranial hemorrhage, conjunctival hemorrhage, Janeway lesions
Immunologic phenomena:	Glomerulonephritis, Osler's nodes, Roth spot, RF
Microbiological criteria:	Positive blood culture not meeting major criterion or serologic evidence of active infection with organism consistent with endocarditis
Echocardiogram:	Consistent with endocarditis but not meeting major criterion

Etiology

Pathogen	Native valve	Prosthetic valve	Narcotic addict
Streptococcus	55–65%		20%
viridans	35–40%		
enterococcus	10–15%		
other	10–15%		
Staphylococcus	15–20%		50%
aureus			
epidermidis		>50% (usually within 2 mos postoperatively)	
Haemophilus, Actinobacillus, Cardiobacterium, Eikenella, Kingella	2–4%	—	—
Gram-negative rods	—	—	20%
Fungus	—	—	10%, especially *Candida*
Culture negative	3–5%	—	—

Source: Adapted from JG Bartlett. *2000 Pocket Book of ID Therapy*. Philadelphia: Lippincott Williams & Wilkins, 2000.

continued

INFECTIOUS DISEASE

Empiric Therapy (Recommendations of the AMA's Drug Evaluations, AMA, II/NF-2:10, 1991)

Native Valve

- Nafcillin or oxacillin 2 g IV q4h + gentamicin 1 mg/kg IV q8h (normal renal function) for peak of 3 µg/ml
- Vancomycin 30 mg/kg/day IV (≤2 g/day) ± gentamicin (above doses)

Prosthetic Valve

- Nafcillin or oxacillin (above doses) ± gentamicin (above doses) ± rifampin 300 mg IV q12h
- Vancomycin (above doses) + gentamicin (above doses) ± rifampin (above doses)

Indications for Cardiac Surgery in Patients with Endocarditis (*Am J Med* 78(suppl 6B):138, 1985)

Indications for Urgent Surgery (Native or Prosthetic Valve)

- Hemodynamic compromise
- Fundal endocarditis
- No effective antimicrobial agents
- Uncontrolled infection
- Unstable prosthetic valve
- Vascular obstruction
- Persistent bacteremia (or persistent signs of sepsis)
- Severe heart failure (especially with aortic insufficiency)

Relative Indications for Surgery in Patient with Native Valve

- Bacterial agent other than susceptible *Streptococcus*
- Abscess shown by echocardiogram/catheter
- Ruptured chordae or papillary muscle
- Relapse (especially if non-*Streptococcus* agent)
- Evidence of intracardiac extension
- Vegetations on echocardiograph
- Rupture of sinus of Valsalva or ventricular septum
- Two or more emboli
- Mitral valve preclosure
- Heart block

Relative Indications for Surgery in Patient with Prosthetic Valve

- Early postoperative endocarditis (≤8 weeks)
- Relapse
- New or increased regurgitation murmur
- Two or more emboli
- Aortic valve involvement
- Periprosthetic leak
- Heart failure
- Non-*Streptococcus* late endocarditis
- Evidence of intracardiac extension
- Mechanical valve as opposed to bioprosthetic valve

MENINGITIS (*N Engl J Med* 336:709, 1997; *Postgrad Med* 103:102, 1998)

Cerebrospinal Fluid Profiles

	Pressure (mm H$_2$O)	Leukocytes (per mm³)	Glucose (mg/dl)	Protein (mg/dl)	Other
Normal	65–195	<5 (1 PMN)	40–80	15–45	CSF/blood glucose ratio >0.6
Bacterial	Increased/ normal	>100 (>80% PMN)	<40	>45	Gram's stain 60% Culture 73% Glucose ratio <0.4
Aseptic	Normal	10–100 (lymphs)	Normal/ decreased	50–100	
TB	180–300	100–400 (lymphs)	30–45	100–500	Stain <33% Culture 50–70%
Fungal	Increased	10–200	<40	50–200	
Traumatic tap	Normal	1 WBC/700 RBC	Normal	Increased	Colorless supernatant
Subarachnoid hemorrhage/intracranial hemorrhage	—	Increased (PMNs)	—	Increased 1 mg/1,000 RBCs	RBCs
Vasculitis	—	Increased (mononuclear)	Normal	Increased	—
Sarcoidosis	—	<100 (mononuclear)	Decreased (in 10%)	Increased	—

Predictors of Bacterial Meningitis (99% positive predictive value)

(*JAMA* 262:2700, 1989)

Each of these criteria have a 99% PPV for bacterial meningitis.

- Glucose <34 mg/dl
- Protein >220 mg/dl
- CSF/serum glucose <0.23
- WBCs >2,000/mm³
- PMNs >1,180/mm³

Check for Papilledema or Focal Neurologic Deficits/Signs

- If absent, obtain blood cultures and LP stat.
- If papilledema or focal neurologic deficits exist, obtain blood cultures and begin empiric therapy while awaiting head CT. LP if no mass lesion.

Etiology

Pathogen	Causative organism (%)	Fatality rate (%)
Streptococcus pneumoniae	30–50	19–46
Neisseria meningitidis	15–40	3–17
Haemophilus influenzae	2–7	3–11
Listeria monocytogenes	1–3	15–40
Other	<5	?

continued **151**

INFECTIOUS DISEASE
Treatment

Likely pathogen	Preferred antibiotic	Dose
CSF Gram's stain		
No stainable organisms	Ceftriaxone or cefotaxime ± Ampicillin	2 g IV q12h 2 g IV q4–6h 2 g IV q4h
Gram-positive cocci	Ceftriaxone or cefotaxime + Vancomycin	As above 1.5 mg/kg q12h (max 2 g/day)
Gram-positive bacilli	Ampicillin + Gentamicin	As above 1.5 mg/kg, then 1 mg/kg q8h
Gram-negative cocci	PCN G	4 mU q4h
Gram-negative bacilli	Ceftriaxone or cefotaxime + gentamicin	As above
Culture results		
S. pneumoniae: PCN MIC <0.06 µg/ml	PCN G, ceftriaxone, or cefotaxime	As above
S. pneumoniae: PCN MIC >0.1 µg/ml	Ceftriaxone or cefotaxime; + vancomycin	As above
N. meningitidis	PCN G	As above
H. influenzae	Ceftriaxone or cefotaxime	As above
L. monocytogenes	Ampicillin + gentamicin	As above
Group B *streptococcus*	PCN G	As above

Duration of Therapy

Pathogen	Duration of therapy (days)
H. influenzae	7
N. meningitidis	7
S. pneumoniae	10–14
L. monocytogenes	14–21
Group B streptococci	14–21
Other gram-negative bacilli	21

Source: Reprinted with permission from *N Engl J Med* 336:709, 1997. Copyright © 1997 Massachusetts Medical Society. All rights reserved.

Adjunctive Corticosteroids

Benefit in neurologic sequelae for children, primarily with *H. influenzae*. The Infectious Diseases Society of America does not support routine use of steroids in adults with meningitis (*J Infect Dis* 165:1, 1992). Consider dexamethasone (0.15 mg/kg IV q6h × 4 days) 30 minutes before antibiotics in high-risk adults (impaired mental status, cerebral edema, very high ICP, or positive Gram's stain) (*Lancet* 346:1675, 1995). Add rifampin empirically to vancomycin if dexamethasone is used (dexamethasone reduces vancomycin levels in CSF).

COMMUNITY-ACQUIRED PNEUMONIA

Inpatient versus Outpatient Management—Point Scoring System

Men: +Age (yrs); Women: +(Age − 10) (yrs); Nursing home resident: +10

Comorbid illnesses:	Cancer	+30	Liver disease	+20	CHF	+10
	Stroke	+10	Renal disease	+10		
Physical exam:	Changed mental state	+20	RR ≥30	+20	Systolic BP <90	+20
	Temperature <35 or ≥40	+15	HR ≥125	+10		
Lab values:	pH <7.35	+30	BUN >10.7	+20	Na <130	+20
	Glucose >13.9	+10	Hct <30%	+10	Pleural effusion	+10
	PaO$_2$ <60 or O$_2$Sat <90%	+10				

Source: Reprinted with permission from University of Chicago Press. JG Bartlett et al. Community-acquired pneumonia in adults: guidelines for management. *Clin Infect Dis* 26:811, 1998.

Risk class	No. of points	No. of patients	Mortality (%)	Recommend
I	No predictors*	3,034	0.1	Outpatient
II	≤70	5,778	0.6	Outpatient
III	71–90	6,790	2.8	Inpatient (briefly)
IV	91–130	13,104	8.2	Inpatient
V	>130	9,333	29.2	Inpatient

*Class I only if age ≤50 years with no associated comorbid illness and no physical exam or lab abnormality.
Source: Reprinted with permission from University of Chicago Press. JG Bartlett et al. Community-acquired pneumonia in adults: guidelines for management. *Clin Infect Dis* 26:811, 1998.

Pathogens

- S. pneumoniae
- Chlamydia pneumoniae
- N. meningitidis
- Gram-negative rods
- RSV
- H. influenzae
- S. aureus
- Moraxella catarrhalis
- Legionella
- Adenovirus
- Mycoplasma pneumoniae
- Streptococcus pyogenes
- Klebsiella pneumoniae
- Influenza virus
- Parainfluenza virus

In prospective studies, most common pathogen is *S. pneumoniae*, 40–60% of cases have no identified etiology, and 2–5% have two or more etiologies.

continued

INFECTIOUS DISEASE

Empiric Therapy

Clinical setting	Preferred	Alternative
Outpatient		
General	Macrolide,[a] fluoroquinolone,[b] or doxycycline	Amoxicillin/clavulanate[c] Some second-generation cephalosporins[c,d]
Suspected PCN-resistant *S. pneumoniae*	Fluoroquinolone[b]	
Suspected aspiration	Amoxicillin/clavulanate	
Young adult (18–40 yrs)	Doxycycline	
Inpatient		
General ward	Cefotaxime/ceftriaxone ± macrolide[a]; or fluoroquinolone[b]	Cefuroxime ± macrolide[a] or azithromycin (alone)
ICU	Erythromycin, azithromycin, or fluoroquinolone[b] + cefotaxime or ceftriaxone or β-lactam/inhibitor[e]	
Structural lung disease (i.e., bronchiectasis)	Antipseudomonal PCN, carbapenem, or cefepime + macrolide[a] or fluoroquinolone[b] + aminoglycoside[f]	
PCN allergy	Fluoroquinolone[b] ± clindamycin	
Suspected aspiration	Fluoroquinolone[b] + clindamycin or β-lactam/inhibitor[e]	

[a]Azithromycin, clarithromycin, or erythromycin.
[b]Levofloxacin, sparfloxacin, grepafloxacin (enhanced activity vs. *S. pneumoniae*).
[c]No atypical coverage.
[d]Cefuroxime, cefpodoxime, cefprozil.
[e]Ampicillin/sulbactam, ticarcillin/clavulanate, piperacillin/tazobactam (in structural lung disease—last two choices).
[f]Aminoglycoside—gentamicin, tobramycin, amikacin.
Source: Reproduced with permission from University of Chicago Press. JG Bartlett et al. Community-acquired pneumonia in adults: guidelines for management. *Clin Infect Dis* 26:811, 1998.

Duration of Therapy
- No controlled trials assess duration
- *S. pneumoniae*: 3 days after patient is afebrile
- Atypical: ≥2 weeks

Change to Oral Antibiotics
- Clinically improving
- Tolerating PO and functioning GI tract
- Hemodynamically stable
- Available drug with adequate bio-availability, activity

154

URINARY TRACT INFECTIONS (*Infect Dis Clin North Am* 11:551, 1997;
Clin Infect Dis 15:S216, 1992)

Urinary Tract Infection Classification

Category	Clinical criteria	Lab criteria
Acute, uncomplicated UTI in women	Dysuria, urgency, frequency, suprapubic pain, no urinary symptoms in last 4 wks, no fever or flank pain	>10 WBC/mm³ >1,000 cfu/ml uropathogen
Acute, uncomplicated pyelonephritis	Fever, chills, dysuria, urgency, frequency, suprapubic pain, costovertebral angle tenderness, flank pain No urologic abnormality, other diagnoses excluded, no other risks for complicated UTI	>10 WBC/mm³ >10,000 cfu/ml uropathogen
Complicated UTI in men, obstruction	Any combination of findings in above categories	>10 WBC/mm³ >100,000 cfu/ml uropathogen

INFECTIOUS DISEASE

TREATMENT REGIMENS FOR URINARY TRACT INFECTIONS

(*Clin Infect Dis* 29:735, 1999; *N Engl J Med* 329:1329, 1993)

Condition	Complications	Empiric treatment
Acute uncomplicated cystitis (*Escherichia coli, Staphylococcus saprophyticus, Proteus mirabilis, K. pneumoniae*)	None	3-day regimen: TMP/SMX, TMP, fluoroquinolones (ofloxacin, norfloxacin, ciprofloxacin; fleroxacin where TMP/SMX resistance >10–20%), cefixime, cefpodoxime 7-day regimen: nitrofurantoin
	For men diabetics, symptoms >7 days, childhood UTI, recent antibiotics, age >65	Consider 7-day regimen: TMP/SMX, TMP, fluoroquinolone
Acute uncomplicated pyelonephritis (*E. coli, P. mirabilis, K. pneumoniae, S. saprophyticus*)	Mild to moderate illness, no nausea and vomiting; outpatient therapy	7–14 days: fluoroquinolone, TMP/SMX, TMP. For known gram-positive infection, amoxicillin or amoxicillin/clavulanic acid alone
	Severe illness or possible urosepsis; hospitalization required	Parenteral fluoroquinolone, an aminoglycoside with or without ampicillin, or an extended-spectrum cephalosporin with or without aminoglycoside. For known gram-positive infection, ampicillin/sulbactam ± aminoglycoside. Follow with oral antibiotics.
Complicated UTI* (*E. coli, Proteus* spp., *Klebsiella* spp., *Pseudomonas* spp., *Serratia* spp., enterococci, staphylococci)	Mild to moderate illness, no nausea/vomiting; outpatient therapy	Oral fluoroquinolone for 10–14 days
	Severe illness or possible urosepsis; hospitalization required	Parenteral fluoroquinolone, ampicillin with an aminoglycoside, or an extended-spectrum cephalosporin ± aminoglycoside. For known gram-positive infection, ampicillin/sulbactam ± aminoglycoside. Follow with oral antibiotics.

*Functionally, metabolically, or anatomically abnormal urinary tract or infection caused by resistant pathogen.

VAGINITIS   (From the Centers for Disease Control. *Sexually Transmitted Diseases Treatment Guidelines 1998.* MMWR 1993;4247-1; and RL Sweet, RS Gibbs. Pelvic inflammatory disease. In: *Infectious Diseases of the Female Genital Tract,* 2nd ed. Baltimore: Williams & Wilkins, 1990.)

Fast Facts

- Vagina has 25 species of bacteria.
- pH is usually 4.0 secondary to lactobacilli.
- Semen, menses, ectropion will alter pH.
- Causes of vaginitis:
      50% bacterial vaginosis
      25% *Trichomonas*
      25% yeast

Evaluation

	pH	Hyphae	Trichomonads	Clue cells
Bacterial vaginosis	>4.5	Absent	Absent	Present
Trichomonas vaginitis	Normal	Absent	Present	Absent
Yeast vaginitis (*Candida*)	Normal	Present	Absent	Absent

Bacterial Vaginosis

- Metronidazole (Flagyl), 2 g PO, repeat in 48 hours
- Metronidazole (Flagyl), 500 mg PO bid for 1 week
- Metronidazole vaginal gel (Metro-Gel), 0.75% PV bid for 5 days
- Clindamycin 1% in acigel PV qhs for 10 days

Trichomonas Vaginitis

- Treat sexual partner as well.
- Metronidazole (Flagyl), 2 g PO, repeat in 48 hours
- Metronidazole (Flagyl), 250 mg PO tid for 1 week

Vulvovaginal Candidiasis

Mystatin (Mycostatin)	Vaginal tablets (150,000 units)	Once daily for 15 days
	Ointment (100,000 units/g)	bid for 15 days for vulvitis
Miconazole (Monistat)	2% vaginal cream	Daily for 7–10 days
	100-mg suppositories	Daily for 7 days
	200-mg suppositories	Daily for 3 days
	2% cutaneous cream	bid for 14 days
Clotrimazole (Gyne-Lotrimin, Mycelex)	1% vaginal cream	Daily for 7–14 days
	100-mg vaginal tablets	Daily for 7 days
	500-mg suppository	Single dose
Butoconazole (Femstat)	2% vaginal cream	Daily for 3 days
Terconazole (Terazole)	0.4% vaginal cream	Daily for 7 days
	80-mg suppository	Daily for 3 days
Ketoconazole (Nizoral)	200- to 400-mg PO tablet	Daily for 5 days
Fluconazole (Diflucan)	150-mg tablet	Single dose
Boric acid	600 mg in size 0 gelatin capsules	Daily for 14 days

INFECTIOUS DISEASE

PELVIC INFLAMMATORY DISEASE   (From the Centers for Disease Control. *Sexually Transmitted Diseases Treatment Guidelines 1998*. MMWR 1993;4247-1; and RL Sweet, RS Gibbs. Pelvic inflammatory disease. In: *Infectious Diseases of the Female Genital Tract*, 2nd ed. Baltimore: Williams & Wilkins, 1990.)

Fast Facts
- Sequela of PID: adhesions, hydrosalpinx, increased risk of ectopic pregnancy (10 times), increased risk of pelvic pair (4 times)
- Starts most often with cervical gonoccocal (or *Chlamydia*) infection and becomes an ascending infection
- 90% with lower abdominal pain
- 75% with mucopurulent cervical discharge
- 75% have ESR >15 mm/hour
- 50% have WBC > 10,000/mm^3
- Have low threshold to treat as inpatient

Diagnosis
All three should be present:
1. History of lower abdominal pain and the presence of lower abdominal tenderness with or without evidence of rebound.
2. Cervical motion tenderness
3. Adnexal tenderness (may be unilateral)

Additional criteria that support a diagnosis of PID include:
- Oral temperature >101°F (>38.3°C)
- Abnormal cervical or vaginal discharge
- Elevated erythrocyte sedimentation rate
- Elevated C-reactive protein, and
- Laboratory documentation of cervical infection with *N. gonorrhoeae* or *C. trachomatis*

The definitive criteria for diagnosing PID in selected cases include:
- Histopathologic evidence of endometritis on endometrial biopsy
- Transvaginal sonography or other imaging techniques showing thickened fluid-filled tubes with or without free pelvic fluid or tubo-ovarian complex, and
- Laparoscopic abnormalities consistent with PID

Treatment
Outpatient
Regimen A
Ofloxacin, 400 mg PO bid for 14 days
  plus
Metronidazole, 500 mg PO bid for 14 days
Regimen B
Cefoxitin, 2 g IM plus probenecid 1 g orally in a single dose, or
Ceftriaxone, 250 mg IM or other parenteral third-generation cephalosporin (e.g., cefotaxime or cefizoxime)
  plus
Doxycycline, 100 mg PO bid for 14 days

Inpatient
Regimen A*
Cefoxitin, 2 g IV q6h, or
Cefotetan, 2 g IV q12h
  plus
Doxycycline, 100 mg PO or IV q12h

*The above regimen should be continued for at least 48 hours after the patient shows significant clinical improvement. After hospital discharge, doxycycline, 100 mg PO bid, should be continued for a total of 14 days.

Regimen B*
Clindamycin, 900 mg IV q8h
  plus
Gentamicin, loading dose IV or IM (2 mg/kg) followed by 1.5 mg/kg IV or IM q8h.

*The above regimen should be continued for at least 48 hours after the patient shows significant clinical improvement. After hospital discharge, doxycycline, 100 mg PO bid, or clindamycin, 450 mg PO 4 times/day, should be continued for a total of 14 days.

Criteria for Hospitalization

- Pregnancy (rare)
- Uncertain diagnosis
- Upper peritoneal signs
- Noncompliant patient
- Consider for acute PID cases
- Suspected pelvic or tuboovarian abscess
- Temperature >38°C
- Nausea and vomiting precluding oral medications
- Failure to respond to oral antibiotics in 48 hours

Other Treatment Guidelines
Uncomplicated Gonococcal Infections
A single dose of
Ceftriaxone 125 mg IM, or
Cefixime 400 mg PO, or
Ciprofloxacin 500 mg PO, or
Ofloxacin 400 mg PO
  plus
A regimen effective against coinfection with *C. trachomatis*, such as doxycycline, 100 mg PO bid for 7 days, or azithromycin, 1 g PO in a single dose.

Chancroid
Recommended:
Azithromycin 1 g PO in a single dose, or
Ceftriaxone 250 mg IM in a single dose, or
Erythromycin base 500 mg PO 4 times/day for 7 days *or*
Ciprofloxacin 500 mg PO bid for 3 days

continued

INFECTIOUS DISEASE

Chlamydia
Recommended:
Doxycycline 100 mg PO bid for 7 days, or
Azithromycin 1 g PO in a single dose
Alternative:
Ofloxacin 300 mg PO bid for 7 days, or
Erythromycin base 500 mg PO 4 times/day for 7 days, or
Erythromycin ethylsuccinate 800 mg PO 4 times/day for 7 days, or
Sulfisoxazole 500 mg PO 4 times/day for 10 days

Genital Herpes
Recommended regimens:
Acyclovir 400 mg PO tid for 7–10 days or
Acyclovir 200 mg PO 5 times/day for 7–10 days or
Famciclovir 250 mg PO tid for 7–10 days or
Valacyclovir 1 g bid for 7–10 days
Recommended regimens for episodic recurrent infection:
Acyclovir 400 mg PO tid for 5 days or
Acyclovir 200 mg PO 5 times/day for 5 days or
Acyclovir 800 mg PO bid for 5 days or
Famciclovir 125 mg PO bid for 5 days or
Valacyclovir 500 mg PO bid for 5 days
Recommended regimens for daily suppressive therapy:
Acyclovir 400 mg PO bid or
Famciclovir 250 mg PO bid or
Valacyclovir 250 mg PO bid or
Valacyclovir 500 mg PO once a day or
Valacyclovir 1,000 mg PO once a day

Syphilis
Patients with primary, secondary, or latent syphilis of <1 year's duration should receive:
Benzathine PCN G 2.4 million units IM in a single dose
Patients with latent syphilis of >1 year's duration should receive:
Benzathine PCN G 7.2 million units IM given as three weekly doses of 2.4 million units

External Genital Warts
Patient-applied:
Podofilox 0.5% solution or gel bid for 3 days followed by 4 days of no therapy. Repeat as needed × 4. Total wart area <10 cm^2, total volume of podofilox <0.5 ml/day.
or
Imiquimod 5% cream; apply qhs three times/week for as long as 16 weeks.
Provider-applied:
Cryotherapy
Podophyllin resin 10–25%
TCA or BCA 80–90%
Surgical removal

TRANSPLANT INFECTIONS

Time Course of Infections   (*Clin Microbiol Rev* 10:86, 1997)

First Month

Postoperative complications:

- Bacterial and candidal wound infections
- UTI
- Catheter-related infection
- Pneumonia
- Line sepsis
- HSV

Two to Six Months

Classic transplant infections:

- PCP
- *Nocardia*
- Listeriosis
- CMV
- Aspergillus
- Toxoplasmosis
- Reactivation of TB, histomycosis, coccidioidomycosis

More Than 6 Months

Common infections:

- Herpes zoster
- Patients with chronic rejection may continue to have infections as listed in 2- to 6-months category
- Patients immunosuppressed with HIV, HBV, HCV
- Pneumonia

INFECTIOUS DISEASE

HUMAN IMMUNODEFICIENCY VIRUS AND ACQUIRED IMMUNODEFICIENCY SYNDROME (J Bartlett. *The Johns Hopkins Hospital Guide to Medical Care of Patients with HIV Infection*, 7th ed. Philadelphia: Lippincott Williams & Wilkins, 1997)

Opportunistic Infections in Human Immunodeficiency Virus

CD4 count	Opportunistic infections	Prophylaxis
>500	Candidal vaginitis	
200–500	Pneumococcal pneumonia, other pneumonias, pulmonary TB, herpes zoster, thrush, *Candida* esophagitis, cryptosporidiosis, B cell lymphoma	
100–200	PCP, disseminated HSV, toxoplasmosis, cryptococcal infections, disseminated histoplasmosis and/or microsporidiosis, extrapulmonary TB	PCP prophylaxis
<50–100	Disseminated CMV, disseminated *Mycobacterium avium-intracellulare*, toxoplasmosis, cryptococcal infection, histoplasmosis/coccidioidomycosis	MAI prophylaxis, toxoplasmosis prophylaxis if seropositive

Prophylaxis in Human Immunodeficiency Virus

Disease	Indications	Regimen
TB	PPD >5 mm, prior positive PPD, high-risk exposure	INH 300 mg/day + pyridoxine 50 mg/day × 12 mos
PCP	Prior PCP, CD4 <200, HIV-associated thrush or FUO × 2 wks	TMP-SMX DS tablet qd
Toxoplasmosis	CD4 <100 + positive serology (IgG)	TMP-SMX DS tablet qd
Mycobacterium avium	CD4 <50–75	Rifabutin 300 mg/day, azithromycin 1,200 mg weekly, or clarithromycin 500 mg bid
S. pneumoniae	All patients	Pneumococcal vaccine (best with CD4 >350)
Influenza	All patients	Influenza vaccine every year
Hepatitis B	Negative anti-HB$_c$ ± risk factors	Hepatitis B vaccine (3 doses)

Source: Adapted from 1997 USPHS/IDSA guidelines for the prevention of opportunistic infections in persons infected with human immunodeficiency virus. *Ann Intern Med* 127:922, 1997.

INFECTIOUS DISEASE

Treatment of Selected Opportunistic Infections in HIV-Infected Patients

Infection	Preferred treatment	Alternative treatment
Pneumocystis carinii, acute	TMP 15 mg/kg/day and SMX 75 mg/kg/day PO or IV in 3–4 divided doses × 21 days In moderate/severe or severe disease with PaO_2 <70 mm Hg, prednisone 40 mg PO bid × 5 days, then 40 mg PO qd × 5 days, then 40 mg PO qd × 5 days, then 20 mg PO qd to completion of treatment	TMP 15 mg/kg/day PO or IV and dapsone 100 mg/day PO × 21 days Pentamidine 4 mg/kg/day IV × 21 days Clindamycin 600 mg IV q8h or 300–450 mg PO q6h and primaquine 30 mg/day base PO × 21 days Atovaquone 750 mg PO with meal bid × 21 days Trimetrexate 45 mg/m²/day IV and folinic acid 20 mg/m² PO/IV q6h ± dapsone 100 mg/day × 21 days
Toxoplasma encephalitis, acute	Pyrimethamine 100–200 mg loading dose, then 50–100 mg/day PO and folinic acid 10 mg/day PO and sulfadiazine or trisulfapyrimidine 4–8 g/day PO for ≥6 wks Dexamethasone 4 mg PO/IV q6h if significant edema/mass	Pyrimethamine + folinic acid (prior doses) and clindamycin 900–1,200 mg IV q6h or 300–450 mg PO q6h for ≥6 wks Azithromycin 900 mg PO × 2 for day 1, then 1,200 mg/day × 6 wks, then 600 mg/day (<50 kg half-dose) Atovaquone 1,500 mg PO bid or 750 mg PO qid and folinic acid for patients who fail or are intolerant of standard therapy (salvage) Azithromycin 500 mg IV × 2 on day 1, then 500 mg/day × 9 days, then PO regimen
Cryptococcal meningitis (initial treatment)	Amphotericin B 0.5–1.0 mg/kg/day IV to complete 0.7–1.0 g or until 15 mg/kg and sterile CSF Amphotericin B 0.7 mg/kg/day IV × 10–14 days ± flucytosine 100 mg/day PO, then fluconazole 400 mg/day × 8–10 wks	Fluconazole 400 mg/day PO × 6–10 wks (only in patients with normal mental status) Itraconazole 200 mg PO tid × 3 days then 200 mg PO bid Fluconazole 400 mg/day PO and flucytosine 100 mg/kg/day PO
Coccidioidomycosis	Amphotericin B 0.5–1.0 mg/kg/day IV × ≥8 wks (2.0–2.5 g) Intrathecal amphotericin B for meningitis	Fluconazole 400 mg PO qd Itraconazole 200-mg tablet PO bid or 100 mg PO suspension bid

Source: Adapted from J Bartlett. *The Johns Hopkins Hospital Guide to Medical Care of Patients with HIV Infection*, 7th ed. Philadelphia: Lippincott Williams & Wilkins, 1997.

continued

INFECTIOUS DISEASE

Postexposure Prophylaxis for Health Care Workers

Risk factors for seroconversion in needle stick (*MMWR Morb Mortal Weekly Rep* 45:468, 1996):

- Deep injury
- Visible blood on device
- Source with late-stage HIV
- Needle placement in vein/artery

AZT prophylaxis reduces transmission rate by 79%.

Chemoprophylaxis after Occupational Exposure to Human Immunodeficiency Virus (*MMWR Morb Mortal Weekly Rep* 45:468, 1996)

Type of exposure	Source material	Antiretroviral prophylaxis	Antiretroviral regimen
Percutaneous	Blood		
	Highest risk	Recommend	ZDV + 3TC + IDV
	Increased risk	Recommend	ZDV + 3TC ± IDV
	No increased risk	Offer	ZDV + 3TC
	Fluid containing visible blood, other potentially infectious fluid, tissue	Offer	ZDV + 3TC
	Other body fluid (e.g., urine)	Do not offer	
Mucous membrane	Blood	Offer	ZDV + 3TC ± IDV
	Fluid containing visible blood, other potentially infectious fluid, tissue	Offer	ZDV ± 3TC
	Other body fluid (e.g., urine)	Do not offer	
Skin, increased risk	Blood	Offer	ZDV + 3TC ± IDV
	Fluid containing visible blood, other potentially infectious fluid, tissue	Offer	ZDV ± 3TC
	Other body fluid (e.g., urine)	Do not offer	

ZDV = zidovudine/AZT 200 mg PO tid or 300 mg PO bid; 3TC = lamivudine 150 mg PO bid; IDV = indinavir 800 mg PO tid or other well-absorbed/tolerated protease inhibitor.
Note: Start prophylaxis as soon as possible (within 1–2 hours).

TUBERCULOSIS TREATMENT *(Am J Resp Crit Care Med 149:1359, 1994; MMWR Morb Mortal Weekly Rep 39RR–8, 9–15, 1990)*

Tuberculosis Classification

Tuberculosis Exposure, No Evidence of Infection
- History of exposure
- Negative PPD
- Treatment: none

Tuberculosis Infection, No Disease
- Positive PPD
- Negative symptoms, CXR
- Treatment: prophylactic/preventative

Tuberculosis Infection, Current Disease
- Positive PPD
- Positive clinical or CXR
- Obtain sputum for smear and culture × 3:
    If smear is positive, perform PCR to confirm *Mycobacterium tuberculosis* (within 48 hours).
    Once culture results are available, therapy can be tailored based on sensitivities.
- Treatment: full

Tuberculosis, No Current Disease
- Positive PPD
- Evidence of old disease on CXR
- No symptoms or active disease on CXR
- Treatment: consider prophylactic/preventative

Tuberculosis Suspected
- Diagnosis pending

Regimen Options for the Initial Treatment of Tuberculosis among Children and Adults

Tuberculosis without Human Immunodeficiency Virus Infection
- **Option 1:** Daily INH, RIF, PZA for 8 weeks followed by 16 weeks of INH and RIF daily or two to three times a week.* Add EMB or SM to the initial regimen until susceptibility to INH and RIF is demonstrated. If sensitive to INH or RIF, may discontinue others. Continue treatment for at least 6 months and 3 months beyond culture conversion. Consult a TB expert if the patient is symptomatic or smear- or culture-positive after 3 months.
- **Option 2:** Daily INH, RIF, PZA, and SM or EMB for 2 weeks followed by twice weekly* administration of the same drugs for 6 weeks (by direct observed therapy) and subsequently with twice weekly* administration of INH and RIF for 16 weeks (by direct observed therapy). If sensitive to INH or RIF, may discontinue others. Consult a TB expert if the patient is symptomatic or smear- or culture-positive after 3 months.
- **Option 3:** Direct observed therapy, three times a week* with INH, RIF, PZA, and EMB or SM for 6 months. If sensitive to INH or RIF, may discontinue others. Consult a TB expert if the patient is symptomatic or smear- or culture-positive after 3 months.

INFECTIOUS DISEASE

Tuberculosis with Human Immunodeficiency Virus Infection

- Option 1, 2, or 3 can be used, but treatment regimen should continue for a total of 9 months and at least 6 months beyond culture conversion.

*All regimens administered twice or thrice weekly should be monitored by direct observation therapy for duration of therapy.

Note: Three-drug treatment with INH, RIF, and PZA is acceptable for pan-sensitive strains and for empiric initial treatment of immunocompetent patients likely to have susceptible strains.

Tuberculosis Treatment Medications

Drug	Daily dose	Adverse reactions
Isoniazid (INH)	5 mg/kg PO or IM, max dose 300 mg (100-, 300-mg tablets)	Elevated hepatic enzymes, hepatitis, peripheral neuropathy, hypersensitivity
Rifampin (RIF)	10 mg/kg, max 600 mg (150-, 300-mg capsules)	Orange discoloration of secretions and urine, nausea, vomiting, fever, hepatitis, purpura
Pyrazinamide (PZA)	15–30 mg/kg, max 2 g PO (500-mg tablet)	Hepatitis, hyperuricemia, arthralgias, rash, GI intolerance
Ethambutol (EMB)	15–25 mg/kg, max 2.5 g PO (100-, 400-mg tablets)	Optic neuritis, skin rash
Streptomycin (SM)	15 mg/kg IM, max 1 g IM	Ototoxicity, possible nephrotoxicity

Preventive Treatment for Tuberculosis

Category	Isoniazid preventive therapy
HIV-positive or abnormal chest x-ray	Treat if PPD ≥5 mm and HIV-positive or chest x-ray evidence of old TB
Risk factor*	Treat if PPD ≥10 mm and age <35 yrs
No known risks	Treat if PPD ≥15 mm and age <35 yrs

*Risk factors: HIV known, or at risk for HIV and suspected but status unknown; close contacts with newly diagnosed cases; IV drug abusers known to be HIV-seronegative; medical conditions increasing the risk of developing TB if infected (silicosis, diabetes, steroids, other immunosuppressive therapy, hematologic and lymphoproliferative diseases, ESRD, and conditions associated with rapid weight loss or chronic malnutrition); foreign-born persons from high-incidence countries (Latin America, Asia, Africa); medically underserved low-income populations; residents of long-term care facilities; staff of facilities who would pose risk to large numbers of susceptible persons.

Usual Regimen

- Isoniazid 300 mg/day for 6–12 months (HIV and stable chest x-ray, 12 months; others, 6–12 months)
- Chest x-rays should be followed up on an annual basis if the PPD is positive and no active disease is present

ANTIBIOTIC SENSITIVITIES*

(Reprinted with permission from L Tompkins, EJ Baron, SD Munro, et al. Antibiotic susceptibility of bacterial isolates. Stanford, CA: UCSF Stanford Health Care: Clinical Microbiology/Virology Laboratory, 1997.)

> **Interpretation of susceptibility results**
> Results are reported as minimum inhibitory concentrations (MICs), the amount of drug needed to inhibit growth. Interpretive criteria are based on achievable serum levels. Thus, for certain antibiotics, the amount excreted into the urine via the kidneys is above the MIC, and may be reported as "resistant," but the agent is effective clinically in this site. Intermediate results (I), especially for beta-lactam agents, indicate that doses higher than standard recommendations may be effective. In other cases, "I" results indicate that the organism may be susceptible or resistant but the in vitro tests are not sensitive enough to determine specifically. For this antibiogram, Intermediate results are NOT included within the "%S" category.

Gram-negative rods (a)

Percent Susceptible by Broth Microdilution MIC 4/1/97 - 12/31/97	No. Tested	PENICILLINS			CEPHALOSPORINS					LACTAMS		AMINOGLYCs			OTHER		URINE ONLY		
		Ampicillin	Piperacillin	Piperacillin/Tazobactam (b)	Cefazolin	Cefotetan (c)	Cefuroxime I.V.	Cefotaxime	Ceftazidime	Aztreonam (d)	Imipenem	Gentamicin	Tobramycin	Amikacin	Ciprofloxacin	TrimethSulfa	1st generation Cephalosporins (see)	Nitrofurantoin	Tetracycline
Acinetobacter baumannii	44	(e)	70						91	34	95	73	95	89	66	91			
Acinetobacter lwoffi	21		86								100	100	100	100	100	90			
Burkholderia cepacia	8		0	17					17		0	0	0	0	0	33			
Citrobacter freundii	51	12	57	78	6	83	65	69	71	73	100	98	100	100	88	73	9	91	83
Citrobacter koseri	21	0	48	100	100	100	100	100	100	100	100	100	100	100	100	90	100	81	88
Enterobacter aerogenes	85	5	64	66	5	66	56	67	66	72	100	99	99	100	96	99		15	88
Enterobacter cloacae	180	3	63	74	2	56	23	63	65	66	99	98	99	100	94	79		16	79
Escherichia coli	1456	61	63	96	88	100	95	99	99	99	100	96	97	100	97	77	48	97	69
Klebsiella oxytoca	65	2	43	97	54	100	88	100	100	95	100	100	100	100	100	92	50	88	75
Klebsiella pneumoniae	324	2	52	93	92	99	90	100	99	100	100	96	98	100	95	89	87	42	84
Morganella morganii	30	0	80	97	0	93	3	90	90	97	90	77	83	97	87	77	0	0	27
Proteus mirabilis	130	88	98	100	92	98	95	100	100	99	91	92	99	95	89	94	86	1	1
Proteus vulgaris (indole +)	17	0	53	100	0	0	0	0	82	100	100	94	100	100	100	100	100	0	
Pseudomonas aeruginosa	669		83	86					76	85	76	61	78	70	65				
Salmonella spp.	30	33						100(c)							100	97			
Serratia marcescens	103	0	72	77	0	94	0	72	95	97	97	85	83	97	89	94	0	0	0
Stenotrophomonas maltophilia	84								37		0				12	96			
Cost($) Inject. Drug only		1.02/g	11.60/4g	15.74/4g	1.96	8.58	3.29/750 mg	7.70	7.95	12.92/g	21.17/500 mg	.07/80 mg	2.79/80 mg	4.75/500 mg	25.00/400 mg	6.07/DS			Doxy 5.07/100mg
Oral		0.11/500 mg													3.17/500 DS tab	0.08/DS 500 tab		0.34/50 tab	Doxy 0.09/100mg

(a) Until final identifications are available, reports describe gram-negative rods as **lactose-fermenters (LF**; such as E. coli, Klebsiella, Enterobacter, Citrobacter); **non-lactose-fermenters (NLF**, such as Proteus, Serratia, Salmonella, Shigella), or **non-fermenters (NF**, such as Pseudomonas, Acinetobacter, Stenotrophomonas, and others, which are intrinsically more resistant to many antibiotics).

(b) Tazobactam adds no increased activity to that of piperacillin against Pseudomonas aeruginosa; pip/tazo should be reserved for mixed aerobic/anaerobic infections with need for broad gram-negative coverage (involving Enterobacteriaceae, Pseudomonas, etc.).

(c) Not all isolates tested against this antibiotic

(d) Aztreonam should NOT be considered as replacement for aminoglycosides in most situations. Aminoglycosides have better in-vitro activity than aztreonam against aerobic gram-negative rods. Unlike aztreonam, aminoglycosides have synergistic activity with β-lactams (ex: piperacillin, ampicillin) against aerobic gram-negative rods and enterococci. Aztreonam should only be used for treating documented infections due to susceptible organisms in patients with anaphylactic reactions to β-lactams. In patients with renal insufficiency, aminoglycosides can be administered safely when doses are adjusted for patient's renal function. For information on dosing, including single daily dosing, please contact Team Clinical Pharmacist (get beeper # from unit secretary).

(e) For Acinetobacter baumannii, ampicillin/sulbactam (93% susceptible) is used instead of ampicillin.

(f) Use of 3rd gen. cephems, such as ceftazidime, for Enterobacter bacteremia has been associated with development of resistance during therapy and subsequent increased mortality. Piperacillin did not show this effect. Therefore, piperacillin + aminoglycoside is treatment of choice for infections due to susceptible strains of Enterobacter spp, and Pseudomonas aeruginosa.

*All decisions about antibiotics should be based on current local antibiotic sensitivities from area hospitals and microbiology laboratories. While the Stanford data may be used as a starting point, it should not be relied on solely, as geographic and temporal resistance patterns may vary.

continued

INFECTIOUS DISEASE

Anaerobes
Anaerobic bacteria not listed have not exhibited resistance. Individual isolates will be tested in cases of therapeutic failure. All 5 fusobacteria tested were uniformly susceptible to all antibiotics. Peptostreptococci and Propionibacterium spp. are susceptible to most antibiotics with anaerobic activity, except that the nonspore-forming gram-positive rods (including Actinomyces and Propionibacterium) do not respond to metronidazole because they are somewhat aerotolerant.

Percent Susceptible by Broth Microdilution MIC 4/1/97 - 12/31/97	No. Tested	Penicillin	Piperacillin	Amp/sulbactam (a)	Ticar/clavulanate	Imipenem	Cefotetan	Chloramphenicol	Clindamicin	Metronidazole
Bacteroides fragilis	14	0	64	100	100	100	71	100	79	100
B.fragilis group (other)	7	0	71	100	100	100	29	100	57	100
Clostridium species	9	89	100	100	100	100	100	100	100	100

(a) Amp/sulbactam costs $10.98/3g

No. Tested	Ampicillin	Amox/Clav	Cefuroxime I.V.	Cefotaxime	Cefaclor	Ciprofloxacin	Trimeth/Sulfa	Chloramphenicol
63	60	100	100	100	100	79	100	89	100

Haemophilus influenzae.
Percent susceptible by Broth Microdilution MIC, 4/1/97-12/31/97, for infections with β-lactamase producing H.influenzae: cefuroxime, cefotaxime, trimethoprim/sulfamethoxazole, amoxicillin/clavulanate, or azithromycin is recommended. Cefotaxime or ceftriaxone is drug of choice for CNS infections.

Mycobacteria
In vitro results of susceptibility tests of M. avium complex isolates have not been shown to correlate with clinical response, particularly since regimens must include combinations and testing is done singly. One exception is clarithromycin (which also predicts azithromycin), for which treatment failures do correlate with in vitro resistance.

Tested by radiometric method Percent Susceptible 4/1/97-12/31/97	No. Tested	Isoniazid 0.1 ug / ml	Streptomycin 2.0 ug / ml	Ethambutol 2.5 ug / ml	Rifampin 2.0 ug / ml	Clarithromycin
M. tuberculosis	10	90	90	100	100	
M. avium complex	15					100

Staphylococci (a)

Percent Susceptible by Broth Microdilution MIC 4/1/97 - 12/31/97	No. Tested	Penicillin (a)	Oxacillin, Nafcillin, Methicillin (b,c)	Cephalosporins 1st generation (c)	Vancomycin	Erythromycin	Clindamycin	Gentamicin	Trimeth/Sulfa	Ciprofloxacin	Tetracycline	Nitrofurantoin (urines only)
Staphylococcus aureus (All;b)	759	12	94	94	100	68	91	97	98	91	93	
MRSA (ONLY) (c)	49	0	0	0	100	16	39	80	89	33		
Staph. coagulase negative	640	18	43	43	100	41	67	72	66	62	72	99
Staph. epidermidis	352	6	24	24	100	23	49	54	48	42	75	100
Staph. haemolyticus	21	19	29	29	100	20	60	62	48	38	73	100
Staph. saprophyticus	19	11	95	95	100			100	100	100	74	100
Cost($) - Drug only Inject.		0.60ml	Naf 1.30/g	1.96/g	5.93/g	1.27/g	3.34/ 600mg	0.70/ 80mg	6.07/ DSamp400mg	25.00/ 400mg	Doxy 5.00/ 100mg	
Oral		0.09/ 250mg	Diclox 0.27/ 500mg	0.13/ 500mg	0.07/ 500mg	0.07/ 500mg	0.95/ 150mg		0.08/ DS tab	3.17/ 500mg	Doxy 0.09/ 100mg	0.34/ 50mg

(a) Penicillin-resistant staphylococci should be considered resistant to all penicillinase-sensitive penicillins, including ampicillin, amoxicillin, mezlocillin, piperacillin, and ticarcillin.

(b) For S. aureus, nafcillin and first generation cephalosporins are recommended drugs of choice at SHC due to low incidence of resistance (6%) to methicillin/nafcillin/oxacillin.

(c) Methicillin resistant staphylococci should be considered resistant to all penicillins, cephalosporins, imipenem, and β-lactams including combinations with clavulanic acid, subbactam and tazobactam. Oxacillin susceptibility predicts susceptibility to all other beta-lactam agents.

continued

Streptococci

Percent Susceptible by Broth Microdilution MIC or disk diffusion 4/1/97 – 12/31/97

	No. Tested	Penicillin or Ampicillin %S	%I	Cefuroxime	Ceftriaxone	Vancomycin	Erythromycin	Clindamycin	Chloramphenicol	Trimethoprim / sulfa	Tetracycline (d)	Gentamicin Synergy with Pen / Amp	Streptomycin Synergy with Pen / Amp	Ciprofloxacin (d)	Nitrofurantoin (d)
Grp. A (Strep pyogenes)	16	100	0	100	100		69	88							
Grp. B (Strep agalactiae) (a)	163	82	18	74	100		66	53	79						
Grp. C, F and G	37	100	0	100	100		70	92							
Grp. D enterococci (b)	345	99	0			99					32	85	77	58	100
Enterococcus faecalis (b)	137	99	0			99					13	84	73	55	100
Enterococcus faecium (b)	126	13	0			25					74	32	32	4	91
Viridans (various species)	36	83	6	86	100		72	100			84				
Strep. pneumoniae (c)	63	70	22	75	88	100	76		91	63	84				
Cost ($) – Drug only — Inject. / Oral		Amp 0.11/500mg (Oral); Amp 1.02/g (Inject.)													

(a) Penicillin is the drug of choice; no clinical pen. resistance has been documented, despite in vitro results.

(b) If susceptible, ampicillin is the drug of choice when enterococci must be treated. Nitrofurantoin or ampicillin are recommended for UTI. Serious infections (septicemia, endocarditis) require both a β-lactam agent and an aminoglycoside. Use vancomycin + aminoglycoside only if strain is ampicillin-resistant or patient is penicillin-allergic. High level resistance to gentamicin also indicates lack of synergy for tobramycin, amikacin, and kanamycin.

(c) Penicillin-susceptible isolates are also susceptible to all other appropriate beta-lactam agents. Beta-lactamase inhibitor combination drugs do not add additional efficacy to penicillin alone. Penicillin-intermediate strains may respond to increased penicillin dosing, except for meningitis for which ceftriaxone should be used if susceptible. Infectious diseases consultation is recommended for meningitis in penicillin-allergic patients or those with intermediate or resistant ceftriaxone / cefotaxime results. Of the 5 penicillin-resistant isolates tested (8% of all strains), 2 were ceftriaxone-intermediate and 3 were ceftriaxone-resistant (88% susceptible).

(d) Urine Enterococcus isolates only.

SITUATIONS FOR WHICH THE USE OF VANCOMYCIN IS APPROPRIATE AND ACCEPTABLE:

---

1. For treatment of serious infections due to β-lactam-resistant gram-positive bacteria. Clinicians should be aware that vancomycin is usually less active and less rapidly bactericidal than β-lactam agents for organisms that are susceptible to the β-lactams.

2. For treatment of infections due to gram-positive organisms in patients with serious allergy to β-lactam antibiotics.

3. Prophylaxis, as recommended by the Amer. Heart Assoc., for endocarditis following certain procedures in patients at high risk for endocarditis.

4. Prophylaxis for major surgical procedures involving implantation of prosthetic materials or devices, e.g., cardiac and vascular procedures and total hip replacements, at institutions with a high rate of infections due to MRSA or MRSE (not currently at SHC). A single dose administered before surgery is sufficient unless the procedure lasts more than 6 hours, in which case the dose should be repeated. Prophylaxis should be dc'd after 2 doses maximum.

Fungi

Although the merits of in vitro antifungal susceptibilities for predicting clinical response are still being studied, the Mycology laboratory has results (by Dr. David Stevens' laboratory) from a few selected isolates from systemic infections. These results agree with those of published series. Additional isolates were tested in numbers too low to report here.

Percent Susceptible by Broth Dilution 1/1/97 - 6/30/98	No. Tested (a)	Amphotericin B	Fluconazole	Itraconazole	5-fluorocytosine
Candida albicans	10	100	67	67	100
Candida (Torulopsis) glabrata	6	100	50	100	
Aspergillus fumigatus	10	100	0	90	17
Scedosporium apiospermum	6	67	0	25	

(a) Not all isolates were tested with each agent.

8. Neurology

DERMATOMES
Anterior View

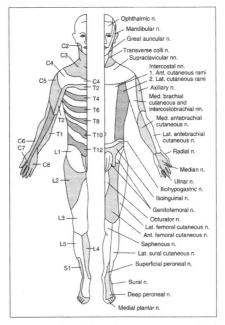

Anterior view of dermatomes (*left*) and cutaneous areas supplied by individual peripheral nerves (*right*). [Reprinted with permission from The McGraw-Hill Companies. AS Fauci, JB Martin, E Braunwald, et al., (eds). *Harrison's principles of internal medicine*, 14th ed. New York: McGraw-Hill, 1998:124.]

Posterior View

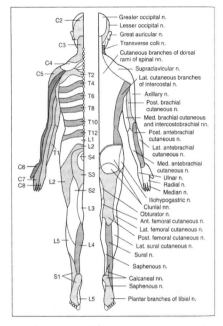

Posterior view of dermatomes (*left*) and cutaneous areas supplied by individual peripheral nerves (*right*). [Reprinted with permission from The McGraw-Hill Companies. AS Fauci, JB Martin, E Braunwald, et al., (eds). *Harrison's principles of internal medicine*, 14th ed. New York: McGraw-Hill, 1998:124.]

NEUROLOGY

PERIPHERAL NERVES

Radial Nerve
- Sensory: dorsolateral surface of upper arm (lateral cutaneous nerve of arm, posterior cutaneous nerve of arm), forearm (posterior cutaneous nerve of arm), wrist, hand, and dorsal surface of first three and a half fingers above the DIP joint
- Motor: extension of thumb at IP, MCP joint; extension of index finger at MCP joint; abduction of thumb at MCP joint; extension of wrist toward radial side

Median Nerve
- Sensory: dorsal surface of first three and a half fingers, lateral two-thirds of palm and palmar three and a half fingers
- Motor: flexion of second and third fingers at DIP; abduction of thumb at MCP joint, thumb opposition with fifth digit

Ulnar Nerve
- Sensory: dorsal and palmar surfaces of medial third of hand; dorsal and palmar surfaces of medial one and a half digits
- Motor: flexion of fourth and fifth fingers at DIP; abduction of fifth digit; finger abduction; adduction of second digit

Femoral Nerve
- Sensory: anterior and medial surface of thigh, medial calf, ankle, and foot
- Motor: extension of leg at knee (quadriceps femoris)

Peroneal Nerve
- Sensory: lateral surface of lower leg and calf; dorsal foot
- Motor: dorsiflexion of foot at ankle; foot eversion at ankle; dorsiflexion of toes

Nylen-Bárány Maneuver
- Equipment: exam table with ability to allow patient's head to drop 30 degrees below horizontal, over the edge of the table, when lying flat.
- Procedure: Sit patient upright on table with head turned to right and lower quickly to supine position with head past the edge of the table, dropped 30 degrees below the horizontal. Observe for symptoms of vertigo or evidence of nystagmus.
- Repeat maneuver with head turned to left and in midline.

GLASGOW COMA SCALE

Criteria	Scale	Score
Eyes open	Never	1
	To pain	2
	To verbal stimuli	3
	Spontaneously	4
Best verbal response	No response	1
	Incomprehensible sounds	2
	Inappropriate words	3
	Disoriented and converses	4
	Oriented and converses	5
Best motor response	No response	1
	Extension (decerebrate)	2
	Flexion (decorticate)	3
	Flexion withdrawal	4
	Localizes pain	5
	Obeys	6
Total possible score		15

NEUROLOGY

INCREASED INTRACRANIAL PRESSURE

Etiology
- CNS tumor/metastasis
- Brain abscess
- Other CNS mass
- Intracranial hemorrhage
- Cerebral infarction

Signs and Symptoms
- Headache (especially if raised ICP is acute)
- Nausea, vomiting
- Focal neurologic findings
- Lethargy
- Fever (in brain abscess, meningitis, or encephalitis)
- Altered level of consciousness
- Papilledema (more common in sub-acute onset)

Diagnosis
- CT scan
- EEG
- MRI
- Blood cultures (for brain abscess)

Management
Consider the following:
- Acute pharmacologic management: mannitol (0.5–2.0 g/kg IV, then 0.25–0.5 g/kg IV q4h to maintain ICP <320 mOsm)
- Surgery
- Antibiotics ± surgery in brain abscesses
- Dexamethasone (4–20 mg IV q6h; primarily for mass effect and shift with intracranial tumors)
- Hyperventilation (post-intubation)
- Chemotherapy or radiotherapy for CNS tumors

COMA: CORRELATING EXAMINATION FINDINGS WITH LEVEL OF BRAIN DYSFUNCTION

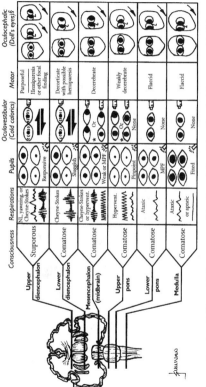

Source: Jonathan Sullivan, M.D., courtesy of the *Detroit Receiving Hospital Emergency Medicine Handbook.*

NEUROLOGY

TRANSIENT INSOMNIA ("SLEEPER") (N Engl J Med 322:239, 1990; J Maldonado. *Delirium, alcohol withdrawal, acute confusional states*. Stanford Health Services, 1997)

Fast Facts
- First, improve sleep hygiene and sleep-wake cycles.
- Remove inciting medications (e.g., caffeine).
- Avoid triazolam (Halcion).
- Avoid agents that alter sleep/wake cycle or exacerbate confusion:
    Medications with high anticholinergic effects (e.g., diphenhydramine)
    Pain medications
    Zolpidem (Ambien) in elderly patients
- In elderly patients, use half-doses and watch for agitation (haloperidol 0.5–1.0 mg PO q6h may work).

Management
Young, Healthy (18–65 Years)
- Trazodone (Desyrel) 50–200 mg PO qhs
- Zolpidem (Ambien) 5–20 mg PO qhs
- Temazepam (Restoril) 15–30 mg PO qhs
- Chloral hydrate (Noctec) 500–2,000 mg PO qhs

Elderly (>65 Years)
- Trazodone (Desyrel) 50–200 mg PO qhs
- Temazepam (Restoril) 15–30 mg PO qhs
- Flurazepam (Dalmane) 15–30 mg PO qhs
- Chloral hydrate 250 mg PO qhs
- Do not use more than one benzodiazepine in the same patient.

ALTERED MENTAL STATUS (Δ-MS)
(N Engl J Med 320:578, 1989; N Engl J Med 335:330, 1996; J Maldonado. *Delirium, alcohol withdrawal, acute confusional states*. Stanford Health Services, 1997)

Features of Delirium
- Disturbance of consciousness
- Change in cognition
- Perceptual disturbances
- Global cognitive impairment
- Attentional abnormalities
- Increased or decreased psychomotor activity
- Sleep-wake cycle disruption
- Waxing and waning pattern

Differential Diagnosis

Mnemonic: I WATCH DEATH:

- **I**nfectious: encephalitis, meningitis, syphilis, septicemia
- **W**ithdrawal syndromes: alcohol, barbiturates, sedative-hypnotics
- **A**cute metabolic encephalopathies: acidosis/alkalosis, electrolyte disturbances, hepatic/renal failure, hypersensitivity reactions
- **T**rauma: head, heat stroke, postoperative status, severe burn
- **C**NS pathology: seizures, neoplasms, abscesses, hemorrhages, stroke, vasculitis, normal pressure hydrocephalus
- **H**ypoxia: pulmonary/cardiac failure, hypoperfusion, anemia, hypotension, intraoperative complications, carbon monoxide poisoning
- **D**eficiencies: vitamin B_{12}, folate, hypovitaminosis, niacin, thiamine
- **E**ndocrinopathies: hyper-/hypoadrenalcorticism, hyper-/hypoglycemia, hyper-/hypothyroidism
- **A**cute vascular: hypertensive encephalopathy, shock
- **T**oxins/drugs: medications (especially anticholinergic), poisons, pesticides, solvents
- **H**eavy metals: lead, manganese, mercury

Diagnosis

- Review time course and medication list
- √SaO$_2$
- √Cultures/LP if suspected infection
- √EEG
- √Neurologic exam
- √CBC/electrolytes
- √Head CT
- √Vitamin B_{12}, folate, TFT, ESR, VDRL, finger-stick blood glucose

Management

- Cocktail of 50 ml D50 + thiamine 100 mg + naloxone 0.4–0.8 mg IV.
- Correct electrolytes, vitamins, nutrition.
- Neuroleptic medication; treatment of choice is haloperidol.
- Combined neuroleptic-benzodiazepines can also be used.
    Haloperidol and lorazepam are favored (no active metabolites).
    Combination allows use of less haloperidol, thus minimizing side effects.
    Act synergistically to control agitation.
    Haloperidol dose is usually at least twice the lorazepam dose.
- "Sundowning":
    Reorient with reassurance, quiet room, calendar, familiar objects.
    Sedation:
        Haloperidol 0.5–1.0 mg PO q4–6h.
        Lorazepam (Ativan) 0.5–1.0 mg PO q6h.
        Watch for ↑agitation in elderly.
- Limit the use of CNS active medications, such as narcotics, antiemetics, and H_2-blockers.

NEUROLOGY

ALCOHOL WITHDRAWAL   (*Am Fam Physician* 54:2, 1996; J Maldonado. *Delirium, alcohol withdrawal, acute confusional states.* Stanford Health Services, 1997)

Early Withdrawal
- Begins on first day of abstinence within 3–6 hours of last drink, peaking 24–48 hours after cessation.
- Tremulousness, irritability, nausea, vomiting.
- Tension, general malaise, hypertension, autonomic hyperactivity, tachycardia, diaphoresis, orthostatic hypotension, insomnia.

Alcohol Hallucinosis
- Auditory (less common, visual) hallucinations with clear sensorium and stable vital signs
- Takes hours to days to resolve, usually within 24–48 hours

Alcohol Withdrawal Seizures ("Rum Fits")
- Generalized motor seizures in absence of known seizure disorder.
- Most common 12–48 hours after last drink (peak 13–24 hours).
- Hypomagnesemia, respiratory alkalosis, hypoglycemia, and increased intracellular sodium are associated.
- Approximately one-third of patients with alcohol withdrawal seizures go on to develop DTs.

Late Withdrawal—Delirium Tremens
- Starts 1–3 days after last drink, peak at days 4–5.
- Mortality usually about 1%, can be as high as 15% if untreated.
- Different from uncomplicated withdrawal by state of delirium/confusion.
- Confusion, disorientation, perceptual disturbances, agitation, insomnia, mild temperature, autonomic hyperactivity.
- Terror, agitation, visual and tactile hallucination (e.g., insects).
- Duration of confusion can be days to weeks, usually with delirious states separated by lucid intervals.
- Death results from infections, arrhythmias, fluid and electrolyte abnormalities, pyrexia, hypertension, suicide.

Treatment
Supportive
- No alcohol
- Adequate nutrition
- Reality orientation in a safe, well-lighted space
- Restraints for combative, agitated patients
- Correct: fluid balance, electrolyte, and BP

continued

Specific
- Correct fluid balance, but do not overcorrect.
- Vitamin supplementation:

  Thiamine 100 mg IV/IM/PO × 3 days   Folate 1 mg PO qd

  Multivitamin PO qd   Vitamin K 5–10 mg PO if INR >1.3
- Monitor fluid balance, electrolytes, vital signs.

Sedation with Benzodiazepines
- Effective in all levels of alcohol withdrawal.
- Dose prn to treat tremor, hypertension, tachycardia.
- Best to use long-acting agents (diazepam, chlordiazepoxide).
- In hepatic dysfunction, use lorazepam and oxazepam, which have no active metabolites.
- In general, avoid short-acting agents.

Degree of alcohol withdrawal	Treatment
Mild	Diazepam 20 mg PO qh × 3.
Moderate/severe	Diazepam 5–10 mg SL/IV q5–10min.
	Repeat until patient is sedated but arousable.
	Average required total dose: 30–160 mg.
	Once symptoms have been controlled, the long half-life allows self-taper.
	Mild re-emergence of withdrawal symptoms.
	Continue to give diazepam (e.g., 10–25 mg PO qh).
	Taper smaller doses over 1–2 wks; may add halo-peridol prn in severely agitated patients or in those experiencing severe hallucinosis.
Mild with liver damage/failure	Lorazepam 1–3 mg SL q4h prn until symptoms are controlled.
	After symptom control achieved, regular standing dose may be required to prevent return of symptoms. Consider lorazepam 2 mg SL/PO q4–6h around the clock, with slow taper of 20% per day.
Moderate/severe with liver damage/failure	Lorazepam 2–4 mg IV/IM q2h until symptom control has been achieved.
	After stabilization, sum total requirement of lorazepam during the first 24 hrs.
	Divide this amount to administer on q4h schedule.
	After 24–48 hrs of complete symptomatic control, initiate slow taper at a rate of no faster than 20% per day. A slightly larger dose may be required at bedtime for insomnia.

NEUROLOGY

DEMENTIA

Definition
- Impairment of cognitive function that does not alter the level of consciousness

Etiology
- Alzheimer's disease
- Multi-infarct dementia
- Parkinson's disease
- Huntington's disease
- Normal-pressure hydrocephalus
- Neoplasm
- Alcohol
- Vitamin B_{12} deficiency
- Wilson's disease
- Hypothyroidism
- Neurosyphilis
- AIDS dementia complex
- Creutzfeldt-Jakob disease
- Pseudodementia/depression

Diagnosis
- CBC
- LFT
- TFT
- Vitamin B_{12} level
- Ceruloplasmin
- FTA for syphilis
- CSF/VDRL for syphilis
- HIV test
- CSF for cytology
- CT or MRI

Management
- Treat correctable cause if one is found on evaluation.
- Neuroleptics to control psychotic features.

FOLSTEIN MINI-MENTAL STATUS EXAMINATION
(*J Psychiatr Res* 12:189, 1975; *JAMA* 269:2386, 1993)

Category	Score	Questions
Orientation	5	What is the year, season, date, day, month?
	5	Where are you? Country, state, town, hospital, floor?
Registration	3	Repeat and remember 3 named objects for later.
Attention/calculation	5	Serial 7 or spell world backward.
Recall	3	Repeat 3 objects from registration.
Language	2	Name 2 objects (point to them).
	1	Repeat, "No ifs, ands, or buts."
	3	Follow 3-stage command (take paper in right hand, fold it, and place it on the table).
	1	Read and obey a sentence (i.e., "close your eyes").
	1	Write any sentence.
	1	Copy figure.
Total possible score	30	

- Median total score:
  - Age 18–24: 29
  - Age ≥80: 25
- Absolute scores no longer generally accepted; score inversely related to age and directly related to years of schooling.

WEAKNESS: DIFFERENTIAL DIAGNOSIS OF ACUTE OR SUBACUTE ONSET

Central Nervous System (Above Spinal Cord)

- Cerebrovascular accident
- Hemorrhage
- Vasculitis
- Mass (neoplasm)
- Infection (abscess)
- Infection (encephalitis)

Spinal Cord

- Infection (polio)
- Infection (abscess)
- Multiple sclerosis
- Transverse myelitis
- Infarction
- Neoplasm
- Disk protrusion

Peripheral Nerve

- Guillain-Barré syndrome
- Heavy metal ingestion (e.g., arsenic)
- Poisoning (organophosphate)
- Porphyria

Neuromuscular Junction

- Myasthenia gravis
- Botulism

Muscle

- Myopathies
- Electrolyte abnormalities
- Hypokalemic periodic paralysis

NEUROLOGY

GUILLAIN-BARRÉ SYNDROME (*Lancet* 352:635, 1998)

Fast Facts
- Peripheral nerve polyneuropathy
- Demyelination of peripheral nerves

Differential Diagnosis of Polyneuropathy
- Diabetes-induced polyneuropathy
- Chronic renal insufficiency–induced polyneuropathy
- Vasculitic neuropathy
- Porphyria
- Nutritional deficiencies
- Heavy metals (gold, mercury, platinum, lead)
- Chronic alcoholism

Symptoms
- Ascending paralysis beginning with paresthesias in the feet
- Absent deep tendon reflexes
- 60% have viral prodrome of URI or diarrhea 2–4 weeks before
- Muscle weakness peaks at 14 days
- Can result in respiratory muscle paralysis

Diagnosis
- CSF, high protein with no pleocytosis
- Nerve conduction studies, slowing of conduction velocities

Management
- Monitor vital capacity and maximum inspiratory force: if less than 15–20 ml/kg, may require intubation and mechanical ventilation.
- IVIG: 400 mg/kg/day × 5 days; begin within 2 weeks of onset.
- Steroids are not helpful and may slow recovery.
- Chest PT/pulmonary toilet.
- DVT prophylaxis.
- ROM and turning to prevent decubiti and contractures.

EMERGENCY HEADACHE EVALUATION (*J Emerg Med* 15:617, 1997)

Diagnostic Clues
- History of trauma
- Location of pain, associated symptoms
- Timing of pain, acuity
- Papilledema
- Neurologic exam, especially cranial nerves
- Fever, neck stiffness

Etiology

Headache	Characteristics/remarks
Subdural/epidural hematoma	History of trauma, anticoagulation
Intracranial hemorrhage/ ischemic stroke	Unilateral, focal neurologic finding
Hypertensive encephalopathy	Diastolic BP >130 mm Hg
Vasculitis/temporal arteritis	Pain over temples, systemic symptoms (arthralgia, myalgia), palpable/tender temporal arteries
Intracranial mass	Chronic, progressive, uni/bilateral, focal neurologic signs (late)
Cavernous sinus disease	Chemosis, proptosis, CN III/IV/V$_{1-2}$/VI, VI deficits
CNS infection	Fever, neck stiffness, change in mental status
Dural vein thrombosis	Papilledema, focal neurologic signs
Pseudotumor cerebri/idiopathic intracranial hypertension	Papilledema
Carotid dissection	Sudden onset, unilateral, nonthrobbing periorbital pain, bruit, focal neurologic signs in carotid distribution
Subarachnoid hemorrhage	Acute onset, worst headache of life/severe pain
Episodic tension headache	≥2 of the following:
	Pressing/tightening (nonpulsating)
	Mild/moderate intensity
	Bilateral
	No ↑ with routine activity
	No nausea/vomiting/photophobia or phonophobia
Cluster headache	Middle-aged men; ≥5 episodes of severe unilateral periorbital pain often accompanied by ≥1 episode of ipsilateral nasal congestion, rhinorrhea, lacrimation, eye redness, and Horner's
Migraine headaches	See Migraine Headache on page 186

NEUROLOGY

MIGRAINE HEADACHE (*Neurol Clin* 8:841, 1990)

Migraine Headache without Aura
- ≥5 attacks
- ≥2 of the following: unilateral, pulsating, moderate/severe intensity, ↑ with routine physical activity
- ≥1 of the following: nausea ± vomiting, phonophobia, photophobia

Migraine Headache with Aura
- ≥2 attacks
- ≥3 of the following:
  - ≥1 reversible aura symptom
  - ≥1 aura symptom developing over 4 minutes or 2 in succession with no aura >60 minutes or headache ≤60 minutes after aura

Migraine Management

Symptoms	Treatment
Early/mild (0–2 hrs)	Quiet/dark room; isometheptene mucate, dichloralphenazone, and acetaminophen (Midrin)/NSAID for headache; metoclopramide (Reglan)/hydroxyzine hydrochloride (Atarax) for nausea
Moderate/severe (0–4 hrs)	No vomiting: oral antiemetic + ergotamine/Indocin
	Vomiting: antiemetic suppository + ergotamine suppository/sumatriptan (Imitrex) SC
Moderate/severe without response (2–6 hrs)	No vomiting: oral combined analgesia (Fiorinal) or codeine
	Vomiting: nasal butorphanol or chlorpromazine suppository
Severe unresponsive to outpatient treatment (6–72 hrs)	IV metoclopramide/Compazine + DHE; IM Toradol; IV dexamethasone; IV opiates
Persistent severe unresponsive (>48 hrs)	Admit to hospital: repetitive DHE protocol (above) with IV hydrocortisone/methylprednisolone; IV lidocaine (100-mg bolus 2 mg/min gtt) with cardiac monitor
Persistent neurologic deficits	Rule out ischemic, structural, inflammatory, metabolic CNS disease
First/worst headache	Exclude bleed with CT, full neurologic exam before potent narcotics; rule out infarction

Source: Reproduced with permission from KL Moore, SL Noble. Drug treatment of migraine. Part I. Acute therapy and drug-rebound headache. *Am Fam Physician* 56:2039, 1997.

Migraine Prophylaxis

Drug	Dosage, increase slowly	Considerations
Propran-olol	40–320 mg/day	If one beta-blocker does not work, another one may
Nortrip-tyline	10–100 mg/day	Especially for migraine with tension head-ache or depression
Diltiazem	90–360 mg/day	Unclear efficacy, good for prolific aura
Depakote	250–1,500 mg/day	Especially with severe migraine
Neurontin	100–800 mg tid	Especially with intolerance to tricyclic anti-depressants
Methyser-gide	2–8 mg/day	Severe/unresponsive to other agents; stop 1 mo q6mo; discontinue if no response after 3 wks
Phenelzine	15 mg tid, titrate up to 60 mg/day (max 90 mg/day)	Severe/unresponsive to other agents; close monitoring necessary given severe MAOI food/drug interactions

Source: Adapted from SL Noble, KL Moore. Drug treatment of migraine. Part II. Preventive therapy. *Am Fam Physician* 56:2279, 1997.

NEUROLOGY

STROKE AND THROMBOLYTICS (*Am Fam Physician* 55:2655, 1997; *Am Fam Physician* 57:1, 1998; *Stroke* 28:8, 1997; *Lancet* 352[Suppl], 1998)

Risk Factors

- TIA or prior cerebrovascular accident
- Carotid disease
- Atrial fibrillation
- Endocarditis
- Cancer

- Hypertension
- Coronary artery disease
- Rheumatic heart disease
- Diabetes mellitus
- Peripheral vascular disease
- Autoimmune disease

Diagnosis

- Time of onset of symptoms (*very* important for thrombolytic therapy; last time patient was without deficit, *not* when symptoms noted if the patient was asleep)
- Physical exam
- Neurologic exam
- ECG
- Pulse oximetry (avoid ABG if thrombolytics possible)
- CBC, chem 7, Ca^{+2}, PT/PTT, fibrinogen, ESR, LFT, cholesterol
- **Noncontrast head CT** (to determine if stroke is ischemic or hemorrhagic)

Management of Ischemic Stroke

- The keys to management are to
    establish the need for thrombolytics
    blood pressure control
    long-term prevention and rehabilitation
- If diastolic BP >140 mm Hg, start Nipride gtt.
- If systolic BP >230 mm Hg ± diastolic BP 121–140 mm Hg, use labetalol 20 mg IV q10min (to max 150 mg). Consider labetalol gtt 2–8 mg/minute.
- If systolic BP 180–230 mm Hg ± diastolic BP 105–120 mm Hg, use labetalol 10 mg IV q10min (to max 150 mg). If labetalol is contraindicated (e.g., in CHF), consider nifedipine.
- If elevated, do not lower blood pressure too quickly—no more than about 25%.

Use of Tissue Plasminogen Activator in Acute
Ischemic Stroke *(Prog Cardiovasc Dis 42:175, 1999; Neurology 53:14, 1999)*

Inclusion Criteria
- ≥18 years old
- Clinical ischemic stroke with significant neurologic deficit
- ≤180 minutes from onset of symptoms to treatment

Contraindications
- Intracranial hemorrhage on CT
- Subarachnoid symptoms (even without CT evidence)
- Active internal bleed
- Known bleeding diathesis (<100,000 platelets, heparin within 48 hours with ↑PTT, PT >15, oral anticoagulation)
- Intracranial surgery/serious head trauma/cerebrovascular accident within 3 months
- Systolic BP >185 mm Hg or diastolic BP >110 mm Hg or difficulty reducing BP to these levels
- History of intracranial hemorrhage; known AVM or aneurysm
- Seizures with symptomatic onset
- History of GI/GU hemorrhage within 3 weeks
- Recent noncompressible arterial puncture
- Recent LP
- Blood glucose <50 or >400 mg/dl
- Minor symptoms or rapidly improving symptoms
- Post-MI pericarditis

Administration (NINDS rt-PA Stroke Study Dosage)
- 0.9 mg/kg tPA (max 90 mg) over 60 minutes, with 10% of total as bolus over 1 minute and remainder over 1 hour within 3 hours of symptom onset
- No acetylsalicylic acid/heparin/warfarin for 24 hours, then check CT

Post–Tissue Plasminogen Activator Infusion
- Monitored bed
- Vital signs/neurologic check q30min × 12 then q1h × 16
- Bleeding precautions/check puncture sites/secretions
- BP control as above
- NPO × 24 hours
- No heparin/coumarin/aspirin × 24 hours
- After 24 hours, CT to exclude intracranial hemorrhage before starting anticoagulants

Comments
- Thrombolysis best administered in centers with 24-hour high-resolution CT and interpretation
- Stroke team for diagnosis and treatment
- Facilities to deal with intra-/extracranial hemorrhage

continued

NEUROLOGY

Management of Hemorrhagic Stroke
- Maintain systolic BP 150–200 mm Hg
- No antiplatelet agents, heparin, or tPA

Common Patterns of Stroke

Lacunar	Contralateral pure motor or pure sensory deficit, ipsilateral ataxia with crural paresis, dysarthria, clumsiness of hand
Anterior cerebral artery	Contralateral leg weakness and cortical sensory loss, possibly contralateral grasp reflexes, paratonic rigidity, abulia, frank confusion, urinary incontinence
Middle cerebral artery	Contralateral hemiplegia, hemisensory loss, homonymous hemianopsia, eyes deviate toward lesion, dominant hemisphere, global aphasia
Vertebro-basilar	Thalamic syndrome/contralateral hemisensory deficit, spontaneous pain, hyperpathia, macular-sparing homonymous hemianopsia
Cerebellar	Vertigo, nausea/vomiting, nystagmus, ipsilateral limb ataxia, contralateral spinothalamic loss including face

QUICK GUIDE TO APHASIA

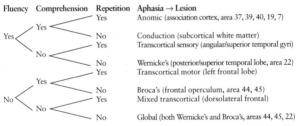

Fluency   Comprehension   Repetition   Aphasia → Lesion

Yes — Anomic (association cortex, area 37, 39, 40, 19, 7)

No — Conduction (subcortical white matter)

Yes — Transcortical sensory (angular/superior temporal gyri)

No — Wernicke's (posterior/superior temporal lobe, area 22)

Yes — Transcortical motor (left frontal lobe)

No — Broca's (frontal operculum, area 44, 45)

Yes — Mixed transcortical (dorsolateral frontal)

No — Global (both Wernicke's and Broca's, areas 44, 45, 22)

SEIZURES   (*Am Fam Physician* 56:1113, 1997; *Postgrad Med* 101:113, 1997; *Emerg Med Clin North Am* 12:4, 1994)

Fast Facts

- Most seizures last only 30–90 seconds (for status epilepticus, see next section)

History

- Previous episodes
- Aura
- Motor/sensory/behavior deficit
- Bowel/bladder incontinence
- Altered mental status
- Duration
- Tongue biting
- Head trauma

Diagnosis

- Precipitants (past seizures, ethanol, diabetes mellitus, infection, trauma)
- Witnessed?
- Workup
    Electrolytes/glucose
    CBC
    Urine toxicology screen
    Antiepileptic drug level
    ABG (if prolonged postictal state)
    ECG
    Head CT and LP to assess infection, subarachnoid hemorrhage

Management

- Oral airway
- Oxygen
- Monitor
- Thiamine 100 mg IV then D50 50 ml IV
- Orders
    Seizure precautions
    Padded bed rails
    Left side down (↓aspiration)

Antiepileptic Medications

- **Dilantin** 1 g IV load (or 18 mg/kg, rate ≤50 mg/minute) then IV 100 mg q8h. Watch for hypotension, ↓HR/contractility, AV block.
- Benzodiazepines (especially if seizures may be alcohol related):
    Lorazepam (Ativan) 2 mg IV q5min (max 8 mg)
    Watch for ↓respiratory rate/BP.
- **Phenobarbital** 10 mg/kg slow IV at <50 mg/minute. Watch for sedation, ↓respiratory rate.
- If initial treatment fails, consider status epilepticus protocol (next section).

NEUROLOGY

STATUS EPILEPTICUS (*N Engl J Med* 338:970, 1998)

Definition
- Tonic/clonic seizures for >30 minutes

Management
- Airway
- Oxygen
- Monitor
- Check finger-stick blood glucose
- Thiamine 100 mg IV, then D50 50 ml IV

Antiepileptic Medications
- At each step in the algorithm, assess whether seizures are controlled and emergency drug therapy can be stopped.
- Immediate treatment: lorazepam (Ativan) 0.1 mg/kg IV at 2 mg/minute.
- 3–4 minutes:
    phenytoin 20 mg/kg IV at 50 mg/minute **or**
    fosphenytoin (less hypotension than phenytoin) 20 mg/kg IV at 150 mg/minute.
- 20 minutes:
    phenytoin 5–10 mg/kg at 50 mg/minute **or**
    fosphenytoin 5–10 mg/kg IV at 150
        mg/minute.

    [If patient develops status epilepticus in ICU, is systemically unstable (e.g., extreme hyperthermia, hypotension), or is seizing >60–90 minutes, proceed directly to protocol for 55 minutes.]

- 35 minutes: phenobarbital 20 mg/kg IV at 50–75 mg/minute.
- 55 minutes: phenobarbital 5–10 mg/kg IV at 50–75 mg/minute.
- 65 minutes: anesthesia with midazolam (Versed) or propofol.

Once patient has received the maximum lorazepam dose and maximum phenytoin dose, consider intubation because the probability of respiratory compromise is high once barbiturates are started.

ACUTE PAIN

Fast Facts

- NSAIDs have an analgesic ceiling, whereas narcotics do not.
- Start with non-narcotics first.
- PO before IV.
- Limit options (dosing, timing). Write "hold for sedation."

Categories

- Acetaminophen (≤4 g/day, normal liver; ≤2 g/day, ↓hepatic function)
- NSAIDs (GI bleeding, renal toxicity)
- Opioids (constipation, addictive potential)
- Neuroactive (e.g., amitriptyline, valproate, gabapentin)

Opioid Drug Equivalencies

Drug	Equi-potent dosage	Route/equiv-alence	Onset of action (mins)	Peak analge-sic effect (mins)	Duration of action (hrs)
Codeine	13 mg	PO: 200 mg IM: 120 mg	PO: 30–45 IM: 10–30	PO: 60–120 IM: 30–60	PO: 4–6 IM: 4
Fentanyl (Sublimaze)	0.01 mg	IM: 0.1 mg	IV:<1 IM: 5–7	IV: 1–2	IV: 0.5–1.0 IM: 1–2
Hydromor-phone (Dilaudid)	0.13 mg	PO: 7.5 mg IM: 1.5 mg	PO: 30 IM: 30–60 IV: 10–15	PO: 90–120 IM: 4–5 IV: <20	PO: 4 IV: 2–3
Levorphanol (LevoDro-moran)	0.2 mg	PO: 4 mg IM: 2 mg	PO: 10–60	PO: 90–120 IM: 30–60 IV: <20	PO: 4–5 IM: 4–5 IV: 4–5
Meperidine (Demerol)	7.5 mg	PO: 300 mg IM: 75 mg	PO: 15 IM: 10–15 IV: 1	PO: 60–90 IM: 60–120 IV 15–30	PO: 2–4 IM: 2–4 IV: 2–4
Methadone (Dolo-phine)	1.0 mg	PO: 20 mg IM: 10 mg	PO: 15 IM: 10–15	PO: 90–120 IM: 60–120 IV: 15–30	PO: 4–6 IM: 4–5 IV: 3–4
Morphine	1.0 mg	PO: 60 mg IM: 10 mg	PO: 15–60 IM: 10–30 IV: <1	PO: 60–120 IM: 30–60 IV: 20	PO: 4–5* IM: 4–5 IV: 4–5
Oxycodone (Percodan)	1.0 mg	PO: 30 mg	PO: 15–30	PO: 60	PO: 4–6

*Morphine-SR (MS-Contin) lasts 8–12 hrs with parenteral equipotent dose of 3 mg/mg.

Source: Reproduced with permission from GM Susla et al. *The Handbook of Critical Care Drug Therapy*, 2nd ed. Philadelphia: Lippincott Williams & Wilkins, 1998. p. 34.

continued

- For acute pain, calculate equivalent dose and taper every week as pain resolves.
- Consider starting laxatives concurrently (e.g., DSS 250 mg PO bid, Senokot 1–2 tablets PO qhs).
- In combination drugs, be sure to consider how much acetaminophen is being given to avoid overdose.

Patient-Controlled Analgesia

- Appropriate for postoperative pain and terminally ill.
- Allows patient control of short-acting agents (MSO_4).
- Set basal rate (e.g., 1–5 mg/hour basal rate).
- Add patient-controlled bolus with timed lockout (e.g., 1 mg q15min lockout).
- Check patient sedation/analgesia and frequency of bolus use.
- Increase or decrease basal rate or bolus based on use and effect.

9. Endocrinology

COMMON SCREENING TESTS IN ENDOCRINE DISORDERS

Cushing's Syndrome
- Dexamethasone suppression test (DST):
  - 1 mg of dexamethasone is given PO at 11 PM
  - √ next 8 AM cortisol (normal <5 µg/dl)
- 24-hour urine for free cortisol (alternative screening or confirmatory study):
  - Cushing's syndrome when ≥100 µg/day free cortisol (>95 mg/mg of creatinine)

Adrenal Insufficiency
- Cosyntropin stimulation:
  - Cortisol is examined at time 0. Cosyntropin 0.25 mg IM or IV is given.
  - Cortisol is rechecked at 60 minutes.
  - (Normal if basal or post-stimulation cortisol ≥18 µg/dl.)

Pheochromocytoma
- 24-hour urine for free catecholamines, metanephrine, vanillylmandelic acid, and creatinine:
  - Normals: total catecholamine (100–150 µg/day), metanephrine (upper limit of normal, 1.3 mg/day), and VMA (upper limit of normal, 7 mg/day)

Diabetes Insipidus
- √Serum osmolarity (sOsm) and urine osmolarity (uOsm):
  - uOsm (<275 mOsm/liter) and sOsm (>290 mOsm/liter) suggests diabetes insipidus (DI).
  - ↓uOsm and sOsm suggests psychogenic polydipsia.
- Water deprivation test:
  1. Baseline uOsm and sOsm.
  2. No further water intake—for mild cases may need to withhold water overnight.
  3. Measure hourly uOsm and weight.
  4. When uOsm stabilizes (a change <30 mmol/kg over two consecutive measures or loss of 3–5% of body weight), give 5 U aqueous vasopressin (AVP) SC.
  5. Repeat uOsm 1 hour later.
- Interpretation:
  1. Normal: uOsm rises to two to four times that of plasma osmolarity, <9% further ↑ with AVP.
  2. Polydipsia: washed out concentration gradient, <9% ↑ with AVP.
  3. Central DI: uOsm does not increase over plasma osmolarity, >50% ↑ with AVP.
  4. Nephrogenic DI: no increase in uOsm; no response to AVP.

continued

ENDOCRINOLOGY

Hypopituitarism (Screen)
- GH ($\downarrow$ or normal)
- LH ($\downarrow$), FSH in women ($\downarrow$), testosterone in men ($\downarrow$)
- TSH ($\downarrow$), FT_4 ($\downarrow$)
- ACTH ($\downarrow$)
- Prolactin ($\uparrow$ if prolactinoma present)
- Urine specific gravity (<1.005)

Pituitary Incidentaloma (Rule Out)
- Oversecretion of growth hormone (100 g oral glucose tolerance test, normal <2 ng/ml at 2 hours)
- Cushing's syndrome (DST or 24-hour urine free cortisol)
- Prolactinoma (normal prolactin 0–20 ng/dl for men and 0–23 ng/dl for women)
- Gonadotroph cell adenoma (FSH/LH, both elevated if tumor present)
- Thyrotroph cell adenoma ($\uparrow T_4$ and T_3, TSH normal or elevated)

Hirsutism
- Rule out ovarian tumors (testosterone >200 ng/dl), adrenal tumors (increased 17-ketosteroid urinary excretion, increased testosterone, increased plasma DHEA without decrease after dexamethasone suppression), polycystic ovarian syndrome.
- If Cushing's syndrome cannot be ruled out, √24-hour urine free cortisol or DST.

Amenorrhea
- Rule out pregnancy ($\uparrow\beta$-hCG), primary gonadal failure ($\uparrow$FSH, $\uparrow$LH), prolactinoma ($\uparrow$prolactin), hyper-/hypothyroidism (TSH).
- Genital outlet atresia: **progestin trial of medroxyprogesterone** 10 mg PO × 5 days. Normal test→withdrawal bleeding.
- Hypothalamic amenorrhea: FSH, LH $\downarrow$ or normal but with low estradiol and failure of progestin withdrawal bleed. Must perform CNS imaging study to rule out abnormality.

THYROID DISEASE (Med Clin North Am 82:103, 1998)

Type of disease	TFTs	Differential diagnosis
Primary hypothyroidism	High TSH; low FT_4	Autoimmune thyroiditis (Hashimoto's disease); post-thyroidectomy; post–radioactive iodine ablation; abnormal thyroid hormone synthesis: iodine deficiency, genetic enzyme defects, anti-thyroid drugs; thyroiditis (transient): silent, subacute, postpartum; infiltrative thyroid disease: sarcoid, amyloid, hemochromatosis
Central hypothyroidism	Low/normal TSH; low FT_4	Hypothalamic/pituitary disease: tumor, infiltrative disease, radiation therapy, postpartum pituitary necrosis, lymphocytic hypophysitis Head trauma
Primary hyperthyroidism	Low TSH; high/normal FT_4; high/normal T_3	High radionuclide uptake: Graves' disease, toxic multinodular goiter, toxic nodule, hCG-induced hyperthyroid Low radionuclide uptake: thyroiditis [transient (subacute, silent, postpartum, radiation)], excessive thyroid ingestion, ectopic thyroid (struma ovarii)
Central hyperthyroidism	High/normal TSH; high FT_4; high T_3	High radionuclide uptake: TSH-secreting pituitary adenoma, thyroid hormone resistance

THYROID NODULE EVALUATION
- Physical examination for lymph nodes, thyroid gland, TFTs.
- Fine-needle aspiration (FNA) should be next step.
- If it is unclear if the nodule is benign or malignant→thyroid uptake scan: TcO4-99m study or 24-hour I^{123}/I^{131}:

    "Hot" (usually benign)→From scan determine diffuse (Graves' disease) versus nodule.

    "Cold" (nonfunctional)→recheck FNA (biopsy) or ultrasound (√size of cyst/nodule/goiter).

ENDOCRINOLOGY

THYROTOXICOSIS (*Med Clin North Am* 79:169, 1995)

Fast Facts
- Usually develops in undiagnosed patient with precipitating illness.
- Thermogenesis leads to shunting of blood to the skin to dissipate heat.

Symptoms
- Fever (101°F), anxiety, agitation, anorexia, nausea and vomiting, abdominal pain, ↑HR, CHF, diarrhea, vision disturbances.
- Elderly may show apathy, confusion, cachexia, and atrial fibrillation.

Evaluation
- Check CBC, electrolytes, TFTs (especially T_3/T_4), cortisol.

Therapy
- Vigorous management of underlying illness
- Antithyroid medications:
    Propylthiouracil 150–250 mg PO q6h or
    Methimazole (Tapazole) 15–25 mg PO q6h
- Beta blockers: esmolol IV drip, titrate to HR <100, or propranolol 10–40 mg PO tid or qid
- Iodine to lower T_4: saturated solution of SSKI 60 mg (1 drop) PO tid or 10% KI in water 0.1–0.3 ml PO tid.
- Hydrocortisone 50 mg IV q6h

MYXEDEMA COMA (*Med Clin North Am* 79:185, 1995)

Fast Fact
- Respiratory failure is the major cause of death in myxedema coma.

Symptoms
- ↓Temperature, ↓respiratory rate, ↓BP, altered mental status, ↓Na, ↑opiate sensitivity, ↓ventilation, ↓DTR

Evaluation
- √CBC, electrolytes, TFTs, cortisol, ABG

Therapy
- Levothyroxine 300–500 μg IVP→50 μg IV qd
- Hydrocortisone 100 mg IVP→25–50 mg IV q8h
- Watch ventilation, √glucose/electrolytes

ADRENAL CRISIS   (*N Engl J Med* 335:1206, 1996)

Symptoms

- Weakness/malaise, ↓PO, ↓weight, abdominal pain, altered mental state, nausea and vomiting, ↓temperature, ↓BP
- Usually in the setting of stress: infarction, trauma, surgery, drugs, cathartics, fasting, sepsis, infection

Evaluation

- Cosyntropin stimulation test: cosyntropin 0.25 mg IV, √cortisol at 0 and 60 minutes (normal ≥18 µg/dl)
- Electrolytes/glucose, serum/urine cortisol, TSH, ACTH
- Lab findings: hyponatremia, hyperkalemia, azotemia
- Less common: anemia, eosinophilia, lymphocytosis, hypoglycemia, hypercalcemia

Therapy

- D5NS: 1–2 liters over 2 hours
- Stress-dose hydrocortisone 100–300 mg IV push→50–100 mg q6h with 5-day taper
- Follow with hydrocortisone 10 mg PO qam and 5 mg PO qpm or fludrocortisone (Florinef) 0.1 mg PO qd

Stress-Dose Steroids

Patient	Stress-dose steroid considerations
Critically ill patients	Most evidence for benefit is in patients in early shock secondary to gram-negative rods and pressor dependence. Stim test is usually unreliable in critically ill who are often "relatively" adrenally insufficient. Consider hydrocortisone 100-mg test dose for response, then 100 mg q8h if responsive.
Chronic autoimmune or inflammatory disease treated with corticosteroids	Minor surgical stress or routine acute illness: continue current steroids or hydrocortisone 25 mg/day. Moderate surgical stress: hydrocortisone 50–75 mg/day. Major surgical stress or complex illness: double or triple current steroids or hydrocortisone 100–150 mg/day × 3 days.
Hypothalamic-pituitary-adrenal insufficiency	Hydrocortisone 100–150 mg/day during illness or surgery.

continued

ENDOCRINOLOGY

Glucocorticoid Therapy

• Hydrocortisone 20 mg = prednisone 5 mg = dexamethasone 0.75 mg

Steroid	GC potency	MC potency	Equivalent dose (mg)	Dura-tion (hrs)
Betamethasone (Celestone)	25	0	0.75 (PO)	36–72
Cortisol/hydrocortisone	1	1.0	20 (IV/IM/PO)	8–12
Cortisone (Cortone)	0.8	0.8	25 (PO)	8–12
Dexamethasone (Decadron)	25	0	0.75 (IV/IM)	36–72
Fludrocortisone (Florinef)	10	125	NA (PO)	8–12
Methylprednisolone (Solu-Medrol)	5	0.5	4 (IV/IM)	12–36
Prednisolone (Prelone)	4	0.8	5 (IV/IM/PO)	12–36
Prednisone (Deltasone)	4	0.8	5 (PO)	12–36
Triamcinolone (Aristocort)	5	0	4 (IM)	12–36

GC = glucocorticoid; MC = mineralocorticoid.

DIABETIC KETOACIDOSIS (*Med Clin North Am* 79:185, 1995)

Definition
- High blood glucose, high serum ketone bodies, metabolic acidosis

Symptoms
- Polyuria, polydipsia, weakness, nausea and vomiting, mental stupor/coma, fruity odor

Causes: Five "I"s
- Infection
- ↓/no Insulin
- Myocardial Infarction
- Surgical Incisions
- Intoxications
- +New diabetes mellitus (DM) diagnosis

Evaluation
- Electrolytes with ketones, CBC, ABG, arterial blood gas, toxicity screen, urinalysis/culture and sensitivity, blood culture, ECG, CXR
- Lab findings: glucose >250, pH <7.3, HCO_3 <15, serum/urine ketones, AG acidosis, DMI >II

Therapy
- Address underlying cause.
- Hyperosmolarity:
  NS 1 liter, then one-half NS at 150–300 cc/hour, follow-up intake and output.
  Watch out for CHF/decreased mental status/CNS edema/hyperchloride acidosis.
- Hyperglycemia:
  Regular insulin 0.15 U/kg IVP, then 0.1 U/kg/hr gtt.
  Check finger-stick blood glucose (FSBG) q1h (should ↓80–200/hour);
    titrate gtt when ketones clear and FSBG 150–200, then change to SC
    and/or previous regimen.
  When glucose ≤200, start D5 one-half NS at 100–250 ml/hour.
  DM diet, diabetes nurse for training.
- Acidosis:
  HCO_3 prn: pH <6.9, 2 ampules; pH 6.9–7.0, 1 ampule; pH >7, no treatment.
  Follow anion gap, ABG, ketones q2–6h until no gap/acidosis/ketones.
- Hypokalemia/electrolytes:
  Check electrolyte panel q2–6h.
  Replace $Mg/PO_4/Ca$ if symptoms.
  Total body K usually low.
  General K scale: K^+ 5–6 mEq/liter, 10 mEq/hour; K^+ 4–5 mEq/liter, 20
    mEq/hour; K^+ 3–4 mEq/liter, 30 mEq; K^+ 2–3 mEq/liter, 40 mEq.

ENDOCRINOLOGY

HYPEROSMOLAR NONKETOTIC COMA (*Med Clin North Am* 79:9, 1995)

Fast Fact
- More common than diabetes ketoacidosis, more insidious, greater free H_2O loss, and *more fatal*

Definition
- pH ≥ 7.3, blood glucose ≥ 600, effective osmolarity ≥ 320

Causes
- Infection, cerebrovascular accident, MI, pancreatitis, uremia with nausea and vomiting, burn, heat stroke, acromegaly, ectopic ACTH, subdural hematoma, dehydration, postoperative, H_2O restriction/bed ridden
- ↑Osmotic load (TPN/enteral feeds, glucose-containing IV fluid)
- Insulin secretion/activity inhibition (beta-blocker, diazoxide, phenytoin, corticosteroids, encainide, cimetidine)

Symptoms
- Tachycardia, low fever, dehydration, hyperpnea/hypertension (autonomic dysfunction)
- Focal/general neurologic findings: seizure, aphasia, homonymous hemianopsia, hemiparesis, Babinski syndrome, myoclonus, nystagmus

Evaluation
- ABG, electrolytes, LFT, CBC, infection workup
- Lab findings: pH ≥ 7.3, ↓total body K, mild AG acidosis, mild ketosis, ↑transaminases/LDH/CK-MM, ↑cholesterol/TG, variable Na^+, CBC

Therapy
- Hyperosmolarity:
  - 1–2 liters NS in 2 hours (as tolerated) to maintain BP/urine output.
  - Then one-half NS to replace free H_2O deficit (one-half in first 24 hours, one-half in second 24 hours).
  - Add D5 when blood sugar ≤ 250.
- Electrolytes:
  - Check electrolyte panel q2–6h, replace $Mg/PO_4/Ca$ if symptoms; total body K low.
- Hyperglycemia:
  - Regulate insulin 0.4 U/kg (one-half IV bolus, one-half SC), then gtt 0.1 U/kg/hour (5–7 U/hr gtt).
  - Check FSBG qhs titrate gtt to response (should ↓80–200/hour).
  - When serum glucose 200 start D5 one-half NS at 100–250 ml/hour.
  - Titrate insulin gtt to FSBG 150–200, then SC and/or previous regimen.
  - DM diet, diabetes nurse for training.

INSULIN THERAPY

- Multiple regimens for initiating insulin therapy exist. Results are affected by injection site, subcutaneous fat and blood flow. All regimens must be tailored to patient and compliance.
- Baseline NPH (approximately two-thirds of total insulin dose split two-thirds in morning, one-third in evening), patient checks FSBG three to four times per day and gives regular insulin 30 minutes before meals and before sleep prn or insulin lispro *immediately* before meals and before sleep prn, **or**
- Regimen divided two-thirds NPH and one-third regular given bid with two-thirds of NPH and regular in morning, one-third of NPH and regular in evening.
- Counsel concerning symptoms of hypoglycemia.

Stanford Sliding Scale Regular Insulin Dosing

FSBG (mg/dl)	Mild scale	Moderate scale	Aggressive scale	Evening dose scale
<60	1 ampule D50 or OJ; call HO	1 ampule D50 or OJ; call HO	1 ampule D50 or OJ; call HO	1 ampule D50 or OJ; call HO
60–150	No insulin	No insulin	No insulin	No insulin
151–200	No insulin	3 U	4 U	No insulin
201–250	2 U	5 U	6 U	2 U
251–300	4 U	7 U	10 U	3 U
301–350	6 U	9 U	12 U	4 U
351–400	8 U	11 U	15 U	5 U
>400	10 U; call HO	13 U; call HO	18 U; call HO	6 U; call HO

Source: Courtesy of Stanford Hospital and Clinics.
HO = house officer.

Stanford Insulin Drip Guidelines for Non-DKA

- Insulin bolus 0.15 U/kg if glucose >300→drip 0.02–0.10 U/kg (2–5 U/hour) keep FSBG 120–200

FSBG (mg/dl)	Adjustments	Action
>300	↑2 U	Bolus 0.15 U/kg; √q15min
>200	↑0.5–2.0 U	√qhs
<150	↑0.5–2.0 U	√qhs
<80	Hold drip	√qhs
<60	Hold drip	Push 1 ampule D50 or OJ, √q15min

ENDOCRINOLOGY

Stanford Diabetes Management Guidelines during Hospitalization (Courtesy of Stanford Hospital and Clinics)

Type I, NPO for >24 hrs	Start insulin drip and IV of D10
Type II on insulin, NPO >24 hrs	Sliding scale, if FSBG >300 mg/dl × 3, start IV insulin
Type I or II on insulin, eating	Resume usual regimen, if ↓FSBG, start one-half to three-fourths of normal
Type I or II initiate insulin	0.25–0.50 U/kg, regular two-thirds AM and one-third PM; alternatively, split dose NPH two-thirds and regular one-third
Type II on orals	Sliding scale (NPO) or orals (eating)
Type I or II on tube feeds	NPH bid, sliding scale prn
Type I or II on TPN	First 24 hrs separate insulin drip, evaluate need, and add to bag

Normal Daily Hormone Requirements
- Thyroxine ≈ 1.6 mg/kg/day (0.83 mg/lb/day)
- Insulin ≈ 24 U (0.3 U/kg/day)
- Cortisol ≈ 30 mg

Oral Hypoglycemics

Generic (trade)	Onset (hrs)	Half-life (hrs)	Dura-tion (hrs)	Start dose	Start dose (elderly)	Max dose daily	Metabolism
Tolbutamide (Orinase)	1	5.6	6–12	1–2 g/day	500 mg qd–bid	2–3 g	Hepatic with renal excretion
Chlorpropamide (Diabinese)	1	35	72	250 mg/day	100 mg/day	500 mg	Hepatic with renal excretion
Glyburide (Micronase)	1.5	2–4	18–24	2.5 mg/day	1.25–2.50 mg/day	20 mg	Hepatic with GI and renal excretion
Glimepiride (Amaryl)	2	9	24	1 mg/day	1 mg/day	8 mg	Hepatic with GI and renal
Glipizide (Glucotrol)	1	3–7	10–24	5 mg/day	2.5–5.0 mg/day	40 mg	Hepatic with renal excretion
Metformin (Glucophage)	1.5	1.5–4.9	16–20	500 mg/day	500 mg/day	2,550 mg	Renal excretion
Regular insulin	0.5–1.0	Peak 2–5	6–8				
NPH insulin	1–2	Peak 4–12	10–16				
Insulin lispro	5–15 mins	0.5–1.5	2–4				

10. Rheumatology

JOINT EXAMINATION

Examination of the range of joint mobility (neutral-null method)

(After recommendations of the German and Swiss Orthopaedic Society)

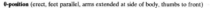

0-position (erect, feet parallel, arms extended at side of body, thumbs to front)

Sagittal plane: Flexion = bending, extension = straightening (plantar flexion = lowering of tip of foot, dorsal extension = elevation of tip of foot)

Frontal plane: Abduction = inclination away from midline, adduction = inclination towards midline

Transverse plane: Outward rotation = turning outwards, inward rotation = turning inwards (shoulder, hip), supination = palm towards front, sole inwards, pronation = palm towards back, lateral border of foot upwards/outwards.

Trans-
verse
plane

Frontal plane

Sagittal plane

Examination of the range of joint mobility (neutral-null method). (After recommendations of the German and Swiss Orthopedic Society.) [Reprinted with permission from M von Planta (ed). *Memorix Innere Medizin* (4th ed). © Chapman & Hall, Weinheim 1996; Hippokrates Verlag, Stuttgart 1999.]

continued

Recording by the null-point transit method
1st Number: Movement towards body (flexion, adduction, inward rotation, anteversion)
2nd Number: 0-position (if not attained, 1st or 3rd number)
3rd Number: Movement away from body (extension, abduction, outward rotation, retroversion)

Normal values shoulder joint

Anteversion/retroversion	150–170/0/40
Adduction/abduction	20–40/0/180

Inward/outward rotation with forearm against body   40–60/0/95

Inward/outward rotation with upper arm elevated sideways to 90 degrees   70/0/70

Normal values elbow joint
Flexion/extension   150/0/5–10
Forearm rotation inwards/outwards   80–90/0/80–90

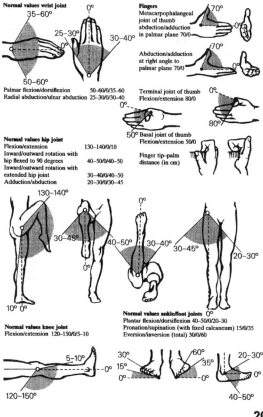

Normal values wrist joint
35–60°
0°
25–30°
30–40°

Palmar flexion/dorsiflexion   50–60/0/35–60
Radial abduction/ulnar abduction   25–30/0/30–40

50–60°

Fingers
Metacarpophalangeal
joint of thumb
abduction/adduction
in palmar plane 70/0   70°
0°

Abduction/adduction
at right angle to
palmar plane 70/0   70°
0°

Terminal joint of thumb
Flexion/extension 80/0   0°
80°

Basal joint of thumb
Flexion/extension 50/0   50°

Finger tip–palm
distance (in cm)

Normal values hip joint
Flexion/extension   130–140/0/10
Inward/outward rotation with
hip flexed to 90 degrees   40–50/0/40–50
Inward/outward rotation with
extended hip joint   30–40/0/40–50
Adduction/abduction   20–30/0/30–45

130–140°
30–45°
0°
40–50°
30–40°
30–45°
20–30°
10° 0°

Normal values ankle/foot joints
Plantar flexion/dorsiflexion 40–50/0/20–30
Pronation/supination (with fixed calcaneum) 15/0/35
Eversion/inversion (total) 30/0/60

0°

Normal values knee joint
Flexion/extension 120–150/0/5–10

5–10°
0°
120–150°

30°
15°
0°
60°
35°
0°
20–30°
0°
40–50°

RHEUMATOLOGY

COMMON PATTERNS OF JOINT INVOLVEMENT IN VARIOUS ARTHRITIDES

Characteristic	Status	Representative disease
Inflammation	Present	RA, SLE, gout
	Absent	Osteoarthritis
Number of joints involved	Monoarticular	Gout, trauma, septic arthritis, Lyme disease
	Oligoarticular (2–4)	Reiter's disease, psoriatic arthritis, inflammatory bowel disease
	Polyarticular (≥5)	RA, SLE
Site of involvement	DIP	Osteoarthritis, psoriatic arthritis (not rheumatoid)
	MCP, wrists	RA, SLE (not osteoarthritis)
	First metatarsal phalangeal	Gout, osteoarthritis

DIP = distal interphalangeal joint; MCP = metacarpophalangeal; RA = rheumatoid arthritis; SLE = systemic lupus erythematosus.
Source: Reproduced with permission from DB Hellmann. Arthritis and musculoskeletal disorders. In LM Tierney, SJ McPhee, MA Papadakis (eds), *Current Medical Diagnosis and Treatment*. East Norwalk, CT: Appleton & Lange, 1997;750–799.

ARTHROCENTESIS AND STEROID INJECTION FOR IDIOTS
(From Andrea Slotkoff Marks, M.D.; and *Postgrad Med* 103:125, 1998.)

1. Obtain verbal consent.
2. Withdraw 0.25–1.00 ml lidocaine using 20-gauge needle and 3-ml syringe; recap with 25- to 27-gauge needle; set aside.
3. Withdraw the desired amount of steroid using same 20-gauge needle with new syringe (lidocaine may be added to this); recap with new 25- or 22-gauge needle.
4. Seat or lay the patient in a comfortable position with a "chuck" underneath area to be injected.
5. Locate the site for injection and mark by pressing with the end of a retracted ballpoint pen. Put on nonsterile gloves.
6. Prepare area with povidone-iodine (Betadine). Allow to dry; then wipe the marked site with alcohol.
7. Infiltrate the skin and tissue with lidocaine at marked site, advancing very slowly, then injecting, then advancing, and so forth. Should not be very painful.
8. Wait 60 seconds.
9. Advance needle with syringe of steroid through same spot. Should not be very painful. Inject the steroid steadily, should be no resistance. For arthrocentesis, aspirate as needle is advanced until joint space is reached. Send fluid for WBC, Gram's stain, culture, and crystal exam.
10. Compress area with gauze. Apply bandage.
11. Advise patient to refrain from strenuous activity for 48–72 hours.
12. Write procedure notes.
13. Nonrheumatologists performing these injections, especially in the ankle, wrist, and elbow, should be properly supervised.

RHEUMATOLOGY

JOINT FLUID ANALYSIS

Arthrocentesis and Steroid Injection Sites
[Reproduced with permission from H. R. Schumacher et al. *Primer on the Rheumatic Diseases* (10th ed). Atlanta: Arthritis Foundation, 1993]

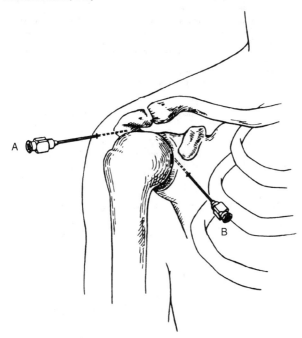

A: Injection of the subacromial bursa or supraspinatus tendon.

B: Anterior approach for injection of the glenohumeral joint.

continued

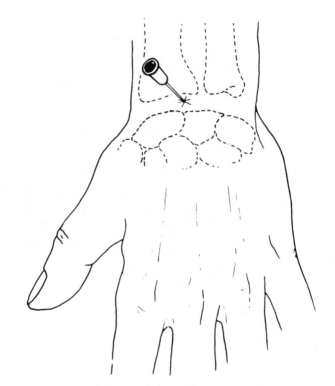

C. Arthrocentesis of the wrist, radial approach.

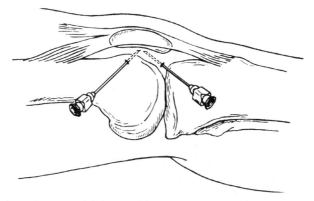

D. Arthrocentesis of the knee, medial approach.

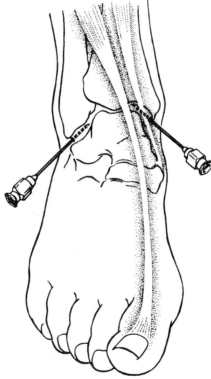

E. Arthrocentesis of the ankle joint, medial and lateral approaches.

SYNOVIAL FLUID ANALYSIS
Differential Diagnoses: Joint Fluid

Test	Normal	Group I (non-inflammatory)	Group II (inflammatory)	Group III (septic)
Color	Clear	Yellow	Yellow to white	Yellow to green
Viscosity	High	Transparent, yellow	Opaque/translucent	Opaque
WBCs/mm^3	<200	<200	5,000–75,000	>50,000–100,000
Neutrophils	<25%	<25%	>50%	>75%
Culture	Negative	Negative	Negative	Positive
Glucose (mg/dl)	≈ Serum	≈ Serum	>25, <serum	>50, <serum
Volume (knee, cc)	<3.5	>3.5	>3.5	>3.5

Source: Modified with permission from DJ McCarty. *Arthritis and Allied Conditions: A Textbook of Rheumatology* (11th ed). Philadelphia: Lea & Febiger, 1989;71, 74. © Lippincott Williams & Wilkins.

Group I
- Degenerative joint
- Trauma
- Neuropathic arthropathy
- Osteochondritis dissecans
- Osteochondroma
- Erythema nodosum
- Hypertrophic osteoarthropathy

Group II
- RA
- Connective-tissue disease (SLE, systemic sclerosis, dermatomyositis/polymyositis)
- Gout/pseudogout
- Reiter's syndrome
- Ankylosing spondylitis
- Rheumatic fever
- Inflammatory bowel

Group III
- Bacterial infection

continued

RHEUMATOLOGY

Crystals in Joints

Crystal	Characteristics	Associated condition
Monosodium urate	Needle shaped, intracellular, strongly negatively birefringent	Gout
Calcium pyrophosphate dihydrate (CPPD)	Rhomboidal, weakly positively birefringent	CPPD deposition diseases (pseudo-gout, pseudo-RA, pseudo–Charcot's joint, pseudo–infectious arthritis, pseudo-osteoarthritis, lanthanic and other syndromes)
Basic calcium phosphate	Nonbirefringent globules and clumps	Calcific periarthritis; acute and chronic arthritis; calcinosis; osteoarthritis
Calcium oxalate	Variable morphology, positively birefringent	Acute, subacute, and dialysis-related arthritis; oxalosis
Cholesterol	Rectangular, Maltese cross, negatively birefringent	Asymptomatic or chronic arthritides
Lipids	Microspheres	Acute and chronic arthritides
Corticosteroids	Irregular	Postinjection flare
Cryoglobulins	Polygonal, positively birefringent	Paraproteinemias and cryoglobulinemias

Source: Reproduced with permission from American College of Physicians, MKSAP 11, Rheumatology.

IMMUNOLOGIC TESTS
Frequency (%) of Autoantibodies in Rheumatic Diseases

Antibody	RA	SLE	Sjögren's	Diffuse sclero-derma	Limited sclero-derma (CREST)	PM/DM	Wegener's
ANA	30–60	95–100	95	80–95	80–95	80–95	0–15
Antinative DNA	0–5	60	0	0	0	0	0
Rheumatoid factor	72–85	20	75	25–33	25–33	33	50
Anti-Sm	0	10–25	0	0	0	0	0
Anti-Ro	0–5	15–20	60–70	0	0	0	0
Anti-La	0–2	5–20	60–70	0	0	0	0
Anti-SCL$_{70}$	0	0	0	20–50	10	10	0
Anti-centromere	0	0	0	1	50–80	0	0
Anti-Jo$_1$	0	0	0	0	0	20–30	0
ANCA	0	0–1	0	0	0	0	93–96

ANCA = antineutrophil cytoplasmic antibodies; CREST = calcinosis cutis, Raynaud phenomenon, esophageal motility disorder, sclerodactyly, and telangiectasia syndrome; PM/DM = polymyositis/dermatomyositis.
Source: Modified from DB Hellmann. Arthritis and musculoskeletal disorders. In LM Tierney, SJ McPhee, MA Papadakis (eds), *Current Medical Diagnosis and Treatment*. East Norwalk, CT: Appleton & Lange, 1997;750–799.

Complement Levels

Test	Range (mg/dl)	Condition
CH50	150–250	Normal
	>250	Inflammation (RA, infection, periarteritis)
	<150	Immune complex disease (SLE, vasculitis)
	<50	Genetic deficiency or active immune complex disease (low C3, C4)
C1q	<35	Vasculitis, hypersensitivity
C4	<28	Immune complex disorder, C4a deficiency
C3	<97	Active immune complex nephritis (SLE)
C2	<1.57	Homozygous C2 deficiency

RHEUMATOLOGY

SYSTEMIC LUPUS ERYTHEMATOSUS (*Arthritis Rheum* 25:1271, 1982; N Engl J Med 330:1871, 1994.)

Note: ≥4 criteria, serially or simultaneously, needed for diagnosis.

Criteria	Definition
Malar rash	Fixed malar erythema sparing nasolabial folds, raised or flat
Discoid rash	Raised erythematous patches with keratotic scaling/follicular plugging
Photosensitivity	Skin rash as reaction to sunlight
Oral ulcers	Usually painless
Arthritis	Nonerosive in ≥2 peripheral joints; tenderness, swelling, effusion
Serositis	Pleuritis, pericarditis
Renal disorder	Proteinuria >0.5 g/day, proteinuria >3+, or cellular casts
Neurologic disorder	Seizures or psychosis (without cause)
Hematologic disorder	Hemolytic anemia, leukopenia (<4,000/µl), lymphopenia (<1,500/µl), or thrombocytopenia (<100,000/µl)
Immunologic disorder	Positive SLE cell preparation, antibody to native DNA, anti-Sm, or false-positive syphilis test
ANA	Elevated titer (not correlated with disease activity)

RHEUMATOID ARTHRITIS (F. C. Arnett et al. The American Rheumatic Association 1987 revised criteria for the classification of rheumatoid arthritis. *Arthritis Rheum* 31:315, 1988.)

Note: Four out of seven criteria needed for diagnosis; must have first four criteria for >6 weeks.

Criteria	Characteristics
Morning stiffness	In and around joints, ≥1 hr before maximum improvement
Arthritis ≥3 joint areas simultaneously	Soft-tissue swelling, PIP, MCP, wrist, elbow, knee, ankle, MTP
Hand joint arthritis	≥1 swollen area in wrist, PIP, MCP
Symmetry	Bilateral PIP, MCP, MTP acceptable without absolute symmetry
Rheumatoid nodules	Subcutaneous nodules, nodules on extensor surface/ bony prominences or juxta-articular areas
Serum rheumatoid factor	Elevated to level + in <5% of normals
X-ray findings	PA hand/wrist x-ray with erosion, juxta-articular decalcification

PIP = proximal interphalangeal; MCP = metacarpophalangeal; MTP = metatarsophalangeal; PA = posterior-anterior.

RHEUMATOLOGY

GOUT   [DB Hellmann. Arthritis and musculoskeletal disorders. In LM Tierney, SJ McPhee, MA Papadakis (eds), *Current Medical Diagnosis and Treatment*. East Norwalk, CT: Appleton & Lange, 1997;750–799]

Fast Facts
- Associated hyperuricemia due to overproduction or underexcretion of uric acid.
- Common in Pacific Islanders (Filipinos and Samoans).
- 90% are men, usually >30 years of age. Women are usually postmenopausal.

Clinical Symptoms
- Acute, painful arthritis typically involving the first metatarsophalangeal joint (podagra).
- May also involve feet, ankles, and knees; more than one joint may be involved.
- Constitutional features: fever, chills.
- Tophi may be found on ears, hands, feet, olecranon, prepatellar bursas.

Laboratory Findings
- Uric acid >7.5 mg/dl in 95% of patients. Butyric acid need not be elevated.
- Leukocytosis and neutrophilia.
- Joint fluid: rod-/needle-shaped, negatively birefringent crystals; synovial WBC 20,000–100,000, predominately PMN.

Acute Management
- NSAIDs are the treatment of choice. Indomethacin, 25–50 mg q8h, until symptoms resolve.
- Corticosteroids are best reserved for patients who are unable to take NSAIDs.
    Monoarticular: inject triamcinolone, 10–40 mg, depending on joint
    Polyarticular: prednisone, 40–60 mg/day tapered off over 7 days
- Analgesics: opioids.

Prophylaxis
- Weight reduction, ↓alcohol consumption, avoid dehydration, avoid purines.
- Avoid hyperuricemic medications: thiazide or loop diuretics.
- Mild hyperuricemia, several attacks: colchicine, 0.6 mg PO bid.
- Reduce serum uric acid:
    Indicated for attacks despite colchicine, tophaceous deposits, and renal damage.
    24-hour urine uric acid: <800 mg/day, use uricosuric agent; >800 mg/day, use allopurinol.
    Uricosuric drugs (may be used with colchicine): probenecid, 0.5 g/day with slow increase to 1 g bid or to goal serum urate <6 mg/dl, *or* sulfinpyra-zone, 50–100 mg bid (up to 200–400 mg bid).
    Allopurinol (especially helpful in cases of urate overproduction), 100 mg/day (up to 300 mg/day; do not start until acute attack under control). *Avoid use with ampicillin, which increases the half-life of probenecid and potentiates azathioprine.*

RHEUMATOLOGY

VASCULITIS
Classification and Selected Clinical Features

Type	Typical host	Vessels involved	Target tissues
Polyarteritis nodosa	40-year-old injection drug users	Medium arteries	Kidney, nerve, gut, heart
Wegener's granulomatosis	40-year-old men	Small and medium arteries; veins	Sinus, lung, kidney
Temporal (giant cell) arteritis	>60-year-old women or men	Large elastic arteries	Eye
Takayasu's arteritis	20-year-old women	Aorta and main branches	Heart, brain, skeletal muscle
Primary angiitis of the CNS	48-year-old women	Arterioles, capillaries	Brain
Hypersensitivity vasculitis	20- to 50-year-old women or men	Capillaries, venules	Skin, kidney, gut, nerve
Vasculitis with connective-tissue disease (SLE, RA)	35-year-old women with SLE	Like polyarteritis nodosa or hypersensitivity vasculitis	Like polyarteritis nodosa or hypersensitivity vasculitis
Churg-Strauss syndrome	45-year-old men with chronic asthma	Like Wegener's granulomatosis	Skin, lung, kidney
Behçet's syndrome	25-year-old women or men	Arterioles, veins	Mouth, genitals, eye, brain
Vasculitis associated with malignancy	70-year-old women or men with lymphoma	Capillaries, veins	Skin

Source: Reproduced with permission from American College of Physicians, MKSAP 11, Rheumatology.

11. Nutrition

NUTRITIONAL REQUIREMENTS

(Nutrition Services, Stanford University Hospital. *Adult TPN Handbook*. Stanford, CA: Stanford University Hospital, 1996; *Surg Clin North Am* 56:1019, 1976)

Caloric Requirements

- Basal energy expenditure (BEE): energy expended under complete rest (in kcal):

  Males = 66 + [13.8 × weight (kg)] + [5 × height (cm)] – [6.8 × age (years)]
  Females = 65 + [9.6 × weight (kg)] + [1.8 × height (cm)] – [4.7 × age (years)]

- Injury factor (IF): used to adjust BEE for effects of disease process

Mild starvation/postoperative	BEE + 10%
Multiple trauma and ventilator or sepsis	BEE + ≥40%
Cancer	BEE + ≥20%
Long-bone fracture	BEE + ≥30%
Fever	BEE + 13%

- Activity factor (AF): used to adjust BEE

Bed rest	1.2
Out of bed	1.3

- Total daily expenditure (TDE): total energy expended per day

  TDE = BEE × IF × AF (kcal/day)

Comments

- Caloric requirements are met from carbohydrates and fat (not protein).
- Dextrose: 3.4 kcal/g.
- Lipids: 9 kcal/g; need to provide at least 4% calories as linoleic acid.
- Amino acids: 4 kcal/g (although usually not included in caloric calculations)

Protein Requirements

Condition	Protein need (g/kg/day)
Minimal	0.5
RDA	0.8
Trauma, sepsis	1.5–3.0
Acute renal failure	0.5–0.8
Hemodialysis	1.0–1.5
Peritoneal dialysis	1.5

Fluid Requirements

- 1.0 ml/calorie/day
- 30 ml/kg/day

NUTRITION

TOTAL PARENTERAL NUTRITION (TPN) (Nutrition Services, Stanford University Hospital. *Adult TPN Handbook*. Stanford CA: Stanford University Hospital, 1996)

Indications
Definite Benefit
- Inability to use the GI tract:

    Massive bowel resection   Diseases of the small   Intractable vomiting
    Severe diarrhea   intestine   Radiation enteritis

- Severely catabolic when the GI tract is unusable for 5–7 days
- Severe malnutrition with a nonfunctional GI tract
- Undergoing high-dose chemotherapy, radiation therapy, bone marrow transplantation
- Moderate to severe acute pancreatitis

Probable Benefit
- Major surgery: NPO expected for 7–10 days
- Moderate stress: enteral feeding not tolerated for 7–10 days
- High-output enterocutaneous fistula (e.g., >500 ml/day)
- Inflammatory bowel disease with nonfunctional GI tract
- Small-bowel obstruction
- Hyperemesis gravidarum

Partial Parenteral Nutrition (PPN) Preferred
- Expected duration of parenteral therapy is <7 days.
- Temporary loss of GI function (e.g., acute ileus).
- Maximum concentration of PPN should not exceed dextrose 10% + amino acids 4.25% and concurrent lipid infusion to decrease vein irritation.

Complications of Total Parenteral Nutrition
- Hyperglycemia
- Hypoglycemia
- Electrolyte disorders (PO_4, K)
- Mineral deficiency (Mg, Zn)
- Vitamin deficiency
- Trace element deficiency
- Essential fatty acid deficiency
- Hyperlipidemia
- Metabolic acidosis
- Heart failure (volume overload)
- Anemia
- Demineralization of bone
- Steatosis
- Cholestasis
- Sepsis (especially fungemia)
- Respiratory failure

Comments
- Determine target caloric protein and fluid requirements (see page 209).
- Start TPN at 40 cc/hour and increase up to desired rate within 24–48 hours.
- Carbohydrates should not exceed 5 g/kg/day to prevent glucose intolerance.
- TPN line should only be used for TPN.
- If TPN must suddenly be stopped, infuse 10% dextrose (D10) at the same rate as TPN.
- Monitor electrolytes, phosphorus, and glucose frequently.
- Monitor triglycerides and LFTs weekly.

ENTERAL NUTRITION

Feeding Tubes

- Check tube placement before initiation of feeds.
- Tips for difficult tube positioning: After initial placement, advance with promotility agent (metoclopramide, cisapride, erythromycin) with right side down for 3–4 hours.
- If all else fails, fluoroscopy can position appropriately.

Feeding

- Start at 10 cc/hour if concerned about tolerability.
- Advance 10–20 cc/hour q8–12h. Check residuals q4h: If >100 cc, hold for 2 hours then recheck residual.
- Note: Feeding tubes may collapse with aspiration and may be inaccurate in providing residuals.

Complications

- Aspiration: Elevation of head of bed >30 degrees is most important in preventing aspiration. Positioning in duodenum is less important.
- Gastric dysmotility
- Diarrhea occurs in ≤20% of patients, usually secretory not osmotic and not an indication to stop feeding. Consider other etiologies.
- Trauma
- Sinusitis/otitis
- Gastroesophageal reflux disease
- Erosion of GI tract
- Volvulus

Condition	Nutritional needs	Enteral feeding preparation
Impaired gut absorption	Peptide formula	Vital, Propeptide
Respiratory failure, ↑CO_2	↓CHO, ↑fat, ↓RQ	Pulmocare
Renal failure	↓Protein, K, Mg, PO_4	Suplena (Nepro if on hemodialysis)
Hepatic failure	↓Aromatic aa, ↑branch aa (only effective in severe encephalitis)	Hepatic-Aid
Diarrhea	↓Osmolarity, ↑fiber	Ultracal, Enrich
Fluid overload	Concentrated	Ensure Plus, Nepro, Pulmocare
Diabetes	↓CHO, ↑fiber	Glucerna, Ultracal, Pulmocare
Sepsis	Immune modulation	Impact, Perative

CHO = carbohydrates; RQ = respiratory quotient; aa = amino acids.

NUTRITION

NUTRITIONAL FEEDING FORMULATION CHART

PRODUCT (MANUF.)	TOTAL KCALS/CC NON-PRO KCALS	PROTEIN SOURCE	gm/L	FAT SOURCE	gm/L	CARBOHYDRATE SOURCE	gm/L
INTACT PROTEIN — LACTOSE FREE — ORAL SUPPLEMENTS							
Citrisource (Sandoz)	0.76 0.61	Whey Protein	37.1	N/A	0	Sucrose, Hydr. Cornstarch	151.2
Ensure® HN (Ross)	1.06 0.88	Sodium/Calcium Caseinate, Soy Protein	44.4	Corn Oil	36.5	Corn Syrup, Sucrose	141.2
Ensure® W/Fiber (Ross)	1.10 0.94	Sodium/Calcium Caseinate, Soy Protein	39.7	Corn Oil	37.2	Hydr. Cornstarch, Sucrose, Soy Fiber	162.0
Ensure Plus® (Ross)	1.50 1.28	Sodium/Calcium Caseinate, Soy Protein	54.9	Corn Oil	53.3	Corn Syrup /Sucrose	200.0
TwoCal® HN (Ross)	2.0 1.67	Sodium/Calcium Caseinate	83.7	Corn Oil, MCT	90.9	Hydr. Cornstarch, Sucrose	217.3
INTACT PROTEIN — LACTOSE FREE — TUBE FEEDING							
Isocal (Mead-Johnson)	1.06 0.92	Sodium/Calcium Caseinate, Soy Protein	34.0	Soy Oil, MCT	44.1	Maltodextrin	134.4
Jevity® (Ross)	1.06 .88	Sodium/Calcium Caseinate	44.4	Safflower Oil, Canola Oil, MCT	35.9	Hydrolyzed Cornstarch, Soy Fiber	151.7
Osmolite® HN (Ross)	1.06 0.88	Sodium/Calcium Caseinate, Soy Protein	44.4	Safflower Oil, Canola Oil, MCT	35.9	Hydrolyzed Cornstarch	141.0
ELEMENTAL/PEPTIDE							
Peptamen (Clintec) unflavored	1.00 0.84	Hydrolyzed Whey	40.0	MCT, Sunflower Oil	39.2	Maltodextrin, Sucrose, Starch	127.2
Vivonex Ten (Sandoz)	1.00 0.95	Free Amino Acids (33% BCAA)	38.2	Safflower Oil	2.77	Maltodextrin, Modified Starch	205.6
SPECIAL FORMULATIONS							
Advera® (Ross)	1.28 1.04	Soy Protein Hydrolysate, Sodium Caseinate	60.0	MCT, Canola Oil, Sardine Oil	22.8	Hydrolyzed Cornstarch, Sucrose, Soy Polysaccharide	215.8
Glucerna® (Ross)	1.00 0.83	Sodium/Calcium Caseinate	41.8	Safflower Oil, Soy Oil	55.7	Hydr.Cornstarch, Soy Fiber, Fructose	93.7
Impact® (Sandoz)	1.00 0.78	Sodium/Calcium Caseinate Arginine	56.0	Structured Lipid (Palm Kernal Oil, Safflower Oil, Refined Menhaden Oil)	28.0	Hydr. Cornstarch	130
Nepro® (Ross)	2.00 1.72	Calcium/ Magnesium & Sodium Caseinate	69.9	Safflower Oil, Soy Oil	95.6	Hydr. Cornstarch, Sucrose	215.2
Pulmocare® (Ross)	1.50 1.25	Sodium/Calcium Caseinate	62.6	Corn Oil	92.1	Sucrose, Hydr. Cornstarch	105.7
Suplena® (Ross)	2.00 1.86	Sodium/Calcium Caseinate	30.0	Safflower Oil, Soy Oil	95.6	Hydr. Cornstarch, Sucrose	255.2
MODULAR COMPONENTS							
Microlipid (Sherwood) 120 cc bottle	4.5/cc	N/A	N/A	Safflower Oil	0.5/cc	N/A	N/A
Polycose® Liquid (Ross)	2.0 cc	N/A	N/A	N/A	N/A	Glucose, Polymers (Cornstarch)	.5/cc
ProMod® (Ross) 1 SCOOP = 5 gm	28/Scoop	Whey Protein	5.0	N/A	0.6	Lactose	0.67

(Adapted from Enteral Nutrition Formulary. Ross Products Division, Abbott Laboratories: 12/94.)

INTACT PROTEIN — LACTOSE FREE — ORAL SUPPLEMENTS									
PRODUCT (MANUF.)	CALCIUM mg/L	PHOS mg/L	Na mg/L	Na meq/L	K mg/L	K meq/L	Osmolality	VOL TO MEET RDA	% FREE WATER
Citrisource (Sandoz)	567	672	210.0	9.1	84	2.2	700	N/A	N/A
Ensure® HN (Ross)	758	758	802	34.9	1564	40.1	470	1321	84.1
Ensure® W/Fiber (Ross)	719	719	846	36.8	1693	43.4	480	1420	82.9
Ensure Plus® (Ross)	705	705	1050	45.7	1940	49.7	690	1420	76.9
TwoCal® HN (Ross)	1052	1052	1310	57.0	2456	63.0	690	947	71.2
INTACT PROTEIN — LACTOSE FREE — TUBE FEEDING									
Isocal (Mead-Johnson)	630.0	525	525	22.8	1302	33.4	300	1890	84.0
Jevity® (Ross)	909	758	930	40.4	1570	40.3	300	1321	83.5
Osmolite® HN (Ross)	758	758	930	40.4	1570	40.3	300	1321	84.2
ELEMENTAL/PEPTIDE									
Peptamen (Clintec) unflavored	800	700	500	21.7	1252	32.1	270	1500	84.0
Vivonex Ten (Sandoz)	500	500	460	20.0	782	20.1	630	2000	84.6
SPECIAL FORMULATIONS									
Advera® (Ross)	845	845	1056	45.9	2827	72.5	680	1184	80.2
Glucerna® (Ross)	704	704	930	40.4	1560	40.0	375	1422	87.4
Impact® (Sandoz)	800	800	1100	48.0	1300	33.0	375	1500	86.0
Nepro® (Ross)	1373	686	829	36.0	1057	27.1	635	947	70.3
Pulmocare® (Ross)	1056	1056	1310	57.0	1730	44.4	465	947	78.6
Suplena® (Ross)	1385	728	783	34.0	1116	28.6	600	947	71.2
MODULAR COMPONENTS									
Microlipid (Sherwood) 120 cc bottle	N/A	N/A	N/A	N/A	N/A	N/A	N/A	80	44.3
Polycose® Liquid (Ross)	.2/cc	.03/cc	.7/cc	.03/cc	06/cc	.002	900	N/A	70.0
ProMod® (Ross) 1 SCOOP = 5 gm	65	33	15	.04	65	1.7	—	—	—

12. Outpatient

HEALTH CARE MAINTENANCE

Test	Ages 19–39	Ages 40–49	Ages 50–64	Ages ≥65
Health maintenance evaluation	q5yr	q2yr	Annually	Annually
Fecal occult blood			Annually	Annually to 75[a]
Sigmoidoscopy[b]			At age 50, then optional q5–10yr	Optional q5–10yr until age 70[a]
Pap smear	q1–3yr	q1–3yr	q1–3yr	Optional q3yr until age 75[a]
Mammogram		q1–2yr (controversial)	q1–2yr	q1–2yr until age 75[c]
Nonfasting total cholesterol	At 35 for men	q5yr	q5yr	q5yr until age 65[a]
Prostate-specific antigen			Optional annually	Optional annually until age 70[a]
Diphtheria-tetanus	Booster q10yr	Booster q10yr	Booster q10yr	Booster q10yr until 75[a]
Influenza				Annually
Pneumococcal				At age 65

Note: Optional recommendations have not been confirmed to be beneficial in long-term, case-controlled studies but are recommended by at least one or more professional organizations.
[a]Discretionary after age indicated.
[b]Sigmoidoscopy has been proven to reduce mortality from colon cancer, although an optimal interval has not been determined. The optional recommendation is based on obtaining annual fecal occult blood tests. Otherwise sigmoidoscopy is recommended q5–10yr.
[c]Mammography in this age group had been confirmed in studies to decrease mortality but is not recommended by all professional organizations due to differing risk-benefit analyses.
Reprinted with permission from M Hufty. *Guidelines for Preventive Health Care*. Palo Alto, CA: Palo Alto Medical Foundation, 1998.

HYPERTENSION (*Arch Intern Med* 157:2413–2446, 1997)

Classification of Blood Pressure for Adults on No Medications

Category	Systolic BP (mm Hg)		Diastolic BP (mm Hg)
Optimal	<120	and	<80
Normal	<130	and	<85
High-normal	130–139	or	85–89
Hypertension			
Stage 1	140–159	or	90–99
Stage 2	160–179	or	100–109
Stage 3	≥180	or	≥110

Risk Stratification and Treatment Choice

BP	Risk group A (no risk factors; no TOD/CCD)	Risk group B (at least 1 risk factor, not including diabetes; no TOD/CCD)	Risk group C (TOD/CCD and/or diabetes, with or without other risk factors)
High normal	Lifestyle modification	Lifestyle modification	Drug therapy
Stage 1	Lifestyle modification (≤12 mos)	Lifestyle modification (≤6 mos)	Drug therapy
Stages 2 and 3	Drug therapy	Drug therapy	Drug therapy

TOD = target organ disease; CCD = clinical cardiovascular disease; cardiac risk factors = diabetes, high cholesterol, smoking, and family history.

Therapy
- Begin or continue with lifestyle modification regardless of stage or risk group.
- For initial drug therapy in a healthy adult, begin with a *beta blocker* or *diuretic*.
- Existing illnesses may dictate an alternative initial drug choice.
- If no response or troublesome side effects are seen, substitute another drug class.
- If inadequate response, add a second agent (*diuretic* if not already used).
- If response continues to be inadequate, continue to add agents.

Compelling Indications and Their Therapies
- Type I diabetes mellitus: ACE inhibitor*
- LV systolic dysfunction: ACE inhibitor, diuretic
- Isolated systolic hypertension: diuretic (preferred), calcium antagonists (long-acting dihydropyridines)
- MI: beta blockers without intrinsic sympathomimetic activity, ACE inhibitors (patients with systolic dysfunction)

*If ACE inhibitor not tolerated (e.g., cough), consider an angiotensin II inhibitor such as losartan/valsartan.

continued **227**

OUTPATIENT

Less-Compelling Indications and Their Therapies
- Diabetes with proteinuria: ACE inhibitor
- Dyslipidemia: alpha blocker
- Osteoporosis: thiazides
- Renal insufficiency (caution in renovascular hypertension and creatinine ≥3 mg/dl): ACE inhibitor

Relative Contraindications and Their Therapies
- Bronchospastic disease: beta blockers (contraindicated)
- Depression: beta blockers, reserpine (contraindicated)
- Gout: diuretics (thiazide or spironolactone)
- Pregnancy: ACE inhibitors (contraindicated), angiotensin II–receptor blockers (contraindicated)

HYPERCHOLESTEROLEMIA

Cholesterol and Lipoprotein Screening

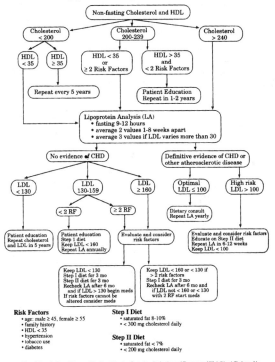

Risk Factors
- age: male ≥ 45, female ≥ 55
- family history
- HDL < 35
- hypertension
- tobacco use
- diabetes

Step I Diet
- saturated fat 8-10%
- < 300 mg cholesterol daily

Step II Diet
- saturated fat < 7%
- < 200 mg cholesterol daily

Adapted from the Second Report of the Expert Panel on Detection, Evaluation and Treatment of High Blood Cholesterol in Adults from the National Cholesterol Education Program (NCEP), NIH Publication No. 93-3096, September 1993.

OUTPATIENT

OUTPATIENT DIABETES MELLITUS GUIDELINES
American Diabetes Association Diagnostic Criteria for Diabetes

	Plasma glucose (mg/dl)			
	Fasting	1 Hour	2 Hours	3 Hours
Normal[a]	<110	—	<140	—
Impaired glucose tolerance[a]	<126	—	140–200	—
Impaired fasting glucose[a]	≥110 to <126	—	—	—
Gestational diabetes[b]	≥105	≥190	≥165	≥145
Diabetes[a]	≥126	No gtt needed	—	—
	<126	—	≥200	—
	Diabetes symptoms and random plasma glucose ≥200			

gtt = glucose tolerance test.
[a]ADA 1999 criteria using 75-g oral glucose load.
[b]100-g oral glucose load; must meet two criteria.
Sources: ADA Clinical Practice Recommendations 1999; *Diabetes Care* 22(Suppl 1).

Treatment Goals

Subject	Goals	Frequency
Hgb A$_{1C}$	Upper limits of normal for Hgb A$_{1C}$, 6% Ideal <7% Action suggested >8%	Biannually Quarterly if treatment changes or patient not meeting goals
Routine blood sugars	Fasting 80–120 Bedtime 100–140	
Cholesterol	LDL <130 (absence of heart disease) LDL <100 (presence of heart disease)	Yearly
Microalbuminuria	Early detection of proteinuria defined as Albumin/creatinine >30 mg/mg *or* 24-hour urine protein 30–300 mg *or* Timed collection >20 µg/min	Yearly
Eye screening	Detection of early diabetic retinopathy	Type II: at diagnosis, then yearly Type I: screen 3–5 yrs from diagnosis, then yearly
Foot screening	Detection of loss of sensory threshold by foot exam including pulses, sensation (monofilament), and inspection	Yearly
Hypertension	≤130/85 mm Hg	Every visit

Hgb = hemoglobin.

TRAVEL MEDICINE   (*Clin Infect Dis* 25:177, 1997)
Malaria

- Chloroquine-resistant *Plasmodium falciparum* regions: Southeast Asia, South America, East and West Tropical Africa
- Chloroquine-resistant *Plasmodium vivax* regions: Papua New Guinea and Indonesia
- Chloroquine-sensitive regions: Central America, the Caribbean, and the Middle East

Malaria Prophylaxis

Drug	Comment	Dosage
Mefloquine	In areas where chloroquine-resistant malaria has been reported	250 mg/wk
Doxycycline hyclate	An alternative to mefloquine	100 mg/day
Chloroquine	In areas where chloroquine-resistant malaria has not been reported	500 mg/wk

Vaccines for the Adult Traveler

Infection	Region/risk	Vaccine	Warnings
Yellow fever	South America, sub-Saharan Africa	Live, attenuated vaccine, single dose	Egg allergy, immunocompromise, pregnant women.
Japanese B encephalitis	Rural Southeast Asia	Three doses	Drug or bee-sting allergy. Reactions every 1/1,000.
HAV	South America, Africa, Eastern Europe	Two versions: Havrix: killed, inactivated virus, single 1-cc dose, boost at 6–12 mos; Vaqta: inactivated whole virus, single 1-cc dose, boost at 6 mos	Patients should be vaccinated at least 1 mo before departure. Otherwise immunoglobulin should also be given.
HBV	Sexual contact, blood; Central Africa, Central America, Southeast Asia, Eastern Europe	Three doses: 0, 1, 6 mos; 0, 2, 4 mos; 0, 1, 4 mos	Ideally 6 mos before travel.
Meningococcal disease	Sub-Saharan Africa, northern India, Nepal	Single-dose quadrivalent vaccine→3-yr immunity	—
Typhoid	Rural South America, Central America, Asia	Two versions: Live oral: 4 doses; Purified capsular polysaccharide: 1 IM dose	Avoid oral in patients with fever, GI disease, pregnancy, or immunocompromise.
Diphtheria	Nonimmunized Americans	Primary series of 3 doses	Prior anaphylactic reaction to vaccine.
Polio	Nonimmunized Westerners	Enhanced inactivated poliovirus series.	—
Influenza	At-risk patients	During flu season or before departure.	Prior anaphylactic reaction to vaccine.

- **Resource:** Centers for Disease Control and Prevention, http://www.cdc.gov/travel

OUTPATIENT

SMOKING CESSATION (*Primary Care* 26:591, 1999; *Primary Care* 26:653, 1999; *Primary Care* 26:633, 1999; *N Engl J Med* 340:685, 1999)

Fast Facts

- Greater counseling intensity correlates with ↑cessation success.
- Pharmacotherapy (nicotine replacement) consistently increases smoking cessation.

Initial Intervention Guidelines

- **Ask** about smoking status.
- **Advise** smokers to stop in a strong, personal message. Convey adverse effects.
- **Assist** cessation. Set quit date. Sign smoking contract. Begin nicotine replacement.
- **Arrange** for follow-up within first week and on days 14, 30, and 60.

Nicotine Replacement Therapy

- Nicotine gum:
  1. Use enough gum to avoid withdrawal symptoms, usually 10–12 pieces per day, 2 mg per piece.
  2. Chew gum before the urge to smoke begins.
  3. Use gum for 2–3 months, then begin to taper.
  4. Chew slowly and leave piece between cheek and gum.
- Nicotine patch:

Proprietary name and dosage	Hours	Delivery control	Duration	Duration of therapy	Cost
Habitrol	24	Rate-limiting membrane		8–12 wks	$216.46
21 mg/day			First 6 wks		
14 mg/day			Next 2 wks		
7 mg/day			Last 2 wks		
Nicoderm	24	Rate-limiting membrane		8–12 wks	$228.72
21 mg/day			First 6 wks		
14 mg/day			Next 2 wks		
7 mg/day			Last 2 wks		
Nicotrol	16	Adhesive		14–20 wks	$208.32
15 mg/day			First 12 wks		
10 mg/day			Next 2 wks		
5 mg/day			Last 2 wks		
ProStep	24	Gel matrix		6–12 wks	$236.64
22 mg/day			4–8 wks		
11 mg/day			2–4 wks		

Source: Kaye. Pharmacologic and behavioral approaches to smoking cessation. *Hosp Med* 34:59, 1998.

- Nicotine nasal spray: more effective nicotine delivery, but may sustain dependence

Non-Nicotine Medication: Bupropion

- Safe and effective in randomized, double-blind, placebo-controlled trial.
- Start 150 mg qd for 3 days, then bid for 7–12 weeks.
- Patients should stop smoking 1 week into therapy.

ORAL CONTRACEPTION
Fast Facts
- Typical failure rate of 3%.
- OCPs start on the fifth day of the cycle (day 1 = first day of menses), followed by 7 days placebo.
- Decrease in estrogen and progestin content has reduced side effects and complications.
- Patients may not be protected fully during first month of use.

Contraindications
- Pregnancy
- Thrombophlebitis or thromboembolic disorders (past or present)
- Stroke or CAD (past or present)
- Cancer of the breast (known or suspected)
- Undiagnosed abnormal vaginal bleeding
- Estrogen-dependent cancer (known or suspected)
- Benign or malignant tumor of the liver

Preparations
- Two types: combination pills (estrogen and progestin) vs. progestin only.
- Combination pills are monophasic (fixed dose) or multiphasic (varying doses).
- Newer progestins may have fewer androgenic side effects.
- For low-dose OCPs, efficacy equivalent; choose OCP by side effect profile.

Androgenic and Estrogenic Activity of Progestins in Oral Contraceptives with Low-Dose Estrogen

Level of activity	Androgenic brand name(s)	Estrogenic brand name(s)
High	Norgestrel: Lo Ovral	Ethynodiol: Demulen 1/35
	Levonorgestrel: Nordette, Levlen, Triphasil, Tri-Levlen	
Middle	Norethindrone: Genora 1/35, Ortho-Novum 1/35, Norinyl 1/35, Ortho 1/11, Tri-Norinyl, Ortho 7/7/7, Modicon, Brevicon, Ovcon 35	
	Norethindrone acetate: Loestrin 1/20, Loestrin 1.5/30	
Low	Ethynodiol: Demulen 1/35	All other progestins
	Norgestimate: Ortho-Cyclen, Ortho-TriCyclen	
	Desogestrel: Desogen, Ortho-Cept	

Source: Reprinted with permission from KJ Carlson, SA Eisenstat (eds). *Primary Care of Women*. St. Louis: Mosby, 1995;202.

- Estrogen effects: menstrual irregularities, breast tenderness, headache, and nausea
- Androgen effects: hirsutism and acne

OUTPATIENT

MENOPAUSE AND HORMONE REPLACEMENT THERAPY (HRT)
(*Med Clin North Am* 82:297, 1998; *Ann Intern Med* 129:551, 1998; *JAMA* 280:605, 1998; *Lancet* 353:571, 1999)

Indications for Hormone Treatment
- Treatment of estrogen deficiency symptoms
- Prevention of CAD:
  Nurses Health Study shows ↓CHD mortality for women on HRT.
  Oral conjugated estrogens ↓total cholesterol and LDL, ↑HDL.
  For women with known CAD, Heart and Estrogen/Progestin Replacement Study (HERS) showed ↑CHD events in first year but ↓CHD decreased in subsequent years.
- Prevention of osteoporosis:
  Calcium, 1,500 mg/day without HRT and 1,000 mg/day with HRT.
  Bone-density study not necessary to start therapy.
  Estrogen and alendronate offer similar degree of protection of bone.
  Maximum benefit achieved within 5 years of menopause; ↑duration ≅ ↑protection against osteoporosis.

Risks of Estrogen Therapy
- Breast cancer (relative risk of 1.1–1.8 at 10–15 years)
- DVT/PE
- Endometrial cancer (risk diminished by concurrent progestin use)
- Gallbladder disease
- SLE

Contraindications
- History of breast cancer.
- Undiagnosed postmenopausal vaginal bleeding.
- Endometrial cancer: HRT may be considered after treatment for stage I cancer.
- Acute liver disease.
- Thromboembolic disease.

Therapy
- Estrogen should be given continuously in most cases, 0.625 mg PO qd.
- Progesterone must be added for patients with uterus.
- Progesterone options:
  Continuous low dose, 2.5 mg qd
  Cyclically 5–10 mg from day 1–12 of every calendar month→mild spotting
- Combination pills such as conjugated estrogens/medroxyprogesterone acetate (Prempro) are also available.

13. Consultative Medicine

Ten Commandments for Effective Medical Consultation
(*Arch Intern Med* 143:1753–1755, 1983)

- Determine the question.
- Establish urgency.
- Look at the case for yourself.
- Be as brief as appropriate.
- Be specific.
- Provide contingency plans.
- Honor thy turf.
- Teach with tact.
- Talk is cheap and effective.
- Follow up.

CONSULTATIVE MEDICINE

PREOPERATIVE EVALUATION: CARDIOVASCULAR
Goldman's Multifactorial Index of Cardiac Risk in Noncardiac Surgery

Risk factor	Point (total 53)
Age >70	5
MI within 6 mos	10
S_3 or JVD on physical exam	11
Significant aortic stenosis	3
Rhythm other than NSR on preoperative ECG	7
>5 PVCs/min at any time preoperatively	7
Po_2 <60 mm Hg or Pco_2 >50 mm Hg	3
K <3.0 or HCO_3 >20	3
BUN >50 or creatinine >3	3
Abnormal SGOT	3
Chronic liver disease	3
Bedridden due to noncardiac disease	3
Intra-abdominal, intrathoracic, or aortic surgery	3
Emergency surgery	4

JVD = jugular venous distention; NSR = normal sinus rhythm; SGOT = serum glutamic-oxaloacetic transaminase.

Risk class	Point total	Minor/no complications	Serious complications*	Cardiac deaths
I	0–5	99%	0.6%	0.2%
II	6–12	95%	3%	1%
III	13–25	86%	11%	3%
IV	>25	49%	12%	39%

*Serious complications include perioperative MI, pulmonary edema, ventricular tachycardia.
Source: Reprinted with permission from *N Engl J Med* 297:845, 1977. Copyright © 1977 Massachusetts Medical Society. All rights reserved.

STEPWISE APPROACH TO PREOPERATIVE CARDIAC ASSESSMENT

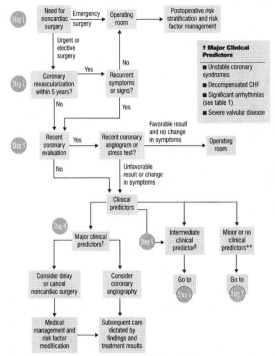

† Major Clinical Predictors

- Unstable coronary syndromes
- Decompensated CHF
- Significant arrhythmias (see table 1)
- Severe valvular disease

(Reprinted with permission. ACC/AHA guidelines for the perioperative cardiovascular evaluation for noncardiac surgery. *J Am Coll Cardiol* 1996;27:910–948. © 1996 by the American College of Cardiology and American Heart Association, Inc.)

continued

CONSULTATIVE MEDICINE

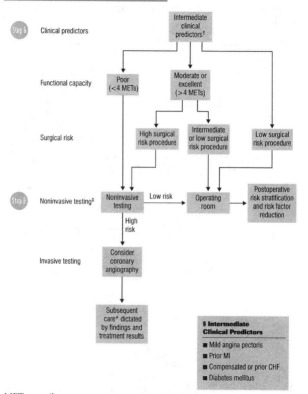

MET = ventilatory oxygen consumption; 1 MET = basal resting requirement; 2–4 METs = 2–4 mph walking on flat ground; 5 METs = activities of daily living; 10 METs = fit/high activity.

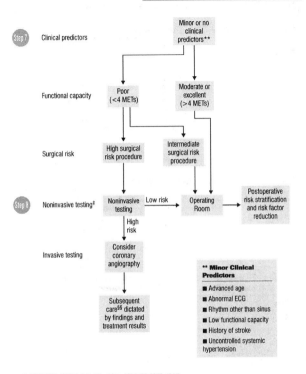

Step 7 — Clinical predictors — **Minor or no clinical predictors****

Functional capacity — **Poor (<4 METs)** / **Moderate or excellent (>4 METs)**

Surgical risk — **High surgical risk procedure** / **Intermediate surgical risk procedure**

Step 8 — Noninvasive testing‡ — **Noninvasive testing** — Low risk → **Operating Room** → **Postoperative risk stratification and risk factor reduction**

High risk ↓

Invasive testing — **Consider coronary angiography**

↓

Subsequent care§§ dictated by findings and treatment results

** Minor Clinical Predictors

- Advanced age
- Abnormal ECG
- Rhythm other than sinus
- Low functional capacity
- History of stroke
- Uncontrolled systemic hypertension

* *JACC* 1996; 27:910-948; *Circulation* 1996; 93:1278-1317.

‡ Myocardial perfusion imaging or stress echocardiography.

§§ Subsequent care may include cancellation or delay of surgery, coronary revascularization followed by noncardiac surgery, or intensified care.

CONSULTATIVE MEDICINE

PREOPERATIVE EVALUATION: PULMONARY (N Engl J Med 340:937, 1999)

Patient-Related Risk Factors

Risk factor	Surgery	Unadjusted relative risk
Smoking	CABG	3.4
	Abdominal	1.4–4.3
ASA class >II (general health status)	Unselected	1.7
	Thoracic or abdominal	1.5–3.2
Age >70	Unselected	1.9–2.4
	Thoracic or abdominal	0.9–1.9
Obesity	Unselected	1.3
	Thoracic or abdominal	0.8–1.7
COPD	Unselected	2.7–3.6
	Thoracic or abdominal	4.7

ASA = American Society of Anesthesiologists.

Procedure-Related Risk Factors

Risk factor	Surgery	Unadjusted relative risk
Surgery >3 hrs	Unselected	1.6–5.2
	Thoracic or abdominal	3.6
General anesthesia	Unselected	1.2–infinity
	Thoracic or abdominal or vascular	2.2–3.0
Intraoperative pancuronium	Unselected	3.2

Risk of Postoperative Pulmonary Complications (Classified by Preoperative Spirometry)

Surgery	Relative risk associated with abnormal findings
Upper abdominal	1.7–2.6
Unselected	1.9–4.0
Abdominal	1.7
Abdominal and thoracic	1.4
Cholecystectomy	3.3
Vascular	3.8
Cardiac	1.0
CABG	0.9

Risk Reduction Strategies

Preoperative
- 8 weeks smoking cessation; baseline treatment of airflow obstruction in COPD/asthma; antibiotics and delay of sugery for pre-existing infection; patient education about lung expansion exercises

Intraoperative
- Limit surgery to <3 hrs; spinal or epidural anesthesia*; avoid pancuronium; laparoscopic procedures when possible; perform less extensive rather than upper abdominal or thoracic surgeries if possible

Postoperative
- Deep breathing/incentive spirometry; continuous positive airway pressure; epidural anesthesia*; intercostal nerve blocks*

Indications for Preoperative Chest X-Ray
- Intrathoracic surgery
- Signs/symptoms of active chest disease

High Pulmonary Risks
- FEV_1/FVC <50% predicted, FVC <70% predicted (*JAMA* 211:787, 1970)
- $PaCO_2$ >45 mm Hg (*Chest* 76:130, 1970)

Additional Strategies
- Early extubation
- Treatment of concurrent infection
- Treatment of underlying lung disease

*Recommended though literature reports variable efficacy.

CONSULTATIVE MEDICINE

PERIOPERATIVE MANAGEMENT: ANTICOAGULATION
Recommendations for Perioperative Anticoagulation
(*N Engl J Med* 336:1506, 1997)

- Withhold four to five warfarin doses to allow INR <1.5 (more doses or INR <1.3 if high risk of bleeding from procedure).
- Check INR 1 day preoperatively. May give vitamin K, 1 mg SC, if INR >1.8.
- For the period during which INR <2.0, alternative pre- and postop prophylaxis should be considered (see table below).

Warfarin indication	Thromboembolism rate (%) without therapy	Recommendations for anticoagulation in patients taking warfarin	
		Preoperative	Postoperative
Acute venous thromboembolism			
Month 1	40	IV heparin	IV heparin
Months 2 and 3	10	No change	IV heparin
Recurrent venous thromboembolism	15	No change	SC heparin
Acute arterial embolism (month 1)	15	IV heparin	IV heparin
Mechanical heart valves	8	No change	SC heparin
Nonvalvular atrial fibrillation	4.5–12.0	No change	SC heparin

Note: Increased DVT rate does not include that associated with therapy; IV heparin = therapeutic dose for anticoagulation; SC heparin = unfractionated or LMHW in recommended prophylactic dose; a vena caval filter should be considered if acute DVT ≤2 weeks postop or high risk of bleeding with IV heparin; IV heparin should be used after surgery only if the risk of bleeding is low.

Prophylaxis against Venous Thromboembolism (*Chest* 108:312S, 1998)

Condition	Risk	Recommendations
General surgery*		
Low risk	3%	No prophylaxis
Moderate risk	29%	Heparin, 5,000 U SC q12h start 2 hrs preoperatively
High risk	39%	Heparin, 5,000 U SC q8h start 2 hrs preoperatively, or dalteparin
Very high risk	80%	Heparin, 5,000 U SC q8h start 2 hrs preoperatively; dalteparin; or perioperative warfarin (INR 2–3)
Total hip replacement	51%	Enoxaparin, 30 mg SC q12h start 12–24 hrs postoperatively, or warfarin (INR 2–3) up to 4 wks postoperatively
Total knee replacement	61%	Postoperative enoxaparin, 30 mg SC q12h, or IPC
Hip fracture surgery	48%	Enoxaparin, 30 mg SC q12h start 2 hrs preoperatively, or warfarin (INR 2–3)
Neurosurgery	24%	IPC, or heparin, 5,000 U SC q12h, and IPC
Acute spinal cord injury	40%	Heparin SC to activated PTT 1.5 × control 6 hrs after dose, or warfarin (INR 2–3), or IPC and heparin, 5,000 U SC q12h
Multiple trauma	53%	IPC until no bleed risk, then enoxaparin, 30 mg SC q12h, or warfarin (INR 2–3)
MI	24%	Heparin, 5,000 U SC q12h
Ischemic stroke	42%	Heparin, 5,000 U SC q12h
Medical patient	20%	Heparin, 5,000 U SC q12h

IPC = intermittent pneumatic compression.
*Classification of risk of postoperative DVT/PE:
    Very high risk: age >40, orthopedic/cancer/hip fracture surgery, prior DVT/PE, spinal cord injury/stroke, coagulopathies (proteins C and S, antithrombin III, anticardiolipin)
    High risk: age >40, major surgery, secondary risks (obesity, immobilized, malignancy, varicose veins, estrogen use, paralysis)
    Moderate risk: age >40, major surgery with no secondary risks
    Low risk: minor surgery with no secondary risks

CONSULTATIVE MEDICINE

PERIOPERATIVE MANAGEMENT: ANTIMICROBIAL PROPHYLAXIS

Fast Facts
- Major component of surgical morbidity and mortality.
- Goal of antimicrobial prophylaxis is to decrease the incidence of wound infection.

Nonantibiotic Interventions
- Minimize preoperative hospitalization or antibiotic uses and treat remote infection sites.
- Resolve malnutrition and obesity, maximize diabetes control, and maintain hydration and nutrition postoperatively.
- Careful skin preparation, aseptic technique.
- Minimize use of postoperative catheters, lines, and drains.

Antibiotic Prophylaxis

Condition	Antibacterial agent	Timing/duration
Clean (cardiac, vascular, neurologic, orthopedic surgery)	Cefazolin or vancomycin	Before and during procedure
Ocular	Topical combinations and subconjunctival cefazolin	During and at the end of procedure
Clean-contaminated: head and neck, high-risk GI/biliary surgery,* emergent C-section, hysterectomy	Cefazolin; clindamycin for head and neck	Before and during procedure
Clean-contaminated: colorectal, appendectomy	Cefoxitin or cefotetan (add oral neomycin and erythromycin for colorectal)	Before and during procedure
Dirty: ruptured viscus	Cefoxitin or cefotetan ± gentamicin (clindamycin + gentamicin) or other broad-spectrum coverage	Before and for 3–5 days after procedure
Dirty: traumatic wounds	Cefazolin, also tetanus prophylaxis	Before and for 3–5 days after trauma

*If cholangitis is a complication, ampicillin-sulbactam may be beneficial for enterococcal coverage.
Source: Modified from AS Fauci, JB Martin, E Braunwald, et al. (eds). *Harrison's Principles of Internal Medicine* (14th ed). New York: McGraw-Hill, 1998;868.

- Antibiotic prophylaxis is *not* generally recommended in
    Routine cardiac catheterization
    Sterile preoperative urine cultures for transurethral surgery
    Elective C-sections, uncomplicated D&C
    Routine breast surgery, inguinal hernia repair, laminectomy/spinal fusion

ENDOCARDITIS PROPHYLAXIS *(Clin Infect Dis 25:1448, 1997)*

Cardiac Conditions Associated with Endocarditis (Prophylaxis Recommended)

- High-risk category:
  - Prosthetic cardiac valves
  - Previous bacterial endocarditis
  - Complex cyanotic congenital heart disease
  - Surgically constructed systemic pulmonary shunts or conduits
- Moderate-risk category:
  - Most other congenital cardiac malformations
  - Acquired valvular dysfunction
  - Hypertrophic cardiomyopathy
  - Mitral valve prolapse with valvular regurgitation and/or thickened leaflets
- Low-risk category: endocarditis prophylaxis not recommended
  - Isolated secundum ASD, or surgical repair of ASD, VSD, or PDA
  - Previous CABG surgery
  - Mitral valve prolapse without valvular regurgitation
  - Physiologic, functional, or innocent heart murmurs
  - Previous Kawasaki disease or rheumatic fever without valvular dysfunction
  - Cardiac pacemakers and implanted defibrillators

Procedures Requiring Endocarditis Prophylaxis

- **Dental:** extraction, periodontal procedures, implant placement, endodontic instrumentation, subgingival placement of strips, initial orthodontic band placement, intraligamentary local anesthetic injection, prophylactic cleaning
- **Respiratory:** tonsillectomy, surgery involving respiratory mucosa, rigid bronchoscopy (not in tympanotomy tube insertion or flexible bronchoscopy)
- **GI:** sclerotherapy, esophageal stricture dilation, ERCP with biliary obstruction, biliary tract surgery, surgery involving intestinal mucosa (not with TEE or routine endoscopy)
- **Genitourinary:** prostatic surgery, cystoscopy, or urethral dilation
- Not in routine cardiac catheterization, pacemaker, defibrillator or stent placement, circumcision

Prophylaxis Regimens

- **Standard:** amoxicillin 2 g PO 1 hour before
- **Penicillin-allergic:** clindamycin 600 mg PO, or cephalexin 2 g PO, or azithromycin/clarithromycin 500 mg PO 1 hour before (vancomycin 1 g IV, if moderate risk)
- **Unable to take oral:** ampicillin 2 g IM/IV, or clindamycin 600 mg IV, or cefazolin 1 g IV 30 minutes before
- **High-risk (genitourinary/GI):** ampicillin 2 g IM/IV, + gentamicin 1.5 mg/kg (≤120 mg) within 30 minutes; then ampicillin 1 g IM/IV 6 hours later (penicillin-allergic: vancomycin 1 g IV, + gentamicin 1.5 mg/kg within 30 minutes)

14. Toxicology

BENZODIAZEPINE OVERDOSE [*American College of Emergency Physicians*. Emergency Medicine (4th ed). New York: McGraw-Hill, 1996]

Symptoms
- CNS effects (drowsy, slurred speech, ataxia, coma)
- Paradoxically excitement/anxiety/aggression
- Headache
- Chest pain
- Nausea and vomiting
- Diarrhea

Diagnosis
- History
- Oxygen saturation
- Consider coingestions
- Toxicology screen (serum levels not useful
- Electrolytes

Treatment
- √ fingerstick glucose. If unable to √ or low glucose, then give 50 ml D50/100 mg thiamine/0.4–2.0 mg naloxone.
- Gastric lavage if within 1 hour of ingestion; charcoal, 1 g/kg
- Forced diureses/hemodialysis not effective
- Monitor for cardiovascular and respiratory depression
- Flumazenil, 0.2 mg IV q1min to response or 3 mg maximum:
  Watch for seizures, especially in patients with coingestion/tricyclic antidepressants or benzodiazepine/alcohol dependence
  Contraindicated with increased intracranial pressure/severe head injury

BENZODIAZEPINE WITHDRAWAL

Fast Facts
- Usually history of prolonged use at high doses.
- May take days to weeks to manifest symptoms.
- Symptoms may appear similar to those for which benzodiazepines originally were prescribed.
- Avoid by slowly tapering dose.

Symptoms
- Anxiety
- Insomnia
- Nausea and vomiting
- Tremor
- Sweating/diaphoresis
- Confusion
- Psychosis
- Seizures

Treatment
- Reintroduce benzodiazepine and taper

OPIOID OVERDOSE [May et al. (eds). *Emergency Medicine* (2nd ed). Boston: Little, Brown, 1992]

Symptoms
- CNS depression (analgesia, sedation, pinpoint pupils, coma, seizures)
- Cardiovascular instability
- Pulmonary edema
- Seizures and respiratory depression

Diagnosis
- History and physical (pinpoint pupils, injection site)
- Toxicology screen
- Oxygen saturation, arterial blood gases, chest x-ray
- Naloxone trial (0.4–2.0 mg IV)
- Consider coingestions

Treatment
- Gastric lavage
- Charcoal, 1 g/kg PO/NG
- Hemodynamic/ventilator support
- Naloxone (0.4–2.0 mg IV up to 10 mg total); may need infusion if large ingestion/synthetic opioids (to rule out other causes of mental status change)

OPIOID WITHDRAWAL [May et al. (eds). *Emergency Medicine* (2nd ed). Boston: Little, Brown, 1992]

Symptoms
- Sympathetic discharge 8–16 hours after cessation (peak in 48–72 hours; resolves in 7–10 days)
- Tachycardia
- Pyrexia
- Hot flashes
- Lacrimation
- Hypertension
- Dilated pupils
- Abdominal cramps
- Diarrhea

Treatment
- Clonidine, 0.1–0.2 mg q8h prn
- Methadone per symptoms:
    - 5 mg: diaphoresis, restless
    - 10 mg: mydriasis, piloerection, fasciculation, myalgia, abdominal pain
    - 15 mg: autonomic instability, anorexia, nausea
    - 20 mg: diarrhea, vomiting, dehydration

TOXICOLOGY

ACETAMINOPHEN OVERDOSE [May et al. (eds). *Emergency Medicine* (2nd ed). Boston: Little, Brown, 1992]

Fast Facts
- Maximum tolerated dose: 4 g/day (normal liver function)
- Toxic >7.5 g/day
- Hepatotoxicity, renal tubular necrosis, myocardial damage, pancreatitis
- Metabolized by liver; toxicity exacerbated by alcohol, liver failure, rapid GI absorption

Symptoms/Diagnosis
- 2–12 hours: nausea and vomiting, diaphoresis, lethargy.
- 24–48 hours: improved symptoms, right upper quadrant pain, elevated transaminases.
- 72–96 hours: maximum increased LFTs (AST, ALT, bilirubin, ammonia, prothrombin time).
- Vomiting, jaundice, hepatic encephalopathy, disseminated intravascular coagulation, coagulopathy, acute tubular necrosis.
- If fatal, usually after 4–18 days due to fulminant hepatic necrosis.
- If recovery, LFTs begin to normalize in 5–6 days.
- Use nomogram (see next section), acetaminophen level at 4 hours, to predict toxicity.

Treatment
- Lavage (within 60–90 minutes)
- Charcoal (1 g/kg PO/NG) within 4 hours (but remove charcoal before N-acetylcysteine administration because charcoal binds it)
- N-Acetylcysteine, 140 mg/kg PO, then 70 mg/kg q4h × 17 doses (discontinue if 4-hour drug level <150 mg/dl)
- Aggressive antiemetics may be required

ACETAMINOPHEN NOMOGRAM

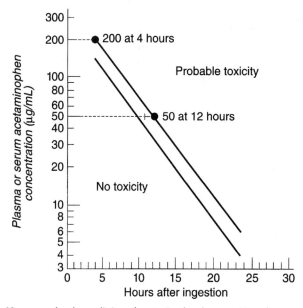

Nomogram for the prediction of acetaminophen hepatotoxicity after acute overdose. The upper line defines serum acetaminophen concentrations known to be associated with hepatotoxicity; the lower line defines serum levels 25% below those expected to cause hepatotoxicity. To give a margin for error, the lower line should be used as a guide to treatment. (Used with permission of the American Academy of Pediatrics. BH Rumack, H Matthew. Acetaminophen poisoning and toxicity. *Pediatrics* 55:871, 1975.)

TOXICOLOGY

ASPIRIN OVERDOSE
[May et al. (eds). *Emergency Medicine* (2nd ed). Boston: Little, Brown, 1992]

Fast Facts
- Toxic: >100 mg/kg
- Severe: >200 mg/kg
- Lethal: 20–25 g
- Respiratory alkalosis secondary to stimulated respiratory center
- Elevated anion gap acidosis due to lactate/ketoacids
- Metabolic alkalosis secondary to vomiting

Symptoms

Level	Severity	Symptoms
30–50 mg/dl	Mild	Tinnitus, vertigo, nausea and vomiting, abdominal pain
>70 mg/dl	Severe	Change in mental status, pulmonary/CNS edema, ulcer/bleed, hyperventilation, oliguria, cardiovascular collapse, seizures

Evaluation
- Check serial levels 2 and 6 hours after ingestion
- ABG
- Electrolytes q2–4h
- Clotting function
- LFTs
- Urine pH q2–4h

Treatment
- Gastric lavage
- Charcoal (1 g/kg PO/NG) + magnesium citrate to decrease transit time
- Hemodynamic/ventilatory support
- IV fluids to increase excretion (watch for CNS edema)
- Correct sodium and glucose
- $NaHCO_3$ [goal urine pH >7.5, add 2 ampules (100 mg of $NaHCO_3$) to 1 liter of D5 0.2% saline and infuse at 150–200 ml/hour]: increase renal excretion
- Hemodialysis if needed: decreased mental status, acute renal failure, uncorrected metabolic abnormalities, repeated levels >100 mg/dl

TRICYCLIC ANTIDEPRESSANT OVERDOSE

[May et al. (eds). *Emergency Medicine* (2nd ed). Boston: Little, Brown, 1992]

Fast Facts

- First 6 hours critical
- Greatest risk for
  - CNS/respiratory depression
  - Atrial/ventricular arrhythmia
  - Seizures
  - Hypotension

Symptoms

- Anticholinergic and peripheral alpha blockade
- Increased HR/temperature
- Dry mouth
- Urinary retention
- Decreased GI motility
- Dilated pupils
- Hallucinations
- Agitation
- Myoclonus
- Pulmonary edema
- QRS >0.1 more likely to have seizure/arrhythmia

Evaluation

- √ ECG for heart block, QRS/PR/QT widths, and ectopy
- Check serum levels:
  - Toxic: >500 ng/ml
  - Life-threatening: >1,000 ng/ml
  - Fatal: >5,000 ng/ml
- CXR, ABG, chem 7 (follow sodium carefully)
- Electrolytes, CK
- Urinalysis

Treatment

- Charcoal, 1 g/kg PO q4h, + cathartics (unless no bowel sounds)
- Lavage if <8 hours
- Alkalinize serum to 7.4–7.5 if ECG changes or hypotension
- Cautious hydration (watch for pulmonary edema)
- Check serial ECGs
- Hemodialysis/diuresis ineffective
- Cardiac monitor
- Treat hypotension with fluid and alpha agonists (norepinephrine, NeoSynephrine)

TOXICOLOGY

ANAPHYLAXIS   (*Am J Emerg Med* 6:456, 1988; *N Engl J Med* 324:1785, 1991)

Fast Facts
- Penicillin is the most common cause of pharmacologic anaphylaxis.
- 75% of fatal drug reactions are due to penicillin.

Treatment for Any Anaphylactic Reaction (Medications, Food, Bites, etc.)
- O_2, monitor, close observation.
- 0.5 ml 1/1,000 epinephrine IM or 3–5 ml 1/10,000 epinephrine IV over 10 minutes (more severe reaction).
- Diphenhydramine (Benadryl), 50 mg IV, + methylprednisolone sodium succinate (Solu-Medrol), 125 mg IV, + famotidine (Pepcid), 20 mg IV.
- Respiratory therapy, albuterol/ipratropium bromide (Atrovent) nebulizers.
- Watch for bradycardia, atropine at bedside.
- 5% have second episode within 72 hours.
- Discharge patient with diphenhydramine (Benadryl) + epinephrine injector (EpiPen) for other reactions; careful counseling about triggers.

15. Clinical Pharmacology

COMPOSITION OF COMMONLY USED INTRAVENOUS SOLUTIONS

Solution	Solute	Concentration (g/100 ml)	Na	K	Ca	Cl	HCO_3	Total mosm/liter
Dextrose in water	Glucose							
5%		5	—	—	—	—	—	278
10%		10	—	—	—	—	—	556
Saline	NaCl							
Half-normal		0.45	77	—	—	77	—	154
Normal		0.90	154	—	—	154	—	308
Hypertonic		3.0	513	—	—	513	—	1,026
		5.0	855	—	—	855	—	1,710
Dextrose in saline								
5% in 0.225%	Glucose	5.0	—	—	—	—	—	—
	NaCl	0.225	38.5	—	—	38.5	—	355
5% in 0.45%	Glucose	5.0	—	—	—	—	—	—
	NaCl	0.45	77	—	—	77	—	432
5% in 0.9%	Glucose	5.0	—	—	—	—	—	—
	NaCl	0.90	154	—	—	154	—	586
Alkalinizing solutions								
Hypertonic $NaHCO_3$ (0.6 M)	$NaHCO_3$	5.0	595	—	—	—	595	1,190
Hypertonic $NaHCO_3$ (0.9 M)	$NaHCO_3$	7.5	893	—	—	—	893	1,786
Polyionic solutions								
Ringer's	NaCl	0.86						—
	KCl	0.03	147	4	5	156		309
	$CaCl_2$	0.03						—
Lactated Ringer's	NaCl	0.60						—
	KCl	0.03						—
	$CaCl_2$	0.02	130	4	3	109	28	274
	Na lactate	0.31						—
Potassium chloride	KCl	14.85		2		2		—

Source: Reproduced with permission from BD Rose. *Clinical Physiology of Acid-Base and Electrolytes Disorders* (4th ed). New York: McGraw-Hill, 1994:405.

CLINICAL PHARMACOLOGY

MONITORING GUIDELINES FOR DRUGS COMMONLY USED IN THE INTENSIVE CARE UNIT

Drug	Elimination	Monitoring guidelines
Antiarrhythmics		
Lidocaine	H, M, and R	TSC: 3–6 µg/ml. Toxicity: muscle twitching and CNS excitation. Common in CHF.
Digoxin	R (60%), H, and B	TSC: 0.8–2.5 ng/ml. Monitor ECG (PR prolongation, T flattening, ST sloping).
Procaina- mide	H, M, and R	TSC: 4–12 µg/ml. Monitor ECG (QRS and QT prolongation).
Anticonvulsants		
Phenytoin	H	TSC: 10–20 µg/ml. Monitor free concentration (1–2 µg/ml) of uremic or hypoalbuminemic patients.
Valproic acid	H	TSC: 30–100 µg/ml.
Phenobarbital	H	TSC: 10–25 µg/ml.
BP medication: Nitroprus- side	H, M (thio- cyanate), and R	Maintain serum thiocyanate concentration <10 mg/dl. Monitor if patient has renal insufficiency and if using >3 days.
Analgesics and sedatives		
Morphine	H, M, and R	Monitor CNS status. Patients with CHF, cirrhosis, and renal failure are at increased risk of toxicity.
Meperidine	H, M, and R	Monitor CNS status. Renal insufficiency increases risk of seizures.
Diazepam (Valium)	H	Avoid large doses and infusions in liver disease. Rapid injections will produce apnea and hypotension.
Midazolam (Versed)	H	Same as for diazepam.
Lorazepam (Ativan)	H	Rapid injection will produce apnea and hypotension.
Haloperidol	H	Rapid injection will produce hypotension. Metabolite accumulation is not a problem with short-term use.
Propofol	H	Monitor BP and cardiac output. For prolonged infusion, monitor lipid profile.
Antiasthmatic: Theophylline	H	TSC: 5–15 mg/ml. Toxicity: tachycardia, hypertension, seizures.

Drug	Elimination	Monitoring guidelines
Antimicrobials		
Aminoglycosides	R	Therapeutic peak serum concentration: 4–8 mg/ml. Amikacin, 20–30 μg/ml. Avoid trough >2 mg/ml and 4–8 μg/ml, respectively.
Vancomycin	R	Therapeutic peak 20–40 μg/ml. Trough <10 μg/ml.
Neuromuscular agents		
Pancuronium	R (30%), M, R, and B	Avoid high doses and prolonged infusions in patients with renal insufficiency. Monitor twitch response.
Vecuronium		See pancuronium.
Antiulcer agent: H₂-blockers	R (65%)	Avoid high doses and prolonged infusions with renal insufficiency. Monitor CNS status.

H = hepatic clearance; M = metabolic clearance; R = renal clearance; B = biliary clearance; TSC = therapeutic serum concentration.
Source: Modified from B Chernow. *Critical Care Pharmacotherapy.* Baltimore: Williams & Wilkins, 1995.

CLINICAL PHARMACOLOGY

DRUGS AND LIVER DISEASE PATIENTS (Chernow, *Critical Care Pharmacotherapy*, 1995)

Group I: Drugs Capable of Causing Hepatic Damage in Normal Subjects

- Acetaminophen
- Chlorpromazine
- Methotrexate
- Acetylsalicylic acid
- Erythromycin estolate
- Methyldopa

Group II: Drugs That Can Compromise Liver Functions

- Anabolic and contraceptive steroids
- Tetracycline
- Prednisone

Group III: Drugs That May Worsen Complications of Liver Disease

- Cyclooxygenase inhibitors (indomethacin)
- Diuretics (Diuretics have been found to be the most common cause of adverse drug reactions and cause the most severe reactions.)
- Meperidine and other CNS depressants
- Morphine
- Pentazocine
- Phenylbutazone

CONSIDERATIONS FOR DRUG DOSAGE ADJUSTMENTS IN LIVER DISEASE

Extent of change in drug dose	Conditions or requirements to be satisfied
No change or minor change in dose	1. Mild liver disease. 2. Extensive elimination of drug by kidneys and no renal dysfunction. 3. Elimination by pathways of metabolism spared by liver disease. 4. Drug is enzyme-limited and given acutely. 5. Drug is flow/enzyme-sensitive and given acutely only by IV route. 6. No alteration in drug sensitivity.
Decrease in dose >25%	1. Elimination by liver does not exceed 40% of the dose; no renal dysfunction. 2. Drug is flow-limited and given by IV route, with no large change in protein binding. 3. Drug is flow/enzyme-limited and given acutely by oral route. 4. Drug has a large therapeutic ratio.
Decrease in dose >0.25%	1. Drug metabolism is affected by liver disease; drug administered chronically. 2. Drug has narrow therapeutic range; protein binding altered significantly. 3. Drug is flow-limited and given orally. 4. Drug is eliminated by kidneys, and renal function is severely affected. 5. Altered sensitivity to drug due to liver disease.

Flow-limited = clearance of drug depends on blood flow to liver; enzyme-limited = clearance depends on intrinsic activity of liver enzymes.

Source: Reproduced with permission from B Chernow. *Critical Care Pharmacotherapy*. Baltimore: Williams & Wilkins, 1995.

NONANTIBIOTIC DRUG DOSAGE ADJUSTMENTS IN RENAL FAILURE

Drug	Dose for ClCr ≥50 ml/min	D or I	Adjustment for renal failure ClCr = 10–50	ClCr = <10	Removed significantly by HD	PD	CAVH/ CVVH	CAVHD/ CVVHD
Acetaminophen	650 mg q4h	I	q6h	q6h	No	No	No	No
Amiodarone	800- to 1,600-mg load, 200–600 mg/day	D	100%	100%	No	No	—	No
Amitriptyline	100–300 mg/day	D	100%	100%	No	No	No	No
Amlodipine	5–10 mg/day	D	100%	100%	No	No	ND	ND
Atenolol	50–100 mg qd	D, I	25–50 mg	25 mg q48h	Yes	No	Yes	Yes
Captopril	25 mg q8–12h	D, I	50–75% q12h	25% q24h	Yes	No	No	No
Chloral hydrate	250 mg tid	D	ND	Avoid	?	ND	ND	ND
Cimetidine	300 mg q6h	D, I	q8–12h	q12h	Yes	No	No	No
Clonidine	0.1–0.6 mg bid	D	100%	100%	No	No	No	No
Diazepam	5–20 mg prn	D	100%	100%	No	ND	No	No
Digoxin	10- to 15-µg/kg load, 0.25–0.50 mg/day	D, I	25–75% q24–48h	25% q48h	No	No	No	No
Diltiazem	60–120 mg q8h	D	100%	100%	No	No	No	No
Enalapril	5–40 mg q24h	D	75–100%	50%	Yes	No	No	No
Esmolol	50–200 µg/kg/min by infusion	D	100%	100%	No	No	ND	ND
Fentanyl	Anesthetic induction	D	100%	100%	NA	NA	NA	NA
Fluoxetine	20–80 mg qAM	D	100%	100%	No	No	No	No
Furosemide	40–80 mg q12h	D	100%	100%	No	No	No	No
Glipizide	2.5–15.0 mg/day	D	100%	100%	ND	ND	ND	ND
Glyburide	2.5–20.0 mg/day	D	Avoid	Avoid	No	No	No	No
Haloperidol	1–5 mg prn	D	100%	100%	No	No	No	No
Hydralazine	20–40 mg q6–8h	D	100%	100%	No	No	No	No
HCTZ	25–50 mg qd	D	100%	Avoid	No	ND	No	No
Insulin	Variable	D	75%	50%	No	No	No	No

continued

CLINICAL PHARMACOLOGY

Drug	Dose for ClCr ≥50 ml/min	D or I	ClCr = 10–50	ClCr = <10	HD	PD	CAVH/ CVVH	CAVHD/ CVVHD
			Adjustment for renal failure		**Removed significantly by**			
Lidocaine	50 mg over 2 mins, repeat q5min × 3, then 1–4 mg/min	D	100%	100%	No	No	No	No
Lisinopril	10–40 mg q24h	D	50–75%	25–50%	Yes	No	ND	ND
Lithium	0.9–2.1 g qd in divided doses	D	50–75%	25–50%	Yes	No	Yes	Yes
Lorazepam	1–2 mg bid/tid	D	100%	100%	No	ND	No	No
Methadone	2.5–10.0 mg q6–8h	D	100%	100%	No	No	ND	ND
Metoprolol	50–200 mg bid	D	100%	100%	Yes	No	No	No
Midazolam	Titrate	D	100%	50–100%	No	ND	No	No
Morphine	2–10 mg q4h	D	75%	50%	No	ND	No	No
Nifedipine	10–30 mg q8h	D	100%	100%	No	No	No	No
Omeprazole	20–40 mg qd	D	100%	100%	No	No	No	No
Paroxetine	20–50 mg qAM	D	50–100%	50%	ND	ND	ND	ND
Phenobarbital	1–3 mg/kg qd	D	100%	75–100%	Yes	Yes	Yes	Yes
Procainamide	Load: 12–17 mg/kg, then individualize	D, I	Load 100%	Load 100%	Yes	No	No	No
Propafenone	150–300 mg q8h	D	100%	100%	No	No	No	No
Ranitidine (IV)	50 mg q8h	I	q12h	q24h	Yes	No	No	No
Sertraline	50–200 mg qAM	D	100%	100%	ND	ND	ND	ND

ClCr = creatinine clearance; D = dose; I = interval; ND = no data; HD = hemodialysis; PD = peritoneal dialysis; CAVH/CVVH = continuous arteriovenous hemofiltration/continuous venovenous hemofiltration; CAVHD/CVVHD = continuous arteriovenous hemodialysis/continuous venovenous hemodialysis; HCTZ = hydrochlorothiazide.

Source: Reproduced with permission from B Chernow. *Critical Care Pharmacotherapy.* Baltimore: Williams & Wilkins, 1995.

DRUG INTERACTIONS WITH DIGOXIN
Increased Digoxin Levels

- Alprazolam
- Amiodarone
- Benzodiazepines
- Captopril
- Diltiazem
- Erythromycin
- Felodipine
- Hydroxychloroquine
- Indomethacin
- Nifedipine
- Propafenone
- Quinidine
- Tetracycline
- Verapamil

- Aminoglycosides
- Anticholinergics
- Bepridil
- Cyclosporine
- Diphenoxylate
- Esmolol
- Flecainide
- Ibuprofen
- Itraconazole
- Omeprazole
- Propantheline
- Quinine
- Tolbutamide

Decreased Digoxin Levels

- Aminoglutethimide
- Aminosalicylic acid
- Antihistamines
- Barbiturates
- Colestipol
- Hypoglycemic agents
- Metoclopramide
- Penicillamine
- Sucralfate
- Rifampin

- Aminoglycosides
- Antacids (aluminum or magnesium)
- Antineoplastics (bleomycin, carmustine, cyclophosphamide, cytarabine, doxorubicin, methotrexate, procarbazine, vincristine)
- Cholestyramine
- Hydantoins
- Kaolin/pectin
- Neomycin
- Sulfasalazine

DRUG INTERACTIONS WITH THEOPHYLLINE
Increased Theophylline Levels

- Allopurinol
- Calcium channel blockers
- Cimetidine
- Disulfiram
- Influenza virus vaccine
- Isoniazid
- Macrolides
- OCPs
- Thiabendazole

- Beta blockers
- Carbamazepine
- Corticosteroids
- Ephedrine
- Interferon
- Loop diuretics
- Mexiletine
- Quinolones
- Thyroid hormones

continued

CLINICAL PHARMACOLOGY

Decreased Theophylline Levels

- Aminoglutethimide
- Carbamazepine
- Hydantoins
- Ketoconazole
- Rifampin
- Sulfinpyrazone
- Thioamines
- Barbiturates
- Charcoal
- Isoniazid
- Loop diuretics
- Smoking (cigarettes or marijuana)
- Sympathomimetics

DRUG INTERACTIONS WITH CYCLOSPORINE
(Reproduced with permission from B Chernow. *Critical Care Pharmacotherapy.* Baltimore: Williams & Wilkins, 1995)

Increased Cyclosporine Levels

- Diltiazem
- Ethanol
- Imipenem/cilastin
- Levonorgestrel
- Methyltestosterone
- Nicardipine
- Prednisolone
- Warfarin
- Erythromycin
- Fluconazole
- Ketoconazole
- Methylprednisolone
- Metoclopramide
- Norfloxacin
- Verapamil

Decreased Cyclosporine Levels

- Carbamazepine
- Phenobarbital
- Rifampin
- Nafcillin
- Phenytoin
- Valproic acid

Enhanced Cyclosporine Nephrotoxicity

- Acyclovir
- Amphotericin B
- Doxorubicin
- Ganciclovir
- Melphalan
- Trimethoprim
- Aminoglycosides
- Digoxin
- Furosemide
- Indomethacin
- Metolazone

DRUG INTERACTIONS WITH COUMADIN:
SEE CHAPTER 5, HEMATOLOGY

SELECTED CLINICAL MANIFESTATIONS OF ADVERSE DRUG REACTIONS (*JAMA* 278:1895, 1997; *N Engl J Med* 331:1272, 1994)

Multisystem

Anaphylactic
- Antimicrobials
- Proteins
- Ethylene oxide

Anaphylactoid
- Radiocontrast media
- Nonsteroidal anti-inflammatory drugs (NSAIDs)
- Opiates
- Polymyxin B
- Tubocurarine
- Dextrans
- Paclitaxel

Stevens-Johnson Syndrome/Toxic Epidermal Necrolysis
- Sulfonamides
- Beta-lactam antibiotics
- Phenytoin
- Carbamazepine

Hypersensitivity Syndrome
- Anticonvulsants
- Sulfonamides
- Allopurinol
- Dapsone

Serum Sickness/Vasculitis
- Proteins
- Antimicrobials
- Allopurinol
- Thiazides
- Pyrazolones
- Phenytoin
- Propylthiouracil

Drug Fever
- Bleomycin
- Amphotericin B
- Sulfonamides

continued

CLINICAL PHARMACOLOGY

- Beta-lactams
- Methyldopa
- Chlorpromazine
- Quinidine
- Anticonvulsants

Dermatologic Patterns

Urticaria/Angioedema
- Same as for anaphylactic reactions, plus opiates

Isolated Angioedema
- Angiotensin-converting enzyme (ACE) inhibitors

Pruritus without Urticaria
- Gold
- Sulfonamides

Morbilliform Rash
- Penicillins
- Sulfonamides
- Barbiturates
- Antituberculous drugs
- Anticonvulsants
- Quinidine

Fixed Drug Eruptions
- Phenolphthalein
- Analgesics/antipyretics
- Barbiturates
- Beta-lactam antibiotics
- Sulfonamides
- Tetracycline

Photoallergic Photosensitivity
- Phenothiazines
- Sulfonamides
- Griseofulvin

Phototoxic Photosensitivity
- Tetracyclines
- Sulfanilamide
- Chlorpromazine
- Psoralens

Contact Dermatitis
- Local anesthetics
- Neomycin
- Paraben esters
- Ethylenediamine
- Antihistamines
- Mercurials

Hepatic Patterns
Cholestasis
- Macrolides
- Phenothiazines
- Hypoglycemics
- Imipramine
- Nitrofurantoin

Hepatocellular
- Valproic acid
- Halothane
- Isoniazid
- Methyldopa
- Quinidine
- Nitrofurantoin
- Phenytoin
- Sulfonylureas

Granulomatous
- Quinidine
- Allopurinol
- Methyldopa
- Sulfonamides

Renal Patterns
Nephrosis (Membranous Glomerulonephritis)
- Gold
- Captopril
- NSAIDs
- Penicillamine
- Probenecid
- Anticonvulsants

Acute Interstitial Nephritis
- Beta-lactams (especially methicillin)
- Rifampin

CLINICAL PHARMACOLOGY

- NSAIDs
- Sulfonamides
- Captopril
- Allopurinol

Respiratory Patterns

Rhinitis

- Reserpine
- Hydralazine
- Alpha-receptor blockers
- Anticholinesterases
- Iodides
- Levodopa
- Triethanolamine

Asthma

- Inhaled proteins (pancreatic extract, psyllium)
- Beta-lactam antibiotics
- Sulfites
- NSAIDs
- Alpha-receptor blockers

Cough

- ACE inhibitors

Pulmonary Infiltrates with Eosinophilia

- Nitrofurantoin
- Methotrexate
- NSAIDs
- Sulfonamides
- Tetracycline
- Isoniazid

Chronic Fibrotic Reactions

- Nitrofurantoin
- Cytotoxic chemotherapeutics

Hematologic Patterns

Eosinophilia

- Gold
- Allopurinol
- Acetylsalicylic acid
- Ampicillin

- Tricyclic antidepressants
- Capreomycin
- Carbamazepine
- Digitalis
- Phenytoin

Thrombocytopenia
- Quinidine
- Sulfonamides
- Gold
- Heparin

Hemolytic Anemia
- Penicillin
- Cisplatin
- Sulfonamides
- Quinines
- Chlorpromazine
- Para-aminosalicylic acid
- Methyldopa
- Penicillin
- Sulfasalazine
- Procainamide
- Penicillins
- Phenothiazines

Neurologic Patterns
Seizures
- Theophylline
- Vincristine
- Lithium
- Tricyclic antidepressants

Deafness
- Aminoglycosides
- Furosemide
- Aspirin
- Bleomycin

Optic Neuritis
- Ethambutol
- Isoniazid
- Aminosalicylic acid

16. Evidence-Based Medicine

HOW TO USE AN ARTICLE ABOUT THERAPY OR PREVENTION
Reader's Guides for an Article about Therapy

(Reprinted with permission from GH Guyatt, DL Sackett, DJ Cook. Users' guides to the medical literature. II. How to use an article about therapy or prevention. B. What were the results and will they help me in caring for my patients? Evidence-Based Medicine Working Group. *JAMA* 271:59–63, 1994. Copyright 1994, American Medical Association.)

Are the Results of the Study Valid?
Primary Guides
- Was the assignment of patients to the treatments randomized?
- Were all the patients who entered the trial properly accounted for and attributed at its conclusion?
- Was follow-up complete?
- Were patients analyzed in the groups to which they were randomized?

Secondary Guides
- Were patients, health workers, and study personnel "blind" to treatment?
- Were the groups similar at the start of the trial?
- Aside from the experimental intervention, were the groups treated equally?

What Were the Results?
- How large was the treatment effect?
- How precise was the estimate of the treatment effect?

Will the Results Help Me Care for My Patients?
- Can the results be applied to my patient care?
- Were all clinically important outcomes considered?
- Are the likely treatment benefits worth the potential harms and costs?

Measures of the effects of therapy	Example
Risk without therapy (baseline risk): X	20/100 = 0.20 or 20%
Risk with therapy: Y	15/100 = 0.15 or 15%
Absolute risk reduction (risk difference): X – Y	0.20 – 0.15 = 0.05
Relative risk: Y/X	0.15/0.20 = 0.75
Relative risk reduction: [1 – (Y/X)] × 100%, or [(X – Y)/X] × 100%	(1.00 – 0.75) × 100% = 25%; (0.05/0.20) × 100% = 25%
Number needed to treat to prevent one event: 1/(X – Y)	1/(0.20 – 0.15) = 20

- Converting odds ratios (OR) to number needed to treat:

$$NNT = \frac{1 - [PEER \times (1 - OR)]}{(1 - PEER) \times PEER \times (1 - OR)}$$

where PEER = patient's expected event rate.

HOW TO USE ARTICLES ABOUT DIAGNOSTIC TESTS

Evaluating and Applying the Results of Studies of Diagnostic Tests

(R Jaeschke, GH Guyatt, DL Sackett. User's guides to the medical literature. III. How to use an article about a diagnostic test. B. What are the results and will they help me in caring for my patients? Evidence-Based Medicine Working Group. *JAMA* 271:703–707, 1994. Copyright 1994, American Medical Association.)

Are the Results of the Study Valid?

Primary Guides

- Was there an independent, blind comparison with a reference standard?
- Did the patient sample include an appropriate spectrum of patients to whom the diagnostic test will be applied in clinical practice?

Secondary Guides

- Did the results of the test being evaluated influence the decision to perform the reference standard?
- Were the methods for performing the test described in sufficient detail to permit replication?

What Were the Results?

- Are the likelihood ratios for the test results presented or the data necessary for their calculation provided?

Will the Results Help Me Care for My Patients?

- Will the reproducibility of the test results and the interpretation be satisfactory in my setting?
- Are the results applicable to my patient?
- Will the results change my management?
- Will patients be better off as a result of the test?

continued

EVIDENCE-BASED MEDICINE

Basic Terms for Evaluating a Diagnostic Test

	Disease positive	Disease negative
Test positive	A	B
Test negative	C	D

Term	Definition	Calculation
Sensitivity	Proportion of subjects with the disease who have a positive test	A/(A + C)
Specificity	Proportion of subjects without the disease who have a negative test	D/(B + D)
Positive predictive value	Likelihood that a positive test indicates disease	A/(A + B)
Negative predictive value	Likelihood that a negative test indicates lack of disease	D/(C + D)
Likelihood ratio	Likelihood that a given test result would be expected in a patient with the target disorder compared to the likelihood that the same result would be expected in a patient without the disorder	$\dfrac{\text{Sensitivity}}{(1\text{-specificity})}$ or $\dfrac{A/(A + C)}{B/(B + D)}$

FAGAN'S NOMOGRAM

Nomogram for interpreting diagnostic test results. (Reprinted with permission from R Jaeschke, GH Guyatt, DL Sackett. User's guides to the medical literature. III. How to use an article about a diagnostic test. B. What are the results and will they help me in caring for my patients? Evidence-Based Medicine Working Group. *JAMA* 271:705, 1994. Copyright 1994, American Medical Association.)

- Anchor a ruler at your patient's pretest probability.
- Rotate until ruler lines up with the LR for the test.
- Find the intersecting post-test probability.

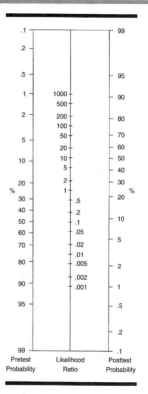

17. Radiology

CHEST RADIOLOGY: CHEST X-RAY

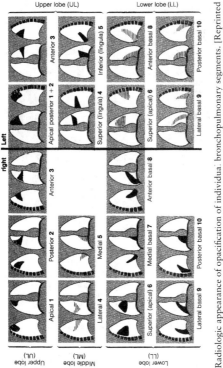

Radiologic appearance of opacification of individual bronchopulmonary segments. [Reprinted with permission from M von Planta (ed). Memorix Innere Medizin (4th ed). © Chapman & Hall, Weinheim 1996; Hippokrates Verlag Stuttgart 1999.]

GASTROINTESTINAL RADIOLOGY: SPECIALIZED IMAGING PROTOCOLS

Procedure	Description	Indications
Barium swallow, upper GI study, SBFT*	Swallow barium in single contrast, addition of effervescent agent and high-density barium, follow multiple images through time. No barium in perforation.	Upper GI contours, mucosal lesions for double contrast
Enteroclysis	IV metoclopramide followed by nasojejunal catheter, balloon inflated with barium/methylcellulose infusion, not in complete obstruction or perforation.	Mucosal details for small bowel better than SBFT
Peroral pneumo-colon*	SBFT with low-density barium reaches colon followed by air via rectal tube to distend cecum. Not in toxic megacolon.	Terminal ileum/colon evaluation
Contrast enema*	Air-contrast barium enema (high-density barium followed by air), glucagon for prior spasm, not in toxic megacolon, suspected or high risk of perforation or biopsy <24 hrs. Water-soluble contrast for perforation.	Colonic mucosa evaluation
Oral cholecysto-gram	Contrast agent absorbed via intestines excreted via biliary tract concentrated in gallbladder (peak 17 hrs after contrast taken).	Adjunct to ultrasound for biliary diseases
Hepatobiliary (^{99m}Tc HIDA) scan, liver-spleen scan	IV injection of contrast (iminodiacetic acid [IDA]) followed by multiple scans (gallbladder visible in 1 hr).	Evaluate cholecystitis, cholestasis, or hepatic function
Gastric-emptying scan	^{99m}Tc sulfur colloid to egg for swallowing followed by multiple scans at sitting position.	Evaluate gastric motility
Meckel's scan	Cimetidine 1–3 days prior, then ^{99m}Tc dye IV followed by multiple scans; pentagastrin IV before dye to stimulate mucosa.	Diagnose 50% Meckel's diverticulum that secretes ^{99m}TcO$_4$
Erythrocytes scan	^{99m}Tc-tagged RBCs injected with imaging up to 24 hrs. (^{99m}Tc sulfur colloid scan only for active bleeding within 15 mins.)	Detects active GI bleeding at 0.05–0.10 cc/min
Arteriography	IV dye injection at localized vessels under fluoroscopy.	Detects active GI bleeding at 0.5 cc/min, also provides therapy and detects ischemia

SBFT = small-bowel follow-through.
*Barium is not water soluble, and should *not* be used if perforation is suspected and should *never* be used for colonic obstruction. Barium also should not be used in suspected aspiration or fistula; if both happen, avoid using contrast or use an NG tube for water-soluble contrast.

RADIOLOGY

SPECIALIZED RADIOLOGIC PROCEDURES PREPARATION (STANFORD PROTOCOL)

Test	Diet	Preparation
Radiologic procedures		
Abdominal/pelvic CT	FL/CL 4 hrs before	Drink contrast ASAP
Chest/extremity CT	No restriction	None
Cystogram	No restriction	Full bladder, plug catheter
Nonfasting oral cholecysto-gram	4 pats of oil after meals day before, NPO after dinner	2 Telepaque tablets after meals day before, water at 9–10 PM, 6 Oragrafin capsules, 2 Telepaque tablets at 3 PM if afternoon study
Fasting oral cholecystogram	NPO	6 Oragrafin capsules 9–10 PM before
Venogram	CL before exam, NPO 1 hr prior	None
Lymphangiogram	Light meal before	Limit fluid (2- to 3-hr exam)
Abdominal ultrasound	NPO 6 hrs before	None
Pelvic ultrasound	No restriction	4 glasses water 1 hr before, no void
T-tube cholangiogram	NPO after MN	No smoking
Barium swallow	NPO 1 hr before	None
Upper GI series; SBFT	NPO after 9 PM	1 glass water qh between 12 and 7 PM, no smoking/chewing after MN
Reflux small-bowel enema (enteroclysis)	CL day before, NPO after 11 PM	1 glass water qh 1–7 PM day before, ? 1. plain water enema at 7 PM, cold Mg citrate at 8 PM, 4 Dulcolax tablets at 11 PM, 1 Dulcolax suppository at 7 AM
Barium enema	CL day before, NPO after 11 PM	Similar to reflux small-bowel enema preparation except no water enema at 7 PM
MRI*	No restrictions	None
Endoscopic procedures		
EGD/ERCP	NPO 6 hrs before	None
Flexible sigmoidoscopy	CL dinner before, NPO after MN, no milk/antacid	Mg citrate at 8 PM, 1 glass water q2h until 10 PM, then 3 Dulcolax tablets at 10 PM, 1 Dulcolax suppository at 6 AM
Colonoscopy	CL day before, NPO after 11 PM	Similar to barium enema
Nuclear imaging: myocardial perfusion scintigraphy	NPO 6 hrs before	No xanthine products (e.g., caffeine, chocolate) × 24 hrs with dipyridamole test

NPO = nothing by mouth; CL = clear liquid; MN = midnight; FL = full liquid; EGD = esophagos-troduodenoscopy.
*Patients scheduled for MRI should be asked about claustrophobia, history of working with metals, brain/cardiac/aneurysm surgery or history of metal fragments/mesh/implants or wire sutures, shunt, and cochlear implants or pacemaker/defibrillators.

- Iodine-sensitive pretreatment: take prednisone 50 mg PO night before, then take diphenhydramine (Benadryl) 50 mg + cimetidine 300 mg + prednisone 50 mg when on call to procedure.

272

18. Procedures

PROCEDURE: CENTRAL VENOUS LINE
Fast Facts
- Indications: delivery of high concentrations of nutrition or medication, inotropic drug, prolonged IV drug delivery, hemodialysis, hemodynamic monitoring, limited access.
- Contraindications: infection/lesion at insertion site, thrombosis, graft site, patient intolerance of exam.
- Precautions: correct coagulopathy (INR <1.5).
- Document all procedures and informed consent with supervision/witness.

Subclavian Vein
- Supine, 15-degree Trendelenburg with head away, place roll under spine between shoulders.
- Sterile preparation and drape, 1% lidocaine local anesthesia, advance aspirating 18-gauge needle at infraclavicular site 1 cm inferior to distal third of clavicle toward suprasternal notch, then below clavicle (total advance ~5 cm).
- Seldinger technique with dilator/catheter over guidewire, saline flush, secure, x-ray.

Internal Jugular Vein
- Supine, 15-degree reverse Trendelenburg with head turned 30 degrees away.
- Sterile preparation and drape, 1% lidocaine local anesthesia, advance aspirating 22-gauge needle at apex of triangle between two sternocleidomastoid muscles toward ipsilateral nipple (or lateral to muscles at 4–5 cm above clavicle toward suprasternal notch ~5 cm), lateral to carotid pulse.
- Seldinger technique with dilator/catheter over guidewire, saline flush, secure, x-ray.

Femoral Vein
- Supine, sterile preparation and drape, 1% lidocaine local anesthesia.
- Advance aspirating 18-gauge needle at halfway between anterior iliac spine and symphysis pubis at 30-degree angle, medial to femoral artery (~4 cm).
- Seldinger technique with dilator/catheter over guidewire, saline flush, secure.

Risks and Complications and Their Treatments
- Venous air embolism: hyperbaric therapy
- Pneumothorax: 100% oxygen, tube thoracostomy if respiratory compromise
- Guidewire embolism: surgery
- Arterial puncture: direct compression, close monitor
- Cardiac tamponade: pericardiocentesis
- Infection: antibiotics, line removal

continued

PROCEDURES

- Vessel thrombosis or thrombophlebitis: line removal, urokinase
- Hemorrhage: direct compression, correct coagulopathy

Remarks

- Line removal: ensure remaining access, place patient supine and prepare site, exhale during removal, culture tip if febrile.
- Pulmonary artery (Swan-Ganz) catheter and pacer require 16-gauge venous sheath.
- Pheresis and hemodialysis require 14-gauge Quinton/Shiley catheters.
- Endomyocardial biopsy (right heart): may have slightly increased risk of perforation (especially during myocarditis) and heart block.

PROCEDURE: LUMBAR PUNCTURE

Indications

- Diagnosis of meningitis, encephalitis, meningeal carcinomatosis, tertiary syphilis, Guillain-Barré syndrome, multiple sclerosis, subarachnoid hemorrhage (with normal CT scan)
- Treatment of pseudotumor cerebri, drug delivery

Contraindications

- Infection at site of LP, increased intracranial pressure (ICP), CNS mass lesion, hemorrhagic diathesis, venous sinus occlusion

Complications

- Headache, persistent leak, bleeding, hematoma, infection, herniation with mass lesion/increased ICP

Procedure

- Patient in lateral decubitus position, spine flexed, knees to abdomen.
- At L4-5 interspace, clean with iodine, anesthetize with 1–2% lidocaine.
- Spinal needle with bevel up in L4-5 interspace, parallel to exam table, toward umbilicus.
- Measure opening pressure; collect four tubes of cerebrospinal fluid.

Tests

- Tube 1: chemistries—protein, glucose
- Tube 2: microbiology—Gram's stain, culture
- Tube 3: cell count with differential
- Tube 4: other diagnostic tests
- Consider: VDRL, cryptococcal antigen, India ink preparation, fungal or viral cultures, cytology, oligoclonal banding

PROCEDURES

PROCEDURE: THORACENTESIS

Indications
- Evaluation of pleural effusion
- Treat large pleural effusion—serial drainage, consider chest tube, pleurodesis

Contraindications
- Bleeding diathesis, thrombocytopenia, patient intolerance of exam

Complications
- Pneumothorax, hemothorax, infection, perforation of liver or spleen, air embolism

Procedure
- Patient in sitting position, arms and head supported on table.
- Identify effusion with percussion/ultrasound, clean with iodine, and anesthetize with 1–2% lidocaine.
- Needle above margin of rib, aspirate fluid.

Tests
- Tube 1: chemistries—protein, LDH, glucose
- Tube 2: if parapneumonic or rule out empyema, pH
- Tube 3: cell count with differential
- Tube 4: other diagnostic tests

Remarks
- In emergent tension pneumothorax, needle decompression can be achieved by inserting a 16-gauge needle into the second or third intercostal space, approaching anteriorly at the midclavicular line on the affected side. Tube thoracostomy may follow if indicated.

PROCEDURE: PARACENTESIS

Indications
- Evaluation of ascites, rule out peritonitis, direct peritoneal lavage
- Treatment of tense ascites, peritoneal dialysis

Contraindications
- Bleeding diathesis, infection at entry site, surgical scars at entry site, bowel distension

Complications
- Persistent leak, perforated bowel, hemorrhage, peritonitis, hypotension from large-volume paracentesis

Procedure
- Patient with empty bladder, position (lateral lower quadrant usually below umbilicus), may use midline approach especially in patients with high bleeding risk.
- Clean with iodine; anesthetize with 1–2% lidocaine.
- Insert needle using z-tracking; remove peritoneal fluid.

Tests
- Tube 1: chemistries—protein, albumin, glucose.
- Tube 2: cell count with differential.
- Tube 3: Gram's stain, other cultures if needed.
- Tube 4: save.
- Inoculate one set of blood culture bottles at bedside with peritoneal fluid to rule out spontaneous bacterial peritonitis.

19. Advanced Cardiopulmonary Life Support

SELECTED ACLS DRUGS

Adenosine	6 mg rapid IV push follow by 20 ml normal saline flush; repeat dose 12 mg IV q1–2 min up to 2 doses
Atropine sulfate	1 mg IV push; repeat dose q3–5min
	Max dose: 0.03–0.04 mg/kg
	Endotracheal dose: 2–3 mg dilute in 10 ml normal saline
Amiodarone	300 mg IV push (after epinephrine in ventricular fibrillation, dose according to ARREST trial [*N Engl J Med* 341:871, 1999])
	Stable VT: 150 mg IV bolus, then 1 mg/min IV drip over next 8 hours, 0.5 mg/min IV drip over next 16 hours
Bretylium	Loading: 5–10 mg/kg (~300–600 mg) IV
	Arrest: bolus, may repeat q5min
	Stable VT: over 8–10 min, may repeat q10–30min
	Drip: 1–2 mg/min IV drip
	Max dose: 30–35 mg/kg over 24 hours
Calcium chloride	8–16 mg/kg (usually 5–10 ml) IV slow push
Epinephrine	1 mg IV push q3–5min (high dose: 0.1 mg/kg IV push)
	Escalating dose: 1 mg, 3 mg, 5 mg IV push
	Endotracheal dose: 2.0–2.5 mg dilute in 10 ml normal saline
Lidocaine	Loading: 1.0–1.5 mg/kg (~100 mg) IV, may repeat q3min Drip: 1–4 mg/min IV drip
	Maximum dose: 3 mg/kg IV
Procainamide	Loading: 30 mg/min (1.0–1.2 g) IV
	Drip: 2–5 mg/min IV gtt
	Max dose: 17 mg/kg IV

VT = ventricular tachycardia.

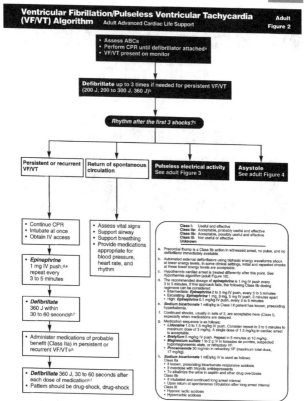

Ventricular Fibrillation/Pulseless Ventricular Tachycardia (VF/VT) Algorithm Adult Advanced Cardiac Life Support

Adult Figure 2

- Assess ABCs
- Perform CPR until defibrillator attached[a]
- VF/VT present on monitor

↓

Defibrillate up to 3 times if needed for persistent VF/VT (200 J; 200 to 300 J; 360 J)[b]

↓

Rhythm after the first 3 shocks?[c]

| Persistent or recurrent VF/VT | Return of spontaneous circulation | Pulseless electrical activity See adult Figure 3 | Asystole See adult Figure 4 |

Persistent or recurrent VF/VT
- Continue CPR
- Intubate at once
- Obtain IV access

- **Epinephrine** 1 mg IV push,[d,e] repeat every 3 to 5 minutes

- **Defibrillate** 360 J within 30 to 60 seconds[b,f]

- Administer medications of probable benefit (Class IIa) in persistent or recurrent VF/VT[g,h]

- **Defibrillate** 360 J, 30 to 60 seconds after each dose of medication[b,f]
- Pattern should be drug-shock, drug-shock

Return of spontaneous circulation
- Assess vital signs
- Support airway
- Support breathing
- Provide medications appropriate for blood pressure, heart rate, and rhythm

---

Class I: Useful and effective
Class IIa: Acceptable, probably useful and effective
Class IIb: Acceptable, possibly useful and effective
Class III: Not useful or effective
Unknown

---

a. Precordial thump is a Class IIb action in witnessed arrest, no pulse, and no defibrillator immediately available.

b. Automated external defibrillators using biphasic energy waveforms shock at lower energy levels. In some clinical settings, initial and repeated shocks at these lower energy levels are acceptable.

c. Hypothermic cardiac arrest is treated differently after this point. *See hypothermia algorithm* (adult Figure 10).

d. The recommended dosage of *epinephrine* is 1 mg IV push every 3 to 5 minutes. If this approach fails, the following Class IIb dosing regimen can be considered:
   - Intermediate: *Epinephrine* 2 to 5 mg IV push, every 3 to 5 minutes
   - Escalating: *Epinephrine* 1 mg, 3 mg, 5 mg IV push, 3 minutes apart
   - High: *Epinephrine* 0.1 mg/kg IV push, every 3 to 5 minutes

e. *Sodium bicarbonate* 1 mEq/kg is Class I if patient has known, preexisting hyperkalemia.

f. Continued shocks, usually in sets of 3, are acceptable here (Class I), especially when medications are delayed.

g. Medication sequence is as follows:
   - *Lidocaine* 1.0 to 1.5 mg/kg IV push. Consider repeat in 3 to 5 minutes to maximum dose of 3 mg/kg. A single dose of 1.5 mg/kg in cardiac arrest is acceptable.
   - *Bretylium* 5 mg/kg IV push. Repeat in 5 minutes at 10 mg/kg.
   - *Magnesium sulfate* 1 to 2 g IV in torsades de pointes, suspected hypomagnesemic state, or refractory VF.
   - *Procainamide* 30 mg/min in refractory VF (maximum total dose, 17 mg/kg).

h. *Sodium bicarbonate* 1 mEq/kg IV is used as follows:
   Class IIa
   - If known, preexisting bicarbonate-responsive acidosis
   - If overdose with tricyclic antidepressants
   - To alkalinize the urine in aspirin and other drug overdoses
   Class IIb
   - If intubated and continued long arrest interval
   - Upon return of spontaneous circulation after long arrest interval
   Class III
   - Hypoxic lactic acidosis
   - Hypercarbic acidosis

ACLS

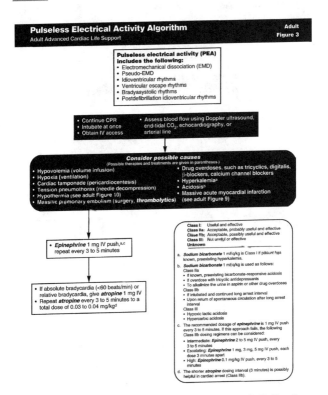

Pulseless Electrical Activity Algorithm
Adult Advanced Cardiac Life Support

Adult
Figure 3

Pulseless electrical activity (PEA) includes the following:
- Electromechanical dissociation (EMD)
- Pseudo-EMD
- Idioventricular rhythms
- Ventricular escape rhythms
- Bradyasystolic rhythms
- Postdefibrillation idioventricular rhythms

- Continue CPR
- Intubate at once
- Obtain IV access

- Assess blood flow using Doppler ultrasound, end-tidal CO_2, echocardiography, or arterial line

Consider possible causes
(Possible therapies and treatments are given in parentheses.)

- Hypovolemia (volume infusion)
- Hypoxia (ventilation)
- Cardiac tamponade (pericardiocentesis)
- Tension pneumothorax (needle decompression)
- Hypothermia (see adult Figure 10)
- Massive pulmonary embolism (surgery, **thrombolytics**)

- Drug overdoses, such as tricyclics, digitalis, β-blockers, calcium channel blockers
- Hyperkalemia[a]
- Acidosis[b]
- Massive acute myocardial infarction (see adult Figure 9)

- **Epinephrine** 1 mg IV push,[a,c] repeat every 3 to 5 minutes

- If absolute bradycardia (<60 beats/min) or relative bradycardia, give **atropine** 1 mg IV
- Repeat **atropine** every 3 to 5 minutes to a total dose of 0.03 to 0.04 mg/kg[d]

Class I: Useful and effective
Class IIa: Acceptable, probably useful and effective
Class IIb: Acceptable, possibly useful and effective
Class III: Not useful or effective
Unknown

a. **Sodium bicarbonate** 1 mEq/kg is Class I if patient has known, preexisting hyperkalemia.

b. **Sodium bicarbonate** 1 mEq/kg is used as follows:
   Class IIa
   - If known, preexisting bicarbonate-responsive acidosis
   - If overdose with tricyclic antidepressants
   - To alkalinize the urine in aspirin or other drug overdoses
   Class IIb
   - If intubated and continued long arrest interval
   - Upon return of spontaneous circulation after long arrest interval
   Class III
   - Hypoxic lactic acidosis
   - Hypercarbic acidosis

c. The recommended dosage of **epinephrine** is 1 mg IV push every 3 to 5 minutes. If this approach fails, the following Class IIb dosing regimens can be considered:
   - Intermediate: **Epinephrine** 2 to 5 mg IV push, every 3 to 5 minutes
   - Escalating: **Epinephrine** 1 mg, 3 mg, 5 mg IV push, each dose 3 minutes apart
   - High: **Epinephrine** 0.1 mg/kg IV push, every 3 to 5 minutes

d. The shorter **atropine** dosing interval (3 minutes) is possibly helpful in cardiac arrest (Class IIb).

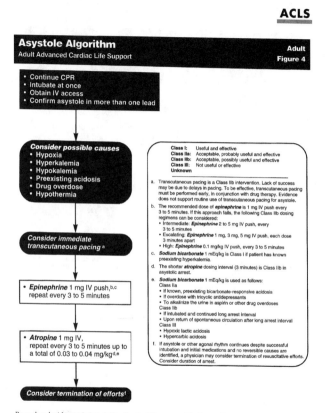

Asystole Algorithm
Adult Advanced Cardiac Life Support

Adult
Figure 4

- Continue CPR
- Intubate at once
- Obtain IV access
- Confirm asystole in more than one lead

Consider possible causes
- Hypoxia
- Hyperkalemia
- Hypokalemia
- Preexisting acidosis
- Drug overdose
- Hypothermia

Consider immediate transcutaneous pacing a

- **Epinephrine** 1 mg IV push,b,c repeat every 3 to 5 minutes

- **Atropine** 1 mg IV, repeat every 3 to 5 minutes up to a total of 0.03 to 0.04 mg/kgd,e

Consider termination of effortsf

Class I:	Useful and effective
Class IIa:	Acceptable, probably useful and effective
Class IIb:	Acceptable, possibly useful and effective
Class III:	Not useful or effective
Unknown	

a. Transcutaneous pacing is a Class IIb intervention. Lack of success may be due to delays in pacing. To be effective, transcutaneous pacing must be performed early, in conjunction with drug therapy. Evidence does not support routine use of transcutaneous pacing for asystole.

b. The recommended dose of **epinephrine** is 1 mg IV push every 3 to 5 minutes. If this approach fails, the following Class IIb dosing regimens can be considered:
   - Intermediate: **Epinephrine** 2 to 5 mg IV push, every 3 to 5 minutes
   - Escalating: **Epinephrine** 1 mg, 3 mg, 5 mg IV push, each dose 3 minutes apart
   - High: **Epinephrine** 0.1 mg/kg IV push, every 3 to 5 minutes

c. **Sodium bicarbonate** 1 mEq/kg is Class I if patient has known preexisting hyperkalemia.

d. The shorter **atropine** dosing interval (3 minutes) is Class IIb in asystolic arrest.

e. **Sodium bicarbonate** 1 mEq/kg is used as follows:
   Class IIa
   - If known, preexisting bicarbonate-responsive acidosis
   - If overdose with tricyclic antidepressants
   - To alkalinize the urine in aspirin or other drug overdoses
   Class IIb
   - If intubated and continued long arrest interval
   - Upon return of spontaneous circulation after long arrest interval
   Class III
   - Hypoxic lactic acidosis
   - Hypercarbic acidosis

f. If asystole or other agonal rhythm continues despite successful intubation and initial medications and no reversible causes are identified, a physician may consider termination of resuscitative efforts. Consider duration of arrest.

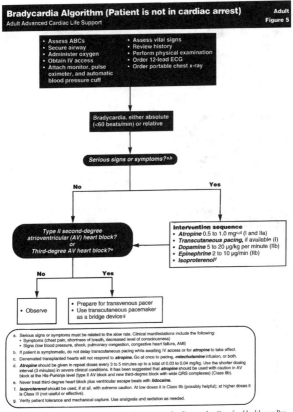

Bradycardia Algorithm (Patient is not in cardiac arrest) — Adult

Adult Advanced Cardiac Life Support — Figure 5

- Assess ABCs
- Secure airway
- Administer oxygen
- Obtain IV access
- Attach monitor, pulse oximeter, and automatic blood pressure cuff

- Assess vital signs
- Review history
- Perform physical examination
- Order 12-lead ECG
- Order portable chest x-ray

Bradycardia, either absolute (<60 beats/min) or relative

Serious signs or symptoms?[a,b]

No | **Yes**

Type II second-degree atrioventricular (AV) heart block?
or
Third-degree AV heart block?[e]

Intervention sequence
- *Atropine* 0.5 to 1.0 mg[c,d] (I and IIa)
- *Transcutaneous pacing,* if available (I)
- *Dopamine* 5 to 20 µg/kg per minute (IIb)
- *Epinephrine* 2 to 10 µg/min (IIb)
- *Isoproterenol*[f]

No | **Yes**

- Observe

- Prepare for transvenous pacer
- Use transcutaneous pacemaker as a bridge device[g]

a. Serious signs or symptoms must be related to the slow rate. Clinical manifestations include the following:
  - Symptoms (chest pain, shortness of breath, decreased level of consciousness)
  - Signs (low blood pressure, shock, pulmonary congestion, congestive heart failure, AMI)
b. If patient is symptomatic, do not delay transcutaneous pacing while awaiting IV access or for *atropine* to take effect.
c. Denervated transplanted hearts will not respond to *atropine.* Go at once to pacing, *catecholamine* infusion, or both.
d. *Atropine* should be given in repeat doses every 3 to 5 minutes up to a total of 0.03 to 0.04 mg/kg. Use the shorter dosing interval (3 minutes) in severe clinical conditions. It has been suggested that *atropine* should be used with caution in AV block at the His-Purkinje level (type II AV block and new third-degree block with wide QRS complexes) (Class IIb).
e. Never treat third-degree heart block plus ventricular escape beats with *lidocaine.*
f. *Isoproterenol* should be used, if at all, with extreme caution. At low doses it is Class IIb (possibly helpful); at higher doses it is Class III (not useful or effective).
g. Verify patient tolerance and mechanical capture. Use analgesia and sedation as needed.

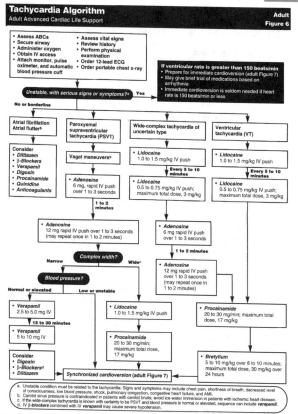

Tachycardia Algorithm
Adult Advanced Cardiac Life Support

Adult
Figure 6

- Assess ABCs
- Secure airway
- Administer oxygen
- Obtain IV access
- Attach monitor, pulse oximeter, and automatic blood pressure cuff

- Assess vital signs
- Review history
- Perform physical examination
- Order 12-lead ECG
- Order portable chest x-ray

If ventricular rate is greater than 150 beats/min
- Prepare for immediate cardioversion (adult Figure 7)
- May give brief trial of medications based on arrhythmia
- Immediate cardioversion is seldom needed if heart rate is 150 beats/min or less

Unstable, with serious signs or symptoms?ª Yes

No or borderline

Atrial fibrillation Atrial flutterᵇ

Consider
- Diltiazem
- β-Blockers
- Verapamil
- Digoxin
- Procainamide
- Quinidine
- Anticoagulants

Paroxysmal supraventricular tachycardia (PSVT)

Vagal maneuversᵇ

- Adenosine
  6 mg, rapid IV push over 1 to 3 seconds

1 to 2 minutes

- Adenosine
  12 mg rapid IV push over 1 to 3 seconds
  (may repeat once in 1 to 2 minutes)

Complex width?

Narrow / Wideᶜ

Blood pressure?

Normal or elevated / Low or unstable

- Verapamil
  2.5 to 5.0 mg IV

15 to 30 minutes

- Verapamil
  5 to 10 mg IV

Consider
- Digoxin
- β-Blockersᵈ
- Diltiazem

Wide-complex tachycardia of uncertain type

- Lidocaine
  1.0 to 1.5 mg/kg IV push

Every 5 to 10 minutes

- Lidocaine
  0.5 to 0.75 mg/kg IV push; maximum total dose, 3 mg/kg

- Adenosine
  6 mg rapid IV push over 1 to 3 seconds

1 to 2 minutes

- Adenosine
  12 mg rapid IV push over 1 to 3 seconds
  (may repeat once in 1 to 2 minutes)

- Lidocaine
  1.0 to 1.5 mg/kg IV push

- Procainamide
  20 to 30 mg/min; maximum total dose, 17 mg/kg

Ventricular tachycardia (VT)

- Lidocaine
  1.0 to 1.5 mg/kg IV push

Every 5 to 10 minutes

- Lidocaine
  0.5 to 0.75 mg/kg IV push; maximum total dose, 3 mg/kg

- Procainamide
  20 to 30 mg/min; maximum total dose, 17 mg/kg

- Bretylium
  5 to 10 mg/kg over 8 to 10 minutes; maximum total dose, 30 mg/kg over 24 hours

Synchronized cardioversion (adult Figure 7)

a. Unstable condition must be related to the tachycardia. Signs and symptoms may include chest pain, shortness of breath, decreased level of consciousness, low blood pressure, shock, pulmonary congestion, congestive heart failure, and AMI.
b. Carotid sinus pressure is contraindicated in patients with carotid bruits; avoid ice-water immersion in patients with ischemic heart disease.
c. If the wide-complex tachycardia is known with certainty to be PSVT and blood pressure is normal or elevated, sequence can include *verapamil*.
d. IV β-blockers combined with IV *verapamil* may cause severe hypotension.

Reproduced with permission. © Handbook of Emergency Cardiovascular Care for Healthcare Providers, 1997. Copyright American Heart Association.

20. Resources

NORMAL LABORATORY VALUES

BLOOD GASES

pH	Arterial:	7.35 - 7.45	
	Venous:	7.32 - 7.43	
pCO2	Arterial:	35 - 45	mmHg
	Venous:	38 - 50	mmHg
pO2	Arterial:	80 - 95	mmHg
	Venous:	about 40	mmHg
HCO3		22.0 - 26.0	mEq/L
tCO2		22.0 - 30.0	mEq/L
Base Excess		no range	mEq/L
O2 Sat'n		95 - 99	%
Hgb	Female:	11.7 - 15.7	g/dL
	Male:	13.5 - 17.7	g/dL
Hct (est)	Female:	35 - 47	%
	Male:	40 - 52	%

GENERAL CHEM

SODIUM		137 - 145	mEq/L
POTASSIUM		3.6 - 5.0	mEq/L
CHLORIDE		98 - 107	mEq/L
CO2		22 - 30	mEq/L
ANION GAP		8 - 16	mEq/L
OSMOL, SERUM		285 - 310	mOsm/kg
GLUCOSE	Fasting:	65 - 110	mg/dL
BUN		7 - 21	mg/dL
CREATININE		0.7 - 1.5	mg/dL
BUN/CREAT		about 10	
CALCIUM		8.4 - 10.2	mg/dL
CA, IONIZED		1.12 - 1.32	mmol/L
LACTIC ACID		0.7 - 2.1	mmol/L
PHOSPHOROUS		2.5 - 4.5	mg/dL
MAGNESIUM		1.4 - 1.8	mEq/L
URIC ACID	Female:	2.5 - 7.5	mg/dL
	Male:	3.5 - 8.5	mg/dL
PROTEIN, TOT		6.3 - 8.2	g/dL
ALBUMIN		3.9 - 5.0	g/dL
GLOBULIN		2.3 - 3.5	g/dL
BILIRUBIN	Adults:	0.2 - 1.3	mg/dL
	Neonates:	1.0 - 10.5	mg/dL
BILI, DIRECT		0.0 - 0.4	mg/dL
BILI, INDIR		no range	mg/dL
ALK PHOS		38 - 126	IU/L
AST (SGOT)	Female:	14 - 36	IU/L
	Male:	17 - 59	IU/L
ALT (SGPT)	Female:	9 - 52	IU/L
	Male:	21 - 72	IU/L
GAMMA GT		8 - 78	IU/L

(Reprinted with permission from Howard H. Sussman, M.D., Professor o
Pathology, Stanford University.)

LIPID PANEL

CHOLESTEROL	Low risk:	< 200	mg/dL
	Moderate risk:	200 - 239	mg/dL
	High risk:	> 239	mg/dL
TRIGLYCERIDE	Normal:	< 200	mg/dL
	Borderline high:	200 - 400	mg/dL
	High:	400 - 1000	mg/dL
	Very high:	> 1000	mg/dL
HDL	Female:	35 - 86	mg/dL
	Male:	29 - 67	mg/dL
VLDL		no range	mg/dL
LDL	Low risk:	< 130	mg/dL
	Moderate risk:	130 - 160	mg/dL
	High risk:	> 160	mg/dL
AMYLASE	Serum:	30 - 110	IU/L
	Plasma:	50 - 130	IU/L
CK TOTAL	Female:	30 - 135	IU/L
	Male:	55 - 170	IU/L
CK-MB (Mass)		< 5.0	ng/mL
CK-MB %RI		0 - 3	%
MYOGLOBIN	Female:	14 - 87	ng/mL
	Male:	22 - 106	ng/mL
TROPONIN I		< 0.5	ng/mL
LD TOTAL		313 - 618	IU/L

CK ISOENZYME

CK 1 (BB)	0	%
CK 2 (MB)	0 - 4	%
	< 10	IU/L
CK 3 (MM)	96 - 100	%

LD ISOENZYME

LD 1	15 - 25	%
LD 2	32 - 41	%
LD 3	18 - 26	%
LD 4	7 - 14	%
LD 5	5 - 17	%

PROT.ELECTPH

PROTEIN, TOT	6.3 - 8.2	g/dL
ALBUMIN	47.5 - 61.0	%
ALPHA 1	2.2 - 6.2	%
ALPHA 2	7.9 - 14.3	%
BETA	9.5 - 17.4	%
GAMMA	11.5 - 23.2	%
MONOCL PK	0	%

continued

SPECIAL CHEM

AFP			0.0 - 8.5	ng/mL
AMMONIA			9 - 33	umol/L
BETA-HCG			less than 5	mIU/mL
CEA			0 - 5	ng/mL
CORTISOL	A.M.		6 - 21	ug/dL
	P.M.		3 - 14	ug/dL
FERRITIN	Female:	Premenopausal:	6 - 81	ng/mL
		Postmenopausal:	14 - 186	ng/mL
	Male:	18 - 30 yrs:	30 - 233	ng/mL
		31 - 60 yrs:	32 - 284	ng/mL
GLUC TT-2 HR			no range	
GLUC TT-3 HR			no range	
GLUC TT-OTHR			no range	
GLYCO HGB			4.0 - 8.0	%
HAPTOGLOBIN			34 - 200	mg/dL
IMMUNOELECT			no range	
IRON	Female:		37 - 170	ug/dL
	Male:		49 - 181	ug/dL
TIBC			250 - 450	ug/dL
% IRON SATN			20 - 50	%
PROLACTIN	Female:		1.9 - 25.9	ng/mL
	Male:		2.2 - 18.5	ng/mL
PSA			0.0 - 4.0	ng/mL
TRANSFERRIN			200 - 380	mg/dL
FOLATE	Normal:		1.5 - 20 6	ng/mL
	Deficient:		0.1 - 1.5	ng/mL
RBC - FOLATE	Normal:		95 - 570	ng/mL
	Deficient:		< or = 60	ng/mL
VITAMIN B$_{12}$	Normal:		130 - 770	pg/mL
	Deficient:		< or = 204	pg/mL

THYROID

Free T$_4$		0.73 - 2.01	ng/dL
TSH		0.4 - 4.0	uIU/mL
T$_3$ Total		100 - 190	ng/dL
T$_4$ Total		6.1 - 11.8	ug/dL
Tg			
	With thyroid gland:	<20	ng/mL
	Athyreotic, on T4:	<2.7	ng/mL
	Athyreotic, off T4:	<5	ng/mL
Anti-M			
	Negative:	< 0.3	U/mL
	Indeterminant:	0.3 - 1.0	U/mL
Anti-Tg	Negative:	< 0.3	U/mL
	Indeterminant:	0.3 - 1.0	U/mL

TDM

ACETAMINOPHEN		lab guide	ug/mL
AMIKACIN		no range	ug/mL
CARBAMAZEPIN		8 - 12	ug/mL
CHLORAMPHEN		10 - 20	ug/mL
CYCLOSPOR-S		75 - 300	ng/mL
CYCLOSPOR-WB			ng/mL
DIGOXIN		0.5 - 2.0	ng/mL
GENTAMICIN		no range	ug/mL
LITHIUM		0.6 - 1.2	mEq/L
LIDOCAINE		1.4 - 6.0	ug/mL
METHOTREXATE		no range	umol/L
NAPA		no range	ug/mL
PENTOBARB		no range	ug/mL
PHENOBARB		10 - 40	ug/mL
PHENYTOIN		10 - 20	ug/mL
PRIMIDONE		5 - 12	ug/mL
PROCAINAMIDE		4 - 8	ug/mL
QUINIDINE		2.5 - 5.0	ug/mL
SALICYLATE		200 - 400	ug/mL
TACROLIMUS (FK506)		no range	ng/mL
THEOPHYLLINE		10 - 20	ug/mL
THIOCYANATE		no range	ug/mL
THIOPENTAL		no range	ug/mL
TOBRAMYCIN		no range	ug/mL
VALPROIC ACD		50 - 100	ug/mL
VANCOMYCIN		no range	ug/mL

IMMUNOLOGY

ANTI-DNA	includes RNP & SM	< 1:10	titer
ANTI-ENA		< 1:100	titer
C3		75 - 140	mg/dL
C4		10 - 34	mg/dL
C-REACT PROT		< 0.5	mg/dL
CUTANEOUS IF		no range	
FANA		< 1:40	titer
IGA	Female:	70 - 370	mg/dL
	Male:	88 - 410	mg/dL
IGG		690 - 1400	mg/dL
IGM	Female:	40 - 240	mg/dL
	Male:	34 - 210	mg/dL
MONO SCREEN		negative	
PREGN,SERUM	Sensitivity:	25	IU/L
RHEUM FACT		< 40	IU/mL

continued

RESOURCES

HEMATOLOGY

CELL COUNTS

HCT	Female:	35 - 47	%
	Male:	40 - 52	%
HGB	Female:	11.7 - 15.7	g/dL
	Male:	13.5 - 17.7	g/dL
PLT		150 - 400	K/uL
WBC		4.0 - 11.0	K/uL
AUTO DIFF	See Notes		
NEUT (ABS)		1.70 - 6.70	K/uL
LYMPH (ABS)		1.00 - 3.00	K/uL
MONO (ABS)		0.30 - 0.95	K/uL
EOS (ABS)		0.05 - 0.55	K/uL
BASO (ABS)		0.00 - 0.25	K/uL
RBC	Female:	3.8 - 5.2	MIL/uL
	Male:	4.4 - 5.9	MIL/uL
MCV		82 - 98	fl
MCH		27 - 34	pg
MCHC		32 - 36	g/dL
RDW		11.5 - 14.5	%
SLIDE DIFF			
POLY		40 - 70	%
BAND		0 - 15	%
META		0 - 1	%
LYMPH		15 - 45	%
MONO		0 - 12	%
EOS		0 - 7	%
BASO		0 - 2	%
REACT LYMPH		0 - 5	%
MYEL		0	%
PROMYEL		0	%
BLAST		0	%
LYMPHOMA		0	%
OTHER		0	%
NRBC		0	/100WBC
MEGA		0	/100WBC

T & B LYMPHS

WBC	4000 - 11000
LYMPH	17.8 - 42.2
T (CD 3)	61 - 84
T (CD 5)	no range
B (CD 20)	7 - 21
HELP (CD 4)	32 - 60
SUPP (CD 8)	13 - 40
T (H+S)	no range
H/S RATIO	0.93 - 4.50
LYMPH ABS	1000 - 3000
T (CD3) ABS	960 - 2580
T (CD5) ABS	no range
B (CD20) ABS	120 - 630
HELPER ABS	540 - 1660
SUPPRES ABS	270 - 930
T (H+S) ABS	no range
CD34 Panel (Blood)	< 5

SPECIAL HEME

ALK P, LEUK		11 - 95	/100 P&B
CRYOPPT			
SERUM 24 HR		0 - 1	%
SERUM 72 HR		0 - 1	%
PLASM 24 HR		0 - 1	%
PLASM 72 HR		0 - 1	%
G-6-PD SCRN	Normal:	0 - 60	min
	Borderline deficient	61 - 90	min
	Deficient:	> 90	min
HEINZ BODIES		0 - 1	%
HGB A2	Normal:	1.5 - 3.0	%
	Borderline:	3.1 - 3.5	%
HGB EPH QUAL		no abnormal Hgb	
HGB EPH QUAN		no abnormal Hgb	
HGB FETAL	Normal:	0.0 - 1.0	%
	Borderline:	1.1 - 2.0	%
HGB H INCLUS		negative	
MALARIA PREP		no parasites seen	
RETIC %-MAN		0.5 - 1.5	%
RETIC %		0.60 - 1.83	%
RETIC (ABS)		29.5 - 87.3	K/uL
SED RATE	Female:	0 - 20	mm/hr
	Male:	0 - 15	mm/hr
	Female: > 50 yrs	0 - 30	mm/hr
	Male: >50 yrs	0 - 20	mm/hr
	F/M: child	0 - 10	mm/hr
SEZARY SCN		none seen	
SICKLE HGB		negative	
	Sensitivity:	20 - 30	% HGB-S
VISCOSITY		1.4 - 1.8	x H2O

continued

COAGULATION

A-2-ANTIPLAS	Adult:	70 - 145	%
	Term neonate:	55 - 115	%
	6-month infant:	70 - 145	%
Anti-Xa/LMWH	Therapeutic	0.5 0 1.2	antiXa U
APC Resist		> 2.0	ratio
Factor V Leiden	by PCR	negative	
APTT		26 - 38	sec
	Heparin range:	1.5 - 2.5	ratio
		times patient baseline	
APTT INH SCR		negative	
AT III	Adult:	86 - 120	%
	Term neonate:	39 - 87	%
	6-month infant:	86 - 120	%
BL TIME	See Notes	2 - 8	min
CLOT LYSIS		no lysis in 24 hrs	
CLOT RETR		4+ in 2 hrs	
D-DIMER		< 250	ng/mL
EUG LYSIS		no lysis in 2 hrs	
FACT II	Adult:	81 - 141	
	Term neonate:	26 - 70	
	6-month infant:	60 - 116	%
FACT V	Adult:	70 - 158	%
	Term neonate:	34 - 108	%
	6-month infant:	55 - 127	%
FACT VII	Adult:	59 - 193	%
	Term neonate:	28 - 104	%
	6-month infant:	47 - 127	%
FACT VIII	Adult:	47 - 192	%
	Term neonate:	47 - 192	%
VIII INHIB		0	units
FACT IX	Adult:	57 - 134	%
	Term neonate:	15 - 91	%
	6-month infant:	36 - 136	%
FACT X	Adult:	68 - 151	%
	Term neonate:	12 - 68	%
	6-month infant:	38 - 118	%
FACT XI	Adult:	54 - 180	%
	Term neonate:	10 - 66	%
	6-month infant:	49 - 134	%
FACT XII	Adult:	60 - 150	%
	Term neonate:	13 - 93	%
	6-month infant:	39 - 115	%
FACT XIII		> 1	%
FIBRINOGEN		190 - 380	mg/dL
FSP		< 10	ug/mL
FITZG SCR		negative	
FLETCHER SCR		negative	
HEPARIN Conc.	Therapeutic	0.2 - 0.4	u/mL

COAGULATION (cont'd)

PASSAV SCR		negative	
PLASMINOGEN		72 - 128	%
P&P		no range	sec
P&P		60 - 100	%
	Coumadin range:	10 - 20	%
PROTEIN C ACTIVITY	Adult:	83 -143	%
	Term Neonate:	17 - 53	%
	6-month infant:	37 - 81	%
PROTEIN S ACTIVITY	Adult:	65- 166	%
	Term Neonate:	12 - 60	%
	6-month infant:	31 - 83	%
PT - INR	See Notes	0.9 - 1.1	INR
	Coumadin range:		
	Low Intensity:	2.0 - 3.0	INR
	High Intensity:	3.0 - 4.5	INR
PT - Seconds	See Notes	10.2 - 13.0	sec
PT INH SCR		negative	
REPTILASE		14.0 - 17.0	sec
RIST COF		> 40	%
THROMBIN T		15.1 - 19.5	sec
VW AG		> 60	%

continued

RESOURCES

CELL COUNTS			
APPEARANCE		colorless/clear	
WBC COUNT	CSF:	0 - 5	/uL
	Synovial:	0 - 150	/uL
RBC COUNT	CSF:	0 - 5	/uL
GRAN	CSF:	0 - 6	%
	Synovial:	0 - 25	%
LYMPH	CSF:	40 - 80	%
MONOCYTOID	CSF:	15 - 45	%
CRYSTALS	Synovial:	negative	
HCT-FLUID		no range	%
THROAT SWAB			
BETA STREP TEST		negative	
NASAL SMEAR			
EOS		none seen	
CHEMISTRY			
ALBUMIN		no range	g/dL
AMYLASE		no range	IU/L
BILI SCAN		no range	
BILIRUBIN		no range	mg/dL
C3		no range	mg/dL
CALCIUM		no range	mg/dL
CHLORIDE-CSF		122 - 132	mEq/L
CHLORIDE-FLD		no range	mEq/L
CHOLESTEROL		no range	mg/dL
CO2		no range	mEq/L
ELECTROPHOR		no range	
OLIGO BAND		no range	
GLUCOSE-CSF		40 - 70	mg/dL
GLUCOSE-FLD		no range	mg/dL
IGA		no range	mg/dL
IGG		no range	mg/dL
IGG (CSF)		1.7 - 3.4	mg/dL
IGG INDEX		< 0.66	
IGM		no range	mg/dL
LD		no range	IU/L
MAGNESIUM-C		no range	mEq/L
MAGNESIUM-F		no range	mEq/L
OSMOL, STOOL		no range	mOsm/kg
POTASSIUM		no range	mEq/L
PROTEIN-CSF		12 - 60	mg/dL
PROTEIN-FLD		no range	
RHEUM FACTOR		no range	IU/mL
SODIUM		no range	mEq/L
SPEC GRAVITY		no range	
TRIGLYCERIDE		no range	mg/dL
UREA NITROGN		no range	mg/dL
URIC ACID		no range	mg/dL

LOCAL RESOURCES

Hospital

General	_____
	_____
Paging	_____
Paging (auto)	_____
Paging (out)	_____
Code	_____
Security	_____
Records	_____
	_____
Transcription	_____

Laboratory

Blood gas	_____
Chemistry	_____
Coagulation	_____
Hematology	_____
Microbiology	_____
Virology	_____
Pathology	_____
Special labs	_____
	_____

Departments/Clinics

Admit (medicine)	_____
(surgery)	_____
(transfer)	_____
Blood bank	_____
Cardiology	_____
CT surgery	_____
Dermatology	_____
Endocrine	_____
ENT	_____
General med.	_____
GI	_____
Hematology	_____
Hepatology	_____
ID	_____
Immunology	_____
Intervent. radiol.	_____
Nephrology	_____

Radiology/Diagnostic Testing

General	_____
X-rays	_____
CT	_____
	_____
Ultrasound	_____
	_____
MRI	_____
	_____
Nuclear med.	_____
	_____
ECG	_____
Treadmill	_____
Echocardio.	_____
Cardiac cath.	_____
Endoscopy	_____
GI radiology	_____

Neurology

Neurosurgery	_____
Nutrition	_____
Obstet./gynecol.	_____
Occup. therapy	_____
Oncology	_____
Orthopedics	_____
Pediatrics	_____

Pharmacy

Inpatient	_____
	_____
Outpatient	_____
	_____
	_____
Drug info.	_____

continued

RESOURCES

Physical therapy		Medicine Department	
Plastic surgery	_____	General	_____
Pulmonary	_____	Chair	_____
Radiotherapy	_____	Library	_____
Surgery	_____	Clinic	_____
Urology	_____	Conference	_____

PERSONAL LOCAL RESOURCES

PERSONAL RESOURCES: SUBSPECIALTY CONSULTANTS

Specialty	Consultant(s)	Contact
Cardiology		
Pulmonary/critical care		
Gastroenterology		
Nephrology		
Endocrinology		
Rheumatology		
Neurology		
Hematology		
Oncology		
Infectious disease/AIDS		
Dermatology		
Ophthalmology		
Otolaryngology		
General surgery		
Cardiothoracic surgery		
Plastic surgery		
Neurosurgery		
Orthopedics		
Urology		
Pediatrics		
Obstetrics/gynecology		

RESOURCES

PERSONAL RESOURCES
Hospital Affiliations

_____
_____
_____
_____

Clinic Affiliations

_____
_____
_____
_____

Colleagues

_____
_____
_____
_____
_____
_____
_____
_____
_____
_____
_____

INTERNET RESOURCES
General Medical Resources
- Medical Matrix: http://www.medmatrix.org/index.asp
- World Health Organization: http://www.who.org/

MEDLINE Database
- PubMed (National Library of Medicine): http://www.ncbi.nlm.nih.gov/PubMed/medline.html

Online Journals
- *American Journal of Medicine*: http://www.meddevel.com/ajm
- *Annals of Internal Medicine*: http://www.acponline.org/journals/annals/annaltoc.htm
- *Archives of Internal Medicine*: http://archinte.ama-assn.org/
- *British Medical Journal*: http://www.bmj.org/
- *Journal of the American Medical Association*: http://www.jama.ama-assn.org/
- *The Lancet*: http://www.thelancet.com
- *New England Journal of Medicine*: http://www.nejm.org/

Subspecialty/Guideline Sites
- General:
    American Medical Association: http://www.ama-assn.org/
    American College of Physicians: http://www.acponline.org/
    National Heart, Lung, and Blood Institute: http://www.nhlbi.nih.gov/index.htm
    National Guidelines Clearinghouse: http://www.guideline.gov/index.asp
- Cardiology:
    American Heart Association: http://www.americanheart.org/
    American College of Cardiology: http://www.acc.org/
- Pulmonary: American College of Chest Physicians: http://www.chestnet.org/
- Gastrointestinal:
    American College of Gastroenterology: http://www.acg.gi.org/
    American Gastroenterological Association: http://www.gastro.org/
- Renal:
    American Society of Nephrology: http://www.asn-online.com/
    National Kidney Foundation: http://www.kidney.org/
- Endocrine:
    American Society of Clinical Endocrinologists: http://www.aace.com/
    American Diabetes Association: http://www.diabetes.org/
- Rheumatology:
    American College of Rheumatology: http://www.rheumatology.org
    The Arthritis Foundation: http://www.arthritis.org/
- Hematology: American Society of Hematology: http://www.hematology.org/

continued **297**

RESOURCES

- Oncology: American Cancer Society: http://www.cancer.org/
- Infectious disease:
    Infectious Disease Society of America: http://www.idsociety.org/
    Centers for Disease Control and Prevention: http://www.cdc.gov/
- Neurology: American Academy of Neurology: http://www.aan.com/
- Emergency medicine:
    American Academy of Emergency Medicine: http://www.aaem.org/
    American College of Emergency Medicine: http://www.acep.org/

Commercial Physician Sites
- WebMD: http://www.webmd.com
- ScienceDirect: http://www.sciencedirect.com
- Ovid (full-text journals): http://www.ovid.com
- MD Consult: http://www.mdconsult.com

Patient Information Sites
- American Academy of Family Physicians: http://www.aafp.org/
- *Journal of the American Medical Association*: http://www.ama-assn.org/

Subject Index

Abdominal pain, bedside diagnosis of, 92
Acanthocyte, 110
Accelerated idioventricular rhythm, 12
Acetaminophen
    hepatoxicity nomogram, 249
    overdose, 248
Acid-base disturbances, 83
Acidosis
    metabolic, 83
        evaluation of, 84
    renal tubular, 85
    respiratory, 83
Acquired immunodeficiency virus syndrome. See Human immunodeficiency virus
Acute coronary syndrome. See Angina, unstable
Adrenal crisis, 199
Adrenal insufficiency, 195
Advanced cardiopulmonary life support, 278–283
    asystole algorithm, 281
    bradycardia algorithm, 282
    drugs for, 278
    pulseless electrical activity algorithm, 280
    tachycardia algorithm, 283
    ventricular fibrillation/pulseless ventricular tachycardia algorithm, 279
Adverse drug reactions, 261–265
    dermatologic, 262–263
    hematologic, 264–265
    hepatic, 263
    multisystem, 261–262
    neurologic, 265–

    renal, 263–264
    respiratory, 264
Agitation, ventilator adjustment in, 54
AIDS. See Human immunodeficiency virus
Alcohol withdrawal, 180–181
Alkalosis
    metabolic, 83
        evaluation of, 86
    respiratory, 83
Alkalosis, metabolic, 68
Alteplase, 30
Altered mental status, 178–179
Alveolar-arterial oxygen gradient, 51
Amenorrhea, 196
Aminoglycoside dosing, 141, 142
Aminotransferase, plasma, changes of in liver disease, 94
Analgesia, patient-controlled, 194
Anaphylactic drug reactions, 261
Anaphylactoid drug reactions, 261
Anaphylaxis, 252
Anemias, 120
Angina, unstable, 26–29
    likelihood of significant coronary artery disease with symptoms suggesting, 26
    management of, 27
        medical, 28–29
Anion gap, 83, 84
Antibiotics
    dosing guidelines, 138
    prophylaxis, 244
    sensitivities, 167–171
        anaerobes, 168
        gram-negative rods, 167
        Haemophilus influenzae, 168

SUBJECT INDEX

Antibiotics—*continued*
    mycobacteria, 168
    staphylococci, 169
    streptococci, 170
Anticardiolipin antibody, 118
Anticoagulation
    in perioperative management, 242
    and prosthetic valves, 7
    for stroke prevention, 16
Antiemetics, 129
Antiepileptic medications, 192
Antimicrobials. *See* Antibiotics
Antithrombin deficiency, 118
Aortic dissection, 45
Aortic regurgitation, chronic, 3
Aortic stenosis, 1
Aphasia, 190
Arrhythmia, as complication of myo-
       cardial infarction, 33
Arterial oxygen content formula, 48
Arteriography
    gastrointestinal, 271
    renal, 70
Arteriovenous oxygen content differ-
       ence, 48
Arthritides, joint involvement in, 208
Arthritis, rheumatoid, 218
Arthrocentesis, 209–214
    ankle, 214
    glenohumeral joint, 211
    knee, 213
    procedure for, 209
    subacromial bursa or supraspina-
       tus tendon, 210
    wrist, 212
Ascites, 103
Aspirin
    overdose, 250
    for stroke prevention, 16
Assist control (AC) ventilation, 53

Asthma
    differential diagnosis of, 64
    exacerbation of, 56
    inhaled steroids for, 58
    NAEPP classification of severity
       of, 57
Asystole algorithm, 281
Atrial fibrillation, 14–17
    and anticoagulation for stroke pre-
       vention, 16
    and cardioversion, 17
    common etiologies of, 15
    rate control in, 15
Atrial flutter, 14
Atrial septal defect, 5
Atrial tachycardia with AV block, 14
Auscultation maneuvers, dynamic, 6
Austin Flint murmur, 3

Barium enema, preparation for, 272
Barium swallow, 271
Basophilic stippling, 110
Beck's triad, 130
Benzodiazepines
    overdose, 246
    withdrawal, 246
Bilevel intermittent positive pressure
       (BIPAP), 51–52
Bilirubin, urinary, 94
Biopsy, renal, 70
Bleeding
    evaluation for, 119
    gastrointestinal, 95–96
Bleeding time, 112
Blister cells, 110
Blood pressure, classification of, 227
Blood urea nitrogen to creatinine
       ratio, 69
Body surface area formula, 48
Bradycardia algorithm, 282

Breast cancer, staging of, 133–134
Bronchitis, chronic, differential diagnosis of, 64
Bronchospasm, and respiratory distress, 50
Brugada criteria for wide complex tachycardia, 12–13
Bundle branch block, and electrocardiography, 9
Bupropion for smoking cessation, 232
Burr cell, 110

CA 19-9, as tumor marker, 127
CA-125, as tumor marker, 127
Calcitonin, as tumor marker, 127
Calcium, 78–79, 80
Caloric requirements, 221
Cancer
  emergencies related to, 130
  evaluation of patient, 126
  staging
    breast, 133–134
    colorectal, 135
    non–small cell lung, 132
    prostate, 136–137
  statistics, 131
Candidiasis, vulvovaginal, 157
Capture beat, 14
Carcinoembryonic antigen, as tumor marker, 127
Cardiac index, 48
Cardiac output formula, 48
Cardiac stenting, 36
Cardiogenic shock
  as complication of myocardial infarction, 33
  pharmacologic interventions for, 34
Cardioversion, 17
Catecholamines, as tumor markers, 127

CD25, as tumor marker, 127
CD30, as tumor marker, 127
Cellulitis, 148
Central venous line, 273–274
Cerebrospinal fluid profiles, 151
Chancroid, treatment of, 159
Chemotherapy, side effects of, 128
Chest pain, differential diagnosis of, 23
Chest x-ray, 270
Child's criteria for cirrhosis, 103
Chlamydia, treatment of, 160
Chloride, 68
Cholangiogram, T-tube, preparation for, 272
Cholangiography, endoscopic retrograde, 93
Cholecystogram, oral, 271
  preparation for, 272
Cholesterol screening, 226, 229
Chronic obstructive pulmonary disease, exacerbation of, 56
Cirrhosis, 103–104
Clostridial cellulitis, 148
Clostridium difficile colitis, 99–100
Clotted Hickman catheter protocol, 126
Coagulation cascade, 112
Coagulation tests, 112
Coarctation of aorta, 5
Colitis, Clostridium difficile, 99–100
Colonoscopy, 93
  preparation for, 272
Colorectal, staging of, 135
Coma, 175, 177
  hyperosmolar nonketotic, 202
  myxedema, 198
Complement levels, 217
Computed tomography
  preparation for, 272
  renal, 70

SUBJECT INDEX

Congenital heart diseases, 5

Constipation, 101

Continuous positive airway pressure (CPAP), 53

Contraception, oral, 233

Contrast enema, 271

COPD, exacerbation of, 56

Coronary artery bypass grafting (CABG), 37

Coronary artery diseases, 23–24. *See also specific diseases*
    risk factors and favorable factors, 23

Coronary care unit formulas, 48

Coronary imaging, 21

Corrigan's sign, 3

Coumadin. *See* Warfarin

Creatinine clearance, calculated, 69

Cryoprecipitate, 122

Crystals, in joints, 216

Cushing's syndrome, 195

Cyclosporine, drug interactions with, 260

Cystogram, preparation for, 272

De Musset sign, 3

Defibrillators, implantable, in myocardial infarction, 32

Delirium, 178–179

Dementia, 182

Dermatomes, 172173

Dexamethasone suppression test, 195

Diabetes insipidus, 195

Diabetes mellitus
    guidelines for outpatients, 230
    management during hospitalization, 204

Diabetic ketoacidosis, 201

Diagnostic tests, evaluating, 267–269

Dialysis, indications for, 88

Diarrhea, acute, 98

Diffusing capacity, 64

Digoxin
    in atrial fibrillation, 16
    drug interactions with, 259

Diphtheria-tetanus immunization, 226

Disseminated intravascular coagulation, 125

Drug fever, 261–262

Drug monitoring guidelines for ICU, 254–255

Duroziez's sign, 3

Ebstein's anomaly, 5

Electrocardiography, 8–10
    bundle branch block and, 9
    diagnostic findings of, 10
    hypertrophy and, 8
    nodal block and, 9
    and presentation of clinical syndromes, 10

Electrolytes, urine, 68

Elliptocyte, 110

Embolism, pulmonary, 59–60

Emphysema, differential diagnosis of, 64

Endocarditis, 149–150
    prophylaxis, 245

Endocrine disorders, screening for, 195–196

Endoscopic procedures, preparation for, 272

Endoscopic retrograde cholangiography, 93

Endoscopic retrograde pancreatography, 93

Endoscopy, gastrointestinal, 93

End-stage renal disease, 90

Enema, contrast, 271

Enteral nutrition, 223
Enteroclysis, 271
  preparation for, 272
Epilepsy. *See* Seizures
Erythrocytes scan, 271
Esophagogastroduodenoscopy
  (EGD), 93
Estrogen therapy, 234
Evidence-based medicine, 266–269
Exercise testing, 38
Extubation, 55

Fagan's nomogram, 269
Fecal occult blood, screening for, 226
Femoral nerve, 174
α-Fetoprotein, as tumor marker, 127
Fever
  and rash, differential diagnosis of,
    144–145
  of unknown origin, 145–147
Fibrinolysis, 118
Fluid requirements, 221
Folstein Mini-Mental Status Examination, 182
Forced expiratory volume in 1 second, 64
Forced vital capacity, 64
Forrester et al. classification of myocardial infarction, 24
Fractional excretion of sodium
  (FENa), 69
Free-wall rupture, as complication of
  myocardial infarction, 33
Fresh frozen plasma, 122
Fulminant hepatic failure, 109

Gallavardin's phenomenon, 1
Gas gangrene, 148
Gastric-emptying scan, 271
Gastrointestinal bleeding, 95–96

Gastrointestinal radiology, 271
Genital herpes, treatment of, 160
Genital warts, external, treatment of,
  160
Gentamicin, 141–142
Glasgow coma scale, 175
Gleason sum, 137
Glucocorticoids. *See* Steroids
Goldman's Multifactorial Index of
  Cardiac Risk in Noncardiac
  Surgery, 236
Gonococcal infections, uncomplicated, treatment of, 159
Gout, 219
Growth factors, in cancer patients,
  126
Guillain-Barré syndrome, 184

Hampton's hump, 59
Headache, emergency, evaluation for,
  185
Health care maintenance, 226
Heart failure, 39–41
  admission criteria for, 39
  medical management of, 40
  reversible etiologies, 40
  surgical management of, 41
Heinz bodies, 110
Hematocrit, 111
Hematuria, 66
Hemodynamic monitoring, 46
Hemoglobin, 111
Hemolytic uremic syndrome, 124
Hemoptysis, 61
Hemothorax, and respiratory distress, 51
Heparin, 242, 243
  low-molecular-weight, 114
    considerations in using, 115
  sliding scale, 60, 114

SUBJECT INDEX

Hepatic encephalopathy, 104
Hepatic failure, fulminant, 109
Hepatitis
    acute, 106–107
    C, 108
    chronic, 103–104
Hepatobiliary scan, 271
Hepatorenal syndrome, 89
HER-2/neu, as tumor marker, 127
Herpes, genital, treatment of, 160
Herpes simplex, in cancer patients, 126
Hill's sign, 3
Hirsutism, 196
HIV. See Human immunodeficiency virus
Hormone replacement therapy, 234
Hormone requirements, daily, 204
Howell-Jolly bodies, 110
β-hCG, as tumor marker, 127
Human immunodeficiency virus, 162–164
    chemoprophylaxis after occupational exposure to, 164
    opportunistic infections in, 162
        treatment of, 163
    postexposure prophylaxis for health care workers, 164
    prophylaxis in, 162
    and tuberculosis, 166
Hyperbilirubinemia, causes of, 94
Hypercalcemia, 78–79
Hypercholesterolemia, 226, 229
Hypercoagulable states, 118
Hyperhomocysteinemia, 118
Hyperkalemia, 75–76
Hypermagnesemia, 82
Hypernatremia, 68, 70
Hyperosmolar nonketotic coma, 202
Hyperphosphatemia, 81

Hyperphosphaturia, 81
Hypertension, 227–228
    pulmonary, 42
Hypertensive crisis, 43–44
    pharmacological management of, 44
Hyperthyroidism, 197
Hypertrophic obstructive cardiomyopathy (HOCM), 4
Hypertrophy, cardiac, and electrocardiography, 8
Hypocalcemia, 80
Hypoglycemics, oral, 204
Hypokalemia, 68, 77
Hypomagnesemia, 82
Hyponatremia, 68, 72–73
Hypophosphatemia, 81
Hypophosphaturia, 81
Hypopituitarism, 196
Hypotension, ventilator adjustment in, 54
Hypothyroidism, 197

Idiopathic hypertrophic subaortic stenosis (IHSS), 4
Imaging. See also Radiology
    coronary, 21
Immunologic tests in rheumatic diseases, 217
Influenza immunization, 226
Insomnia, transient, 178
Insulin therapy, 203–204
Intermittent mandatory ventilation (IMV), 53
Internet resources, 297–298
Interstitial lung disease, differential diagnosis of, 64
Intra-aortic balloon pump, in myocardial infarction, 32
Intracranial pressure, increased, 176
Intravenous pyelogram, 70

Intravenous solutions, composition of, 253

Intubation, indications for, 53

Iron studies and microcytic anemias, 120

Joint examination, 205—207

Junctional rhythm, 14

Karnofsky scale, 126

Killip and Kimball classification of myocardial infarction, 24

Laboratory values, normal, 284–292
    blood gases, 284
    cell counts, 292
    chemistry, 292
    coagulation, 290–291
    CK isoenzyme, 285
    general chemistry, 284
    hematology, 288–289
    immunology, 287
    LD isoenzyme, 285
    lipid panel, 285
    nasal smear, 292
    special chemistry, 286
    throat swab, 292
    thyroid, 286

Lactated Ringer's solution, composition of, 253

Landolfi's sign, 3

Left ventricular aneurysm, as complication of myocardial infarction, 33

Left ventricular dysfunction, as complication of myocardial infarction, 33

Left ventricular pseudoaneurysm, as complication of myocardial infarction, 33

Left ventricular thrombus, as complication of myocardial infarction, 33

Liver disease, drug adjustments in, 256–257

Liver failure, fulminant, 109

Liver function tests, 94

Low-molecular-weight heparin, 114
    considerations in using, 115

Lumbar puncture, 275

Lung cancer, non–small cell, staging of, 132

Lupus anticoagulant, 118

Lymphangiogram, preparation for, 272

Macro-ovalocyte, 110

Magnesium, 82

Magnetic resonance imaging, preparation for, 272

Malaria, 231

Mammogram, 226

Mean cell hemoglobin, 111

Mean cell hemoglobin concentration, 111

Mean corpuscular volume, 111

Mechanical ventilation, 53–55
    adjustment considerations, 54
    indications for intubation, 53
    initial settings, 53
    modes of, 53
    weaning and extubation, 55

Meckel's scan, 271

Median nerve, 174

Meleney's synergistic gangrene, 148

Meningitis, 151–152

Menopause, 234

Metabolic acidosis, 83
    evaluation of, 83

Metabolic alkalosis, 68, 83
    evaluation of, 86

SUBJECT INDEX

Metastasis, 127

Microalbuminuria, 66

β_2-Microglobulin, as tumor marker, 127

Migraine, 186–187

Mini-Mental Status Examination, Folstein, 182

Minimum mandatory ventilation (MMV), 53

Mitral regurgitation
  chronic, 2
  as complication of myocardial infarction, 33

Mitral stenosis, 2

Mitral valve prolapse, 4

Mixed venous oxygen formula, 48

Monoclonal immunoglobulin, as tumor marker, 127

Mouth care, for cancer patients, 126

Muller's sign, 3

Multifocal atrial tachycardia, 14

Murmur characteristics, 7

Myocardial infarction
  adjunctive medical therapy in, 31
  classification of, 24
  complications of, 33
  ECG changes in, 25
  nonmedical therapeutic interventions in, 32

Myocardial ischemia, enzymes for, 24

Myocardial perfusion scintigraphy, preparation for, 272

Myxedema coma, 198

Narrow complex rhythm, 14

Nausea, 97

Necrotizing fasciitis, 148

Nephrolithiasis, 91

Nephrotic syndrome, 66, 118

Neuron-specific enolase, as tumor marker, 127

Neutropenic fever, 130

New York Heart Association Classification for Systolic heart failure, 39

Nicotine replacement therapy, 232

Nodal block, and electrocardiography, 9

Noninvasive positive pressure ventilation (NIPPV), 52

Non–small cell lung cancer, staging of, 132

Nuclear imaging, preparation for, 272

Nutrition
  enteral, 223
  total parenteral, 223

Nutritional feeding formulation chart, 224–225

Nutritional requirements, 221

Nylen-Bárány maneuver, 174

Obesity, differential diagnosis of, 64

Oncology. See Cancer

Opioids
  drug equivalencies, 193
  overdose, 247
  withdrawal, 247

Ortner's syndrome, 2

Osmolality, 68

Oxygen, for respiratory support, 51

Oxygen delivery formula, 48

Pacemakers, 19–20
  modes, 19
  permanent, indications for, 20
  settings, 19

Nonanion gap, 84

temporary, in myocardial infarction, 32
Pain, acute, 193–194
Palla's sign, 59
Palmar click, 3
Pancreatitis, 102
Pancreatography, endoscopic retrograde, 93
Pancytopenia, 121
Pap smear, 226
Pappenheimer bodies, 110
Paracentesis, 277
Partial thromboplastin time, 112
Patent ductus arteriosus, 5
Pelvic inflammatory disease, 158–160
diagnosis of, 158
treatment of, 158–159
Percutaneous transluminal coronary angioplasty (PTCA), 35
vs. coronary artery bypass grafting, 37
Pericardial effusion and tamponade, 130
Pericarditis, as complication of myocardial infarction, 33
Perioperative management
anticoagulation, 242–243
antimicrobial prophylaxis, 244
Peripheral blood smear, 110
Peripheral nerves, 174
Peritonitis, spontaneous bacterial, 105
Peroneal nerve, 174
Peroral pneumocolon, 271
pH, 68
Pheochromocytoma, 195
Phosphate, 81
Pigment nephropathy, 89
Pituitary incidentaloma, 196
Plasminogen deficiency, 118

Platelets, transfusion of, 122
Pleural effusion, 62–63
and respiratory distress, 51
Pleural fluid, analysis of, 62
Pneumococcal immunization, 227
Pneumonia, community-acquired, 153–154
Pneumothorax, and respiratory distress, 51
Poikilocyte, 110
Polyneuropathy, differential diagnosis of, 184
Positive end expiratory pressure (PEEP), 51, 53
Postinfarct angina, as complication of myocardial infarction, 33
Potassium, 68, 75–77
Preoperative evaluation
cardiovascular, 236–239
pulmonary, 240–241
Pressors, 49
Pressure control ventilation (PCV), 53
Pressure support (PS) ventilation, 53
Prostate cancer, staging of, 136–137
Prostate-specific antigen
as tumor marker, 127
screening for, 226
Prostatic acid phosphatase, as tumor marker, 127
Prosthetic valves, 7
Protein C deficiency, 118
Protein requirements, 221
Protein S deficiency, 118
Proteinuria, 66
Prothrombin time, 112
Pseudohypocalcemia, 80
PTCA, 35
vs. CABG, 37

SUBJECT INDEX

Pulmonary artery catheter, in myocardial infarction, 32
Pulmonary artery catheterization, 46
Pulmonary artery pressures, 46–47
Pulmonary disease, differential diagnosis of, 64
Pulmonary edema, and respiratory distress, 50
Pulmonary embolism, 59–60
Pulmonary function testing, 64
Pulmonary hypertension, 42
Pulmonary regurgitation, 4
Pulmonary stenosis, 4
Pulmonary vascular resistance formula, 48
Pulse oximetry, 51
Pulseless electrical activity algorithm, 280
Pulsus parvus et tardus, 1

Quincke's sign, 33

Radial nerve, 174
Radiology procedures
    gastrointestinal, 271
    preparation for, 272
Radionuclide scintigraphy, renal, 70
Ranson's prognostic criteria, 102
Rash, differential diagnosis of, 144–145
Reciprocal beat, 14
Red blood cells
    count, 111
    distribution width, 110
    indices, 111
    nucleated, 110
    packed, 122
Reentrant supraventricular tachycardia, 14

Renal failure
    acute, 68, 87–88
        drugs associated with, 88
    chronic, 90
Renal imaging, 70
Renal tubular acidosis, 68, 85
Reptilase time, 112
Residual volume, 64
Respiratory acidosis, 83
Respiratory alkalosis, 83
Respiratory distress, 50–51
Respiratory support, 51
Reteplase, 30
Reticulocyte count, 110
Reticulocyte index, 111
Reticulocytes, 110, 120
Revascularization, 35–36
Rhabdomyolysis, 89
Rheumatic diseases, immunologic tests in, 217
Rheumatic fever, 3
Rheumatoid arthritis, 218
Right ventricular dysplasia, 5
Right ventricular infarction, as complication of myocardial infarction, 33
Ringer's solution, composition of, 253
Rosenbach's sign, 3
Rouleaux of red blood cells, 110
rPA, 30
"Rum fits," 180

Saline, composition of, 253
Schistocytes, 110
Seizures, 191
    antiepileptic medications, 192
Sensitivities, antibiotic. *See* Antibiotic sensitivities
Shunt ratio formula, 48

Sickle cells, 110

Siderocytes, 110

Sigmoidoscopy, 226
  preparation for, 272

Small-bowel follow-through, 271

Smoking cessation, 232

Sodium, 68, 70, 72–73

Soft-tissue infections, severe, 148

Spherocytes, 110

Spinal cord compression, 130

Spontaneous bacterial peritonitis, 105

Staging, cancer. *See* Cancer staging

Status epilepticus, 192

Stenting, cardiac, 36

Steroids, 199–200
  inhaled, 58
  stress-dose, 199

Stomatocytes, 110

Streptokinase, 30

Stress testing, 38

Stroke, 188–190
  common patterns of, 190
  diagnosis of, 188
  hemorrhagic, management of, 190
  ischemic, management of, 188
  risk factors for, 188
  t-PA and, 189

Superior vena cava syndrome, 130

Supraventricular tachycardia with aberrant tachycardia, 12

Swan-Ganz catheter, 46

Synchronized intermittent mandatory ventilation (SIMV), 53

Syndrome of inappropriate antidiuresis (SIAD), 74

Synovial fluid analysis, 215–216
  crystals in joints, 216

Syphilis, treatment of, 160

Systemic lupus erythematosus, 218

Systemic vascular resistance formula, 48

Tachycardia
  algorithm, 283
  wide complex, 12–13

Target cells, 110

Tetralogy of Fallot, 5

Theophylline, drug interactions with, 259–260

Thoracentesis, 276

Thrombin time, 112

Thrombocytopenia, etiologies of, 121

Thrombolytic therapy, 30

Thrombotic thrombocytopenic purpura, 124

Thrush, in cancer patients, 126

Thyroid disease, 197

Thyroid nodule evaluation, 197

Thyrotoxicosis, 198

Tissue plasminogen activator, 30, 189

Tobramycin, 141

Total lung capacity, 64

Total parenteral nutrition (TPN), 222

t-PA, 30, 189

Transfusions, 122–123
  reactions to, 123

Transplant infections, 161

Traube's sign, 3

Travel medicine, 231

Trichomonas vaginalis, 156

Tricuspid regurgitation, 4

Tricuspid stenosis, 4

Tricyclic antidepressant overdose, 251

Tuberculosis, 165–166

Tumor lysis syndrome, 130

Tumor markers, 127

Ulnar nerve, 174

SUBJECT INDEX

Ultrasonography
  preparation for, 272
  renal, 70
Uric acid stone disease, 68
Urinalysis, 65
Urinary tract infections, 155–156
Urine electrolytes, 68
Urine net charge, 69
Urine protein electrophoresis (uPEP), 67
Urine tests, 67
Urine urea nitrogen test, 67
Urobilinogen, 94

Vaccines for travelers, 231
Vaginitis, 156
Valves, prosthetic, 7
Valvular diseases, congenital, 5
Valvular heart disease, 1–4
  aortic stenosis, 1
  chronic aortic regurgitation, 3
  chronic mitral regurgitation, 2
  hypertrophic obstructive cardi-
    omyopathy (HOCM), 4
  mitral stenosis, 2
  rheumatic fever, 3
Vancomycin dosing, 141
Vasculitis, 118, 220
Vasopressors, 49
Venogram, preparation for, 272
Venous thromboembolism prophy-
  laxis, 243
Ventilation. See Mechanical ventilation

Ventricle, left, American Society of
    Echocardiography 16-seg-
    ment model of, 22
Ventricular fibrillation/pulseless ven-
    tricular tachycardia algo-
    rithm, 279
Ventricular septal defect, 5
Ventricular septal rupture, as compli-
    cation of myocardial infarc-
    tion, 33
Ventricular tachycardia, 12
Vomiting, 97
Vulvovaginal candidiasis, 157

Warfarin, 116–117, 242, 243
  drugs that affect, 117
  reversal of, 116
  for stroke prevention, 16
Warts, external genital, treatment of, 160
Watermark's sign, 59
Watter-hammer sign, 3
Weakness, differential diagnosis of, 183
Weaning from mechanical ventila-
    tion, 55
Wide complex tachycardia, 12–13
Wolff-Parkinson-White syndrome, 11
Wood's lamp test, 67

Xerostomia, in cancer patients, 126

Zubrod scale, 126

Drug Index

Abciximab, 28, 35, 36
Acetaminophen, 123, 186, 248, 257
Acetazolamide, 130
Acyclovir, 126, 138, 160
Adenosine, 278
Aggrastat, 36
Albuterol, 56, 76, 252
Aldactone, 104
Allopurinol, 130, 219
Alteplase, 30
Amaryl, 204
Ambien, 178
Amikacin, 138, 154, 255
Aminophylline, 56
Amiodarone, 17, 257, 278
Amitriptyline, 257
Amlodipine, 257
Amoxicillin, 155, 245
Amoxicillin/clavulanate, 154, 155
Amphotericin B, 130, 138, 163
Ampicillin, 138, 152, 245
Ampicillin/sulbactam, 138, 154, 155
Aristocort, 200
Aspirin, 16, 28, 31, 35, 250
Atarax, 186
Atenolol, 257
Ativan, 97, 179, 191, 192, 254
Atovaquone, 163
Atropine, 31, 278
Atrovent, 56, 252
Attapulgite, 98
Azithromycin, 138, 154, 159, 160,
    162, 163, 245
Aztreonam, 138

Beclomethasone, 58
Benadryl, 97, 129, 252, 272
Benzathine, 160

Betamethasone, 200
Bisacodyl, 101
Bismuth subsalicylate, 98
Boric acid, 157
Bretylium, 278
Budesonide, 58
Bupropion, 232
Butoconazole, 157
Butorphanol, 186

Calcitonin, 79
Calcium chloride, 278
Captopril, 257
Carbapenem, 154
Cefazolin, 138, 244, 245
Cefepime, 154
Cefixime, 155, 159
Cefotaxime, 105, 138, 152, 154
Cefotetan, 138, 159, 244
Cefoxitin, 158, 159, 244
Cefpodoxime, 154, 155
Cefprozil, 154
Ceftazidime, 130
Ceftriaxone, 138, 152, 154, 158, 159
Cefuroxime, 138, 154
Celestone, 200
Cephalexin, 245
Chloral hydrate, 178, 257
Chlorpheniramine, 126
Chlorpromazine, 186
Chlorpropamide, 204
Cimetidine, 257, 272
Ciprofloxacin, 105, 138, 155, 159
Clarithromycin, 138, 162
Clavulanic acid, 130
Clindamycin, 139, 154, 157, 159,
    163, 244, 245
Clonidine, 247, 257

DRUG INDEX

Clopidrogel, 36
Clotrimazole, 126, 157
Codeine, 186, 193
Colace, 101
Compazine, 97, 186
Cortisol/hydrocortisone, 200
Cortisone, 200
Cortone, 200
Cyclosporine, 260

Dalmane, 178
Dalteparin, 28
Dapsone, 163
Decadron, 97, 129, 200
Deltasone, 200
Demerol, 102, 123, 193
Depakote, 187
Desyrel, 178
Dexamethasone, 97, 129, 130, 152, 163, 176, 186, 200
Diabinese, 204
Diazepam, 181, 254, 257
Diazoxide, 44
Dichloralphenazone, 186
Diflucan, 157
Digoxin, 2, 16, 90, 254, 257, 259
Dihydroergotamine, 186
Dilantin, 191
Dilaudid, 193
Diltiazem, 15, 29, 187, 257
Dioctyl sodium sulfosuccinate, 29
Diphenhydramine, 97, 123, 129, 178, 252, 272
Diphenoxylate HCl, 98
Dobutamine, 34, 44
Docusate sodium, 101
Dolophine, 193
Dopamine, 34, 44
Doxycycline, 139, 154
Doxycycline, 158, 159, 160

Dulcolax, 101
Dyclonine, 126

Enalapril, 257
Enalaprilat, 44, 45
Enoxaparin, 24, 28, 114, 123
Epinephrine, 44, 56, 123, 278
Epoetin α, 90
Eptifibatide, 28, 36
Ergotamine, 186
Erythromycin, 139, 154, 159, 160, 244
Esmolol, 44, 45, 15, 198, 257
Ethambutol, 139, 165, 166

Famciclovir, 160
Famotidine, 252
Femstat, 157
Fentanyl, 193, 257
Fiorinal, 186
Flagyl, 157
Flecainide, 17
Fleroxacin, 155
Fluconazole, 126, 139, 157, 163
Flucytosine, 139
Fludrocortisone, 200
Flumazenil, 246
Flunisolide, 58
Fluoxetine, 257
Flurazepam, 178
Fluticasone, 58
Fosphenytoin, 192
Furosemide, 34, 50, 76, 79, 89, 104, 257

Ganciclovir, 139
Gentamicin, 130, 139, 141, 142, 150, 152, 154, 159, 244, 245
Glimepiride, 204

Glipizide, 204, 257
Glucophage, 204
Glucotrol, 204
Glyburide, 204, 257
GoLYTELY, 93, 101
Granisetron, 129
Grepafloxacin, 154
Gyne-Lotrimin, ,157

Halcion, 178
Haloperidol, 178, 179, 254, 257
HCTZ, 257
Heparin, 28, 31, 32, 35, 60, 112,
    114–115, 125, 242, 243
Hydralazine, 44, 257
Hydrocortisone, 123, 126, 186, 198,
    199
Hydromorphone, 193
Hydroxyzine hydrochloride, 186

Ibutilide, 17
Imipenem, 130, 139
Imiquimod, 160
Imitrex, 186
Imodium, 98
Indinavir, 164
Indocin, 186
Indomethacin, 219
Integrilin, 36
Interferon, 108
Ipratropium bromide, 56, 252
Isometheptene mucate, 186
Isoniazid, 139, 162, 165, 166
Itraconazole, 139, 163

Kaopectate, 98
Kayexalate, 76, 89
Ketoconazole, 139, 157
Ketorolac, 91
K-Phos, 81

Kytril, 129

Labetalol, 44, 45, 188
Lamifiban, 28
Lamivudine, 164
Lanoteplase, 30
Lasix, 34, 104
Lasix, 34
LevoDromoran, 193
Levofloxacin, 139, 154
Levorphanol, 193
Levothyroxine, 198
Lidocaine, 126, 186, 254, 258, 278
Lisinopril, 258
Lithium, 258
Lomotil, 98
Loperamide HCl, 98
Lorazepam, 97, 179, 181, 191, 192,
    254, 258
Losartan, 227
Lovophed, 44

Magnesium citrate, 101
Mannitol, 35, 89, 109, 176
Meperidine, 102, 193, 254
Meropenem, 139
Metamucil, 101
Metformin, 204
Methadone, 193, 247, 258
Methimazole, 198
Methylprednisolone, 56, 124, 186,
    200
Methylprednisolone sodium succi-
    nate, 252
Methysergide, 187
Metoclopramide, 97, 129, 186
Metoprolol, 15, 45, 258
Metronidazole, 99, 100, 139, 157,
    158
Miconazole, 157

DRUG INDEX

Micronase, 204
Midazolam, 192, 254, 258
Midrin, 186
Milrinone, 44
Misoprostol, 101
Mithramycin, 79
Monistat, 157
Morphine, 29, 50, 193, 254, 258
Mycelex, 126, 157
Mycostatin, 157
Mystatin, 157

Nafcillin, 139, 150
Naloxone, 179, 247
Na-Phos, 81
Neomycin, 104, 244
NeoSynephrine, 44, 251
Nephrocaps, 90
Neurontin, 187
Neutro-Plus, 81
Nicardipine, 44
Nifedipine, 3, 42, 258
Nipride, 44, 188
Nitrofurantoin, 139, 155
Nitroglycerin, 29, 31, 35, 44
Nitroprusside, 2, 44, 45, 254
Nizoral, 157
Noctec, 178
Norepinephrine, 44, 251
Norfloxacin, 155
Nortriptyline, 187
nPA, 30
Nystatin, 126

Ofloxacin, 155, 158, 159, 160
Omeprazole, 258
Ondansetron, 97, 129
Orinase, 204
OsCal, 80
Oxacillin, 150

Oxycodone, 193

Pamidronate, 79
Pancuronium, 255
Paregoric, 98
Paroxetine, 258
Penicillin G, 139, 152
Pentamidine, 139, 163
Pepcid, 95, 252
Pepto-Bismol, 98
Percodan, 193
Phenelzine, 187
Phenergan, 97
Phenobarbital, 191, 192, 254, 258
Phentolamine, 44
Phenylephrine, 44
Phenytoin, 192, 254
PhosLo, 89, 90
Phospho-Soda, 81
Piperacillin, 130, 139
Piperacillin/tazobactam, 139, 154
Pneumovax, 56
Podofilox, 160
Podophyllin resin, 160
Prednisolone, 200
Prednisone, 56, 79, 200, 219, 272
Prelone, 200
Probenecid, 219
Procainamide, 11, 17, 254, 258, 278
Prochlorperazine, 97
Promethazine, 97
Propafenone, 17, 258
Propofol, 192, 254
Propranolol, 15, 45, 187, 198
Propylthiouracil, 198
Prostacyclin, 42
Pyrazinamide, 139, 165, 166
Pyridoxine, 162
Pyrimethamine, 163

Ranitidine, 258
Reglan, 97, 129, 186
ReoPro, 36
Restoril, 178
Reteplase, 30
Ribavirin, 108
Rifabutin, 162
Rifampin, 140, 150, 152, 165, 166
Rolaids, 80
rPA, 30

Senokot, 194
Sertraline, 258
Solu-Medrol, 56, 200, 252
Sorbitol, 89
Sotalol, 17
Sparfloxacin, 154
Spironolactone, 104
Streptokinase, 30
Streptomycin, 165, 166
Sublimaze, 193
Sulfinpyrazone, 219
Sulfisoxazole, 160
Sumatriptan, 186

Tapazole, 198
Tazobactam, 130
Temazepam, 178
Tenecteplase, 30
Terazole, 157
Terconazole, 157
Tetracycline, 126
Theophylline, 56, 254, 259–260
Ticarcillin, 130
Ticarcillin/clavulanate, 140, 154

Ticlopidine, 35, 36
Tirofiban, 28
Tirofiban, 36
Tissue plasminogen activator, 189
TNK-tPA, 30
Tobramycin, 140, 141, 154
Tolbutamide, 204
Toradol, 186
t-PA, 30, 189
Trazodone, 178
Triamcinolone, 58, 200, 219
Triazolam, 178
Trimethoprim/sulfamethoxazole,
    105, 140, 155, 162, 163
Trimetrexate, 163
Tums-EX, 80

Urokinase, 126

Valacyclovir, 160
Valium, 254
Valproic acid, 254
Valsartan, 227
Vancomycin, 130, 140, 141, 150,
    152, 244, 245, 255
Vancomycin, 99–100
Vecuronium, 255
Verapamil, 15
Versed, 192, 254

Warfarin, 16, 116–117, 242, 243

Zidovudine, 164
Zofran, 97, 129
Zolpidem, 178

NOTES

NOTES

NOTES

NOTES